Based on the *New York Times* bestselling diet—
lose up to 11 pounds in 2 WEEKS

400 CALORIE FIX *Cookbook*

400 ALL-NEW, SIMPLY SATISFYING MEALS

Liz Vaccariello,
coauthor of *Flat Belly Diet!*

WITH MINDY HERMANN, RD,
AND THE EDITORS OF **Prevention** MAGAZINE

RODALE.

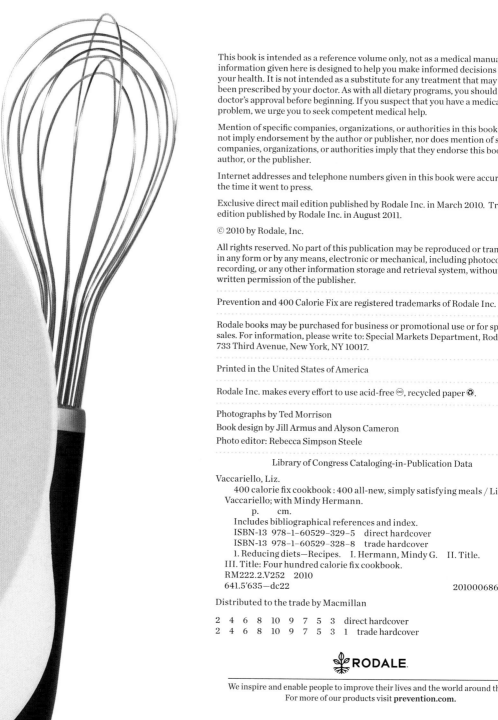

Exclusive direct mail edition published by Rodale Inc. in March 2010. Trade edition published by Rodale Inc. in August 2011.

© 2010 by Rodale, Inc.

Prevention and 400 Calorie Fix are registered trademarks of Rodale Inc.

Rodale books may be purchased for business or promotional use or for special sales. For information, please write to: Special Markets Department, Rodale Inc., 733 Third Avenue, New York, NY 10017.

Printed in the United States of America

Rodale Inc. makes every effort to use acid-free ♾, recycled paper ♻.

Photographs by Ted Morrison
Book design by Jill Armus and Alyson Cameron
Photo editor: Rebecca Simpson Steele

Library of Congress Cataloging-in-Publication Data
Vaccariello, Liz.
    400 calorie fix cookbook : 400 all-new, simply satisfying meals / Liz
Vaccariello; with Mindy Hermann.
        p.   cm.
    Includes bibliographical references and index.
    ISBN-13 978–1–60529–329–5   direct hardcover
    ISBN-13 978–1–60529–328–8   trade hardcover
    1. Reducing diets—Recipes.   I. Hermann, Mindy G.   II. Title.
III. Title: Four hundred calorie fix cookbook.
RM222.2.V252   2010
641.5′635—dc22   2010006862

Distributed to the trade by Macmillan

2   4   6   8   10   9   7   5   3   direct hardcover
2   4   6   8   10   9   7   5   3   1   trade hardcover

RODALE

We inspire and enable people to improve their lives and the world around them.
For more of our products visit **prevention.com**.

DEDICATION

For all the 400 Calorie Fixers who wanted more

CONTENTS

CONTENTS

1

THE STORY OF CALORIE CREEP

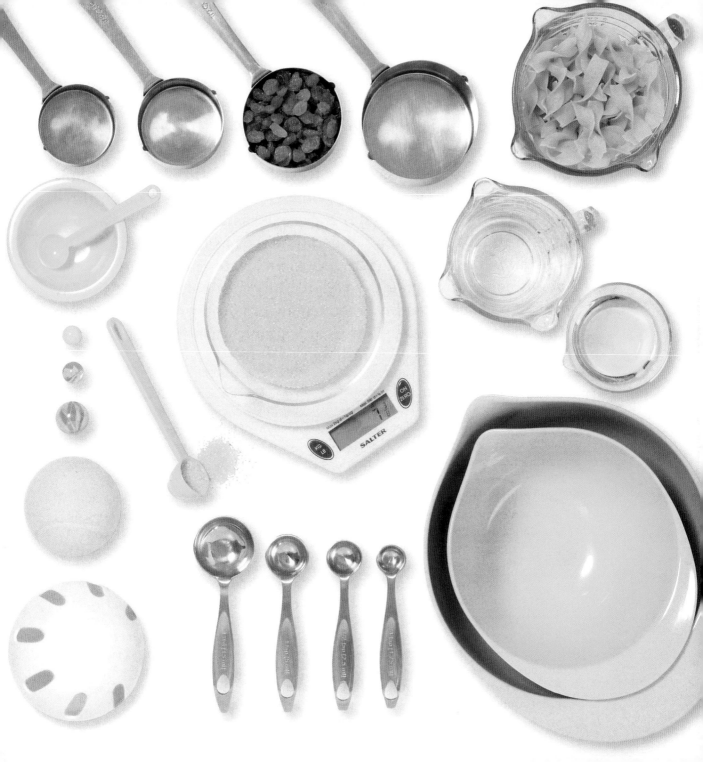

"Where did this extra weight suddenly come from?" That's what I found myself thinking a few years ago when I realized that I was about 10 pounds heavier than I wanted to be. Now, 10 pounds isn't cause for alarm, but it still made me wonder what I was doing wrong. I was eating fresh fruits and vegetables, whole grains, lean proteins, and lots of low-fat dairy. (I was good for three glasses of skim milk a day!) I was exercising regularly. And as a health and fitness editor, I understood the basic principles of nutrition and exercise—it was my *job* to motivate and educate women about achieving a healthy weight. But the scale doesn't lie. My weight had been steadily creeping upward. And when I sat down to think about it, the cause was clear: I simply wasn't paying attention to the calories I was consuming.

Weight gain and obesity are big problems in our country, and it's not entirely our fault. We live in an environment where food is supersized and most of us eat more calories than our bodies need. In fact, in 2007 the average American ate close to 2,800 calories per day, compared to about 2,200 in 1970, according to the USDA's Economic Research Service. That daily difference can add up to an extra pound of body fat every week! Growing portion sizes are partially to blame, explains Cornell University professor Brian Wansink, PhD, in a 2007 study published in the *Journal of the American Dietetic Association*, which shows that when plates, packages, and portions are larger, we eat more. Even cookbook portions have been upsized: A recent study in the *Annals of Internal Medicine* found a 42 percent increase in recipe portion size since 1931. (A *portion* is the amount of food that you serve yourself, while a *serving* is the measured amount recommended on the label and contains the displayed number of calories.)

Not only are we presented with giant piles of food at every turn, but most of us don't even know the basics: how many calories we need or consume. In a study in the *American Journal of Public Health*, close to 200 survey respondents who were asked to estimate the calories and fat in nine restaurant entrées were off by more than 100 percent—they thought that a meal with more than 1,300 calories had only 642 calories! Do me a favor. Take the quiz on pages 4 and 5 to find out how your calorie savvy stacks up.

Why Calories Count

When it comes to managing weight, there is one clear, simple truth: Calories count. And they count more than fat or carbs, sugar or sodium. We've all tried the many diet trends of the past 20 years, but the latest scientific research backs up plain and simple calorie control as the smartest means to losing weight and keeping it off. In a 2009 study in the *New England Journal of Medicine*, more than 800 overweight adults were assigned to one of four different low-calorie diets. Each diet group lost about the same amount of weight over 2 years, *regardless of which diet the group was on.*

Counting calories isn't a new idea, but if the answer is so simple, why are so many of us still struggling with the scale? It's about more than just willpower, that much I can tell you. The truth is, most of us don't know how many calories we really should be eating or how many calories are in the foods we eat. (How did you do on the quiz?) And even if we do, we don't really want to count calories anyway. That's why I wrote the *400 Calorie Fix*: We all need delicious, portion-controlled meals *and* the tools to choose food through a healthy calorie lens. We want to control calories, not count them. And that's what the *400 Calorie Fix* is all about.

400: The Magic Number

Why 400 calories? That calorie count is the perfect per-meal "fix," with enough food to provide the energy you need and keep you satiated until your next meal. Plus, 400 calories allows for a variety of tastes, textures, and nutrients at each meal. Go any lower and it would be difficult to get a good mix of filling and fun foods on your plate to satisfy your stomach and your taste buds.

SUCCESS STORY

Patti Robbins, 53

LOST 10½ POUNDS, 7¾ INCHES IN 2 WEEKS!

Gladys DiSisto, 54

LOST 5½ POUNDS, 6¼ INCHES IN 2 WEEKS!

Tennis partners Patti and Gladys are long used to supporting each other on the court. So when it came time to finally lose those last 10 to 15 pounds they'd each been complaining about, the two once again joined forces. "Having the support of a friend made a big difference in keeping up the plan," notes Patti. "We'd check in on the phone almost every day to see how it was going," adds Gladys. Their teamwork paid off: After 2 weeks, Patti had lost more than 10 pounds; Gladys dropped 5½. ("She's very competitive!" Gladys says with a laugh.) Both continued to lose weight on the plan even after the 2 Week Quick Slim: Patti was down more than 17 pounds at 8 weeks and Gladys more than 10.

TEST YOUR CALORIE SAVVY!

HOW MANY CALORIES ARE IN...

CHICKEN

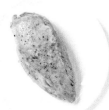

3 OZ COOKED
BONELESS, SKINLESS
CHICKEN BREAST

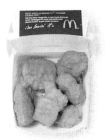

6 COOKED
CHICKEN NUGGETS

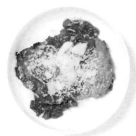

3 OZ COOKED CHICKEN
CUTLET PARMESAN WITH
3 TBSP MOZZARELLA AND
¼ CUP MARINARA SAUCE

POTATOES

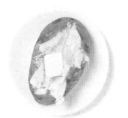

MEDIUM BAKED POTATO
WITH 2 PATS OF BUTTER

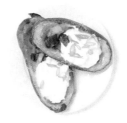

2 BACON & CHEDDAR
BAKED POTATO SKINS

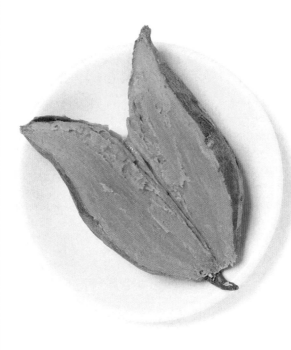

MEDIUM BAKED
SWEET POTATO

LOBSTER

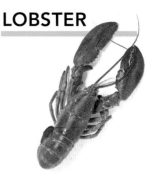

1 LB STEAMED LOBSTER

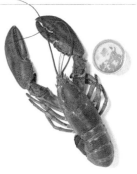

1 LB STEAMED LOBSTER
WITH ¼ CUP MELTED
BUTTER

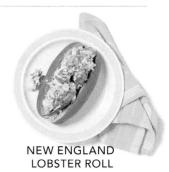

NEW ENGLAND
LOBSTER ROLL

CHEESE

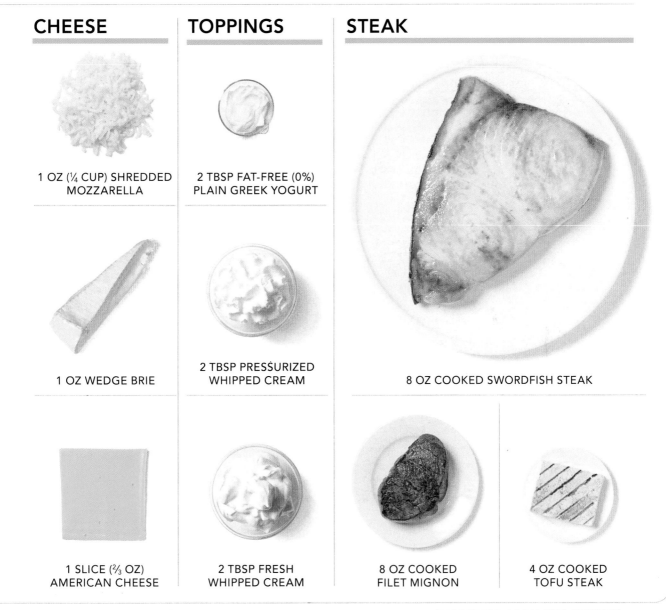

1 OZ (¼ CUP) SHREDDED
MOZZARELLA

1 OZ WEDGE BRIE

1 SLICE (⅔ OZ)
AMERICAN CHEESE

TOPPINGS

2 TBSP FAT-FREE (0%)
PLAIN GREEK YOGURT

2 TBSP PRESSURIZED
WHIPPED CREAM

2 TBSP FRESH
WHIPPED CREAM

STEAK

8 OZ COOKED SWORDFISH STEAK

8 OZ COOKED
FILET MIGNON

4 OZ COOKED
TOFU STEAK

TURN THE PAGE FOR THE ANSWERS. >>>>>

AND THE CALORIE COUNTS ARE...

1. CHICKEN

	calories
3 oz cooked boneless, skinless chicken breast	140
6 cooked chicken nuggets	280
3 oz cooked chicken cutlet Parmesan with 3 Tbsp mozzarella and ¼ cup marinara sauce	310

Coating the naturally ultralean chicken breast with breading for nuggets or chicken Parmesan can more than double the calories.

2. POTATOES

	calories
Medium baked potato with 2 pats of butter	230
2 Bacon & Cheddar Baked Potato Skins	280
Medium baked sweet potato	100

The sweet potato deserves to be promoted from the Thanksgiving menu into a year-round treat. It is relatively low in calories and has plenty of key nutrients. Not only is the sweet potato lower in calories than a regular potato, it also is so moist and sweet that it doesn't need butter (30 calories per teaspoon) or sour cream (25 calories per tablespoon).

In our Bacon and Cheddar Baked Potato Skins (page 275), we slimmed down the classic stuffed potato skins by using just modest amounts of filling.

3. LOBSTER

	calories
1 lb steamed lobster	110
1 lb steamed lobster with ¼ cup melted butter	520
New England Lobster Roll	260

It's the high-fat condiments that make lobster so indulgent—a small dish of melted butter adds more than 400 calories! Our New England Lobster Roll (page 102) uses just enough light mayo to moisten the lobster meat, compared to a typical lobster roll oozing with mayo and over 500 calories.

4. CHEESE

	calories
1 oz (¼ cup) shredded mozzarella	80
1 oz wedge Brie	90
1 slice (⅔ oz) American cheese	70

Shred your cheese whenever possible to make a small amount, such as 1 ounce of mozzarella, go a long way. Since most regular cheeses have close to the same number of calories, it's all about portion control—a slice of American on a burger, a couple of tablespoons of shredded mozzarella on a salad, or a slim wedge of Brie paired with low-cal partners like sliced apple or chilled grapes.

5. TOPPINGS

	calories
2 Tbsp fat-free (0%) plain Greek yogurt	15
2 Tbsp pressurized whipped cream	20
2 Tbsp fresh whipped cream	50

Greek yogurt is thicker and creamier than regular yogurt, giving it a decadent feel. For a sweet topping, flavor with a bit of sugar and a dash of vanilla extract. The extra air in pressurized whipped cream makes it surprisingly low in calories.

6. STEAK

	calories
8 oz cooked swordfish steak	350
8 oz cooked filet mignon	500
4 oz cooked tofu steak	100

Both size and fat content affect the number of calories. Cut the size of your filet mignon or swordfish steak in half to fall well within the parameters of a 400-calorie meal. Tofu steaks tend to be smaller—they're delicious but lack the indulgent allure.

A 400-calorie meal also fits neatly into the daily calorie needs of women and men. A woman at a healthy weight and activity level who wants to maintain her weight needs about 1,600 calories per day; that's four 400-calorie meals a day. The average man needs about 2,000 calories a day, or five 400-calorie meals.

Women and men who are trying to lose weight may need fewer meals and calories. If you follow our 2 Week Quick Slim, described in *400 Calorie Fix,* you'll eat three 400-calorie meals a day.

We asked 16 men and women to try the 2 Week Quick Slim. All of them were surprised by how satisfied they felt on just 1,200 calories a day. And they got results! They lost an average of 6 pounds and 8 inches, with some dropping as many as 11 pounds and more than 15 inches overall. You'll continue to see some of their stories throughout these pages.

Consult the chart on the next page to determine the number of 400-calorie meals you should eat per day—and hence, your daily calorie count. (To find out more about your daily calorie needs, visit www.prevention.com/healthtracker.)

400 Calorie Fix Toolbox

The 400 Calorie Fix was created to fit all sorts of food personalities and dieting lifestyles. If you want structure, we give you meal plans to follow. If you prefer more flexibility, you can mix and match any of the meals on these pages or in the original *400 Calorie Fix* book. Above all, food should be fun. You should be able to enjoy a bowl of ice cream or a glass of red wine and still maintain a healthy weight. The secret is moderation. Here's an overview of the five main tools we created to help you customize the 400 Calorie Fix to your life and your tastes.

✦ *400 Calorie Meals.* Choose from prepared foods, takeout, casual dining, quick fix, or recipes.

✦ *4 Star Nutrition System.* A simple way to ensure you get a healthy balance of protein, fiber, good fats, and fruits and vegetables throughout the day.

✦ *400 Calorie Lens.* Learn how to use simple visual tricks and shortcuts to help you gauge how much food really adds up to 400 calories.

✦ *2 Week Quick Slim.* A 14-day jumpstart of planned meals to help you drop pounds quickly and get you motivated and excited about the 400-calorie frame of mind.

✦ *400 Calorie Menus.* Ready-made meal plans designed to match your tastes and lifestyle, based on specific health needs or eating challenges.

You should certainly feel free to use all the tools you find helpful. Some of these are more applicable to cooking than others, so in the *400 Calorie Fix Cookbook*, I focus on the 400 Calorie Meals, 4 Star Nutrition System, and 400 Calorie Lens. Here's more detail on how to adapt these three tools to your kitchen.

FOUR HUNDRED 400 CALORIE MEALS

I'm so proud to offer 200 delicious new recipes in the *400 Calorie Fix Cookbook*—everyday dishes such as Mushroom-Stuffed Turkey Burgers (page 92), as well as foods to make for parties and entertaining. Try the Peking Duck Quesadillas (page 94)—it's a crowd-pleaser! We drew on cuisines from around the world to develop these scrumptious recipes, including Mexican, Asian, and, my favorite, Italian. The recipes are

---

"HOW MANY MEALS SHOULD I EAT?"

WOMEN

WEIGHT GOAL	SEDENTARY	SOMEWHAT ACTIVE/ ACTIVE	VERY ACTIVE
Lose	3 meals	3–4 meals	4 meals
Maintain	3–4 meals	4 meals	4–5 meals

MEN

WEIGHT GOAL	SEDENTARY	SOMEWHAT ACTIVE/ ACTIVE	VERY ACTIVE
Lose	3–4 meals	4 meals	4–5 meals
Maintain	4 meals	4–5 meals	5+ meals

SEDENTARY: You sit most of the day and drive everywhere, and you log plenty of hours of screen time each day.

SOMEWHAT ACTIVE: You get about 30 minutes of physical activity daily. Nothing too strenuous, generally the equivalent of walking about 1½ to 3 miles daily, or 3,000 to 6,000 steps on a pedometer.

ACTIVE: You like to move around and clock 30 to 60 minutes of daily physical activity by hitting the gym, climbing stairs at the office, and parking farther away at the market, along with moderate exercise, the equivalent of walking more than 3 miles per day, or more than 6,000 steps on a pedometer.

VERY ACTIVE: You're more than a weekend warrior; you thrive on high-intensity sports and rigorous activities that total more than 60 minutes per day.

simple to follow and include right-size portions, plus side dishes to make sure you get 400 calories per meal. (Just for the record, I should note that a complete meal weighs in at 380 to 420 calories.) Easy, right?

But it gets better. On each recipe page, Mindy and I have given you two different meals per recipe—200 recipes, each with two meal options, equals four hundred 400-calorie meals! In most cases, the side dishes to "Make It a Meal" change while the main recipe stays the same. For example, the Sicilian Pizza "Squares" (page 283) are accompanied by either an antipasto side dish or grilled zucchini and a glass of wine, all for 400 calories. Yum! In some cases, the main recipe is a meal in itself, but we've provided a variation to give you a second option—for example, our Holiday Cherry Turkey Meat Loaf (page 234) and its cranberry variation. And in a few cases, you'll see that the main recipe has one set of side dishes to "Make It a Meal" while the variation of the recipe, which may have a different calorie count, has a different set of side dishes. For example, our Summer Chopped Salad with Grilled Shrimp (page 106) is paired with vanilla ice cream. The variation is made with chicken (higher in calories than shrimp) and the side dish is a grilled banana (lower in calories than ice cream).

4 STAR NUTRITION SYSTEM

The 4 Star Nutrition System helps you eat for health and nutrition while following a 400-calorie lifestyle. (Technically, I suppose you could eat four 400-calorie servings of ice cream every day, but your arteries, energy level, and digestive system would pay the price.) As in the *400 Calorie Fix*, the four important components of healthy meals are each assigned a colored star—blue for

SUCCESS STORY

Sandi Hill, 37

LOST 11 POUNDS, 9½ INCHES IN 2 WEEKS!

Over the years Sandi had tried everything from point plans to liquid fasts, with the same result: She'd lose the weight, then quickly gain it back. But her experience on the 2 Week Quick Slim, part of the 400 Calorie Fix, opened her eyes to a new way of eating. "I never really felt like I was on a diet. I always felt satisfied, and it didn't feel like I was making too many sacrifices," Sandi says. "I was really surprised that I could lose weight while eating real food." After 2 weeks, Sandi dropped 11 pounds and had significantly more energy, for herself and her 3-year-old daughter. "I want to be healthier so I can keep up with her!" she says with a laugh. More than a year later, she happily reported that she was "down 75 pounds and still going."

protein, orange for fiber, red for good fats, and green for fruits and veggies.

★ *Protein—at least 20 grams*
Protein-rich foods hold off hunger best and actually stimulate the hormones and neurotransmitters that signal fullness. Research also suggests that protein might cause the body to rev up metabolism as well as maintain muscles, which burn more calories than body fat does. Our Mexican Eggs Benedict (page 38) and Grilled Steak Burgers with Onion Compote (page 90) are two examples of the dozens of meals marked with a blue star.

★ *Fiber—at least 7 grams*
Foods that are highest in fiber—typically fruits and vegetables, legumes such as chickpeas and kidney beans, and whole grains—are highly filling so they help make a meal more satisfying. The 400 Calorie Meals that are highest in fiber, such as Vegetable Stew with Quinoa (page 82), are marked with an orange star.

★ *Good fats—a significant source of monounsaturated fats or omega-3s*
Thanks to studies done by researchers such as Purdue University's Richard Mattes, MPH, PhD, RD, and others, peanuts, almonds, and other nuts, all high in monounsaturated fats (MUFAs), are now considered important parts of a healthy diet and healthy weight management. Olives, fatty fish such as salmon and tuna, and even dark chocolate are also rich in good fats. In fact, you get a double benefit from some of these foods,

which contain not only MUFAs but also heart-healthy omega-3 fatty acids.

Spanish researchers found that MUFAs in a meal can help you feel fuller longer. A group of overweight men and women in a Harvard study found it easy to stick with a healthy eating plan that included a bit more fat, mainly as MUFAs, and they lost more weight as compared to men and women on a low-fat diet. Omega-3 fatty acids, found in fatty fish, flaxseed, and other foods, can help lower blood pressure, as shown in a 2009 study conducted in three European countries.

You'll find the red healthy fats star on meals such as the Vegetable Dumplings with Dipping Sauce (page 168) and the Salmon Pasta Primavera (page 191).

★ *Fruits/veggies—1 cup*
Fruits and vegetables help you feel full because they are naturally high in water and fiber. They also are packed with vitamins and minerals and are relatively low in calories. Meals that are particularly high in vegetables or fruits include our Pasta with Spinach and Parsley-Cheese Sausage (page 262) and Thai Beef Salad (page 112).

Meals (as well as foods listed in the appendix) that meet the criteria for each category are awarded stars accordingly. You will notice that some meals have just one star while others have two, three, even four stars because they qualify in more than one category. The handful of meals with no stars—

STAR SYSTEM
★ PROTEIN
★ FIBER
★ GOOD FATS
★ FRUITS / VEGGIES

our fun meals—still have a place in a healthy (real) life. Collect each star at least once during the day—the more stars, the better—and you'll be on the road to healthy eating.

THE 400 CALORIE LENS

Estimating food portions and calories is tough, no matter how many diets you've been on. And estimating ingredient amounts rather than measuring when you're cooking can have disastrous results. I know from experience! So while you will be measuring out ingredients for each recipe—look for more information on measuring tools in Chapter 2—you will also be learning to use visual cues and other tricks to help you view the meals you create through a 400 Calorie Lens. It's a whole new way of looking at food.

Weigh and Measure

I know that weighing and measuring meals isn't terribly fun—plus it's inconvenient, boring, and tough to keep up for more than a couple of days. But it's the most accurate way to tell how much food you're eating. We've given you a hand by calling for common, standard measurements, such as 1 cup of cereal, $\frac{1}{2}$ cup of fruit, 1 tablespoon of salad dressing, 1 teaspoon of butter. Items from each traditional food group—grains, fruits, vegetables, dairy, and meats and other proteins—follow general portion standards, although in some cases we adjust portions to keep calories within our range of 380 to 420 calories per meal.

See the Visual Cues

You don't need any special gadgets or gizmos. The 400 Calorie Lens is literally in your mind's eye. It's a way to use common visual references, such as a golf ball or the palm of your hand, to eyeball amounts of food.

You'll notice that almost all of these are volume measurements (teaspoons, tablespoons, and cups), which is the easiest way to visualize most foods. But some foods,

SUCCESS STORY

Janet Sartorius, 50

LOST 10¼ POUNDS, 9 INCHES IN 2 WEEKS!

A few years ago, Janet lost an amazing 90 pounds through a popular weight-loss plan. She even took a new career direction—walking dogs—to help her stay more active. But after a couple of years, she regained about two-thirds of the weight and was starting to worry that she was doomed to obesity. But after starting the 2 Week Quick Slim, Janet was surprised to see that the needle on the scale was once again moving downward. "Suddenly I had hope again!" she says. "I realized I could be at a healthy weight and stay there." A bonus? Her family loved the 400 Calorie Fix foods, too. "I know I'm moving in the right direction; I'm so much more motivated now to get healthier, both for myself and my family."

It's a ball, it's a hand, it's a portion

	BALL	HAND	PORTION	EXAMPLES
	Small marble	Tip of the thumb	1 teaspoon	oil, butter, margarine, sugar
	Large marble	Thumb to the first knuckle	1 tablespoon	chopped nuts, honey, ketchup
	Two large marbles	Whole thumb	2 tablespoons/ 1 ounce liquid	salad dressing, grated cheese, raisins
	Golf ball	Cupped handful	¼ cup, 1 ounce shredded cheese	beans, chopped vegetables, salsa, hummus
	Hockey puck	Palm of the hand	½ cup/ 4 ounces (¼ pound) raw meat, poultry, fish	burger patty, beef, pork, chicken, turkey, fish
	Tennis ball	Open handful	½ cup	rice, pasta, fruit salad, melon balls, small roll, scrambled eggs
	Wiffle ball	Very loose cupped handful	1 cup/ 1 to 2 ounces chips	potato chips, tortilla chips, popcorn, pretzels
	Baseball	Whole fist	1 cup	cereal, lettuce, vegetables, strawberries, soup

such as chips and pretzels, as well as meat, poultry, and fish, are awkward shapes and don't fit neatly into either a real or an imaginary spoon or cup. You'll usually see such foods measured by weight. Also, we've listed 4 ounces here as a serving size for meat, poultry, or fish, even though the most frequently recommended serving size for meat is 3 ounces. It's not a mistake: 4 ounces refers to the raw weight, 3 ounces to the cooked weight. For more details on how weight measurements match up to volume measurements, see the Conversion Chart on page 348.

It's also important to use these visual cues when grocery shopping, particularly for foods such as apples, potatoes, and other fresh fruits and vegetables that are not typically marked with their weight and recommended serving size. In Chapter 3, you will learn how these shortcuts can guide you in the grocery store.

Know Your Common Foods

You probably know the calorie counts of your favorite foods. Memorizing the calorie counts of all the different foods you eat and ingredients you use, however, is virtually impossible. The appendix lists dozens of foods and ingredients, along with a standard portion, number of calories, and star (when applicable), to help you create your own meals while staying within the 400-calorie framework.

Learn to Divide Your Plate

It is unlikely that you will cook three meals a day (I'm lucky if I cook one!), so we've also included an easy system for putting together quick-fix meals that don't require a recipe. The 1-2-3-400-Calorie trick shows you how to put together a balanced 400-calorie meal—one that has important nutrients such as protein, fiber, vitamins, and minerals, as well as the right combination of foods to keep you satisfied and therefore less likely to overeat.

Mentally divide your plate into six sections:

- Fill **ONE** section with one portion of a protein. For meat, chicken, or fish, that's 3 ounces cooked (4 ounces raw), about the size of a hockey puck. One cup of milk or yogurt; 2 extra-large or 3 large eggs; up to a cup of beans; or a couple tablespoons of peanut butter also equal one portion. (We had to keep the peanut butter portion small because it's pretty high in calories.)
- Fill **TWO** sections with two portions of a grain food such as rice, pasta, or bread. For rice and pasta, that is ⅔ cup, or slightly less than a baseball-size scoop. For bread, it's two slices (no butter, though!).
- Fill **THREE** sections with three portions of vegetables or fruit. You'll have a total of 1 cup, or a baseball-size heap of greens, other veggies, or fruit.

You may notice that not all of our four hundred 400 Calorie Meals follow this 1-2-3-400-Calorie trick. Although it's important to get a good balance of nutrients, meals could get boring if they all had to have exactly the same proportion of meat to

DIVIDE YOUR PLATE

Here are a few sample 1-2-3-400-calorie meals using calorie information from the list of foods in Appendix A:

	PORTIONS		CALORIES
	1	3 ounces grilled London broil	170
	2	⅔ cup mashed potato	90
	3	1 cup steamed broccoli (60), ½ cup fruit salad (50)	110
	BONUS	1 teaspoon unsalted whipped butter (25) + 2 tablespoons low-fat milk (15) in the mashed potato	40
	TOTAL:		410
	1	2 ounces deli-sliced ham (60) + 1 slice American cheese (70)	130
	2	2 slices wheat bread	140
	3	1 large banana (1 cup sliced)	130
	TOTAL:		400
	1	1 cup low-fat plain yogurt	150
	2	⅔ cup raisin bran	130
	3	1 cup sliced strawberries	50
	BONUS	2 tablespoons walnut halves	80
	TOTAL:		410

grain to fruits and vegetables. In addition, the system isn't always precise because of the way that foods are prepared. Specifically, many dishes have hidden calories from fats and sugars. And often, foods within the same food group can have very different calorie counts. For example, 1 cup of sliced banana has 130 calories, but 1 cup of sliced strawberries has only 50 calories.

If your 1-2-3-400-Calorie meal falls short of the 400-calorie mark, you can add an extra food as a bonus. Or you can use the extra calories for calories from fats and sugars in ingredients such as mayonnaise, salad dressing, or sweeteners that have calories. If your meal goes over 400 calories, try a different combination of foods to bring the calories down or choose foods based on how they're prepared, for example, grilled instead of fried.

Spy Hidden Calories

Fats such as oil and butter, and sweeteners such as sugar, honey, jam, and syrup, create particular challenges when you're trying to eat 400-calorie meals. A little pat of butter can add 40 calories to a serving of steamed broccoli. Regular Caesar salad dressing douses your otherwise skinny salad with 80 calories per tablespoon. The difference between a regular and a diet soft drink is about 100 calories per cup, all of them from sugars. The first challenge: High-fat and high-sugar ingredients add calories, so using them can mean that your portions have to be smaller in order to stay near the 400-calorie mark. The second

challenge: Fats and sugars can be hidden in certain packaged ingredients; if you don't read the label carefully and compare different brands of the same ingredient, you might end up with more calories than you expect. In Chapter 3, you'll learn tips for finding the fat and spotting the sugar when you're shopping.

SUCCESS STORY

Melody Rubie, 48

LOST 5 POUNDS, 9 INCHES IN 2 WEEKS!

Like many moms, Melody found it difficult to lose the weight she'd gained with the birth of her son, Benjamin, now 6½. Melody is also no ordinary working mom: She's a regular cast member in Broadway's famed *Phantom of the Opera*, where she says her excess weight often slowed her down. "On the days where we do both a matinee and an evening performance, I really would be dragging at the end. We work hard on stage and off." But after just 2 weeks on the program, she says her energy levels are at an all-time high. "I feel like I can keep going as long as I need to." Even after the 2 Week Quick Slim was over, Melody continued to lose weight, dropping nearly 10 more pounds at 8 weeks and getting close to her final goal weight of 135 pounds. "I feel so empowered," she says. "I have a much greater sense of control, and it's spilling into other areas of my life—work, home. I feel like I can do almost anything now!"

2

400 CALORIES IN THE KITCHEN

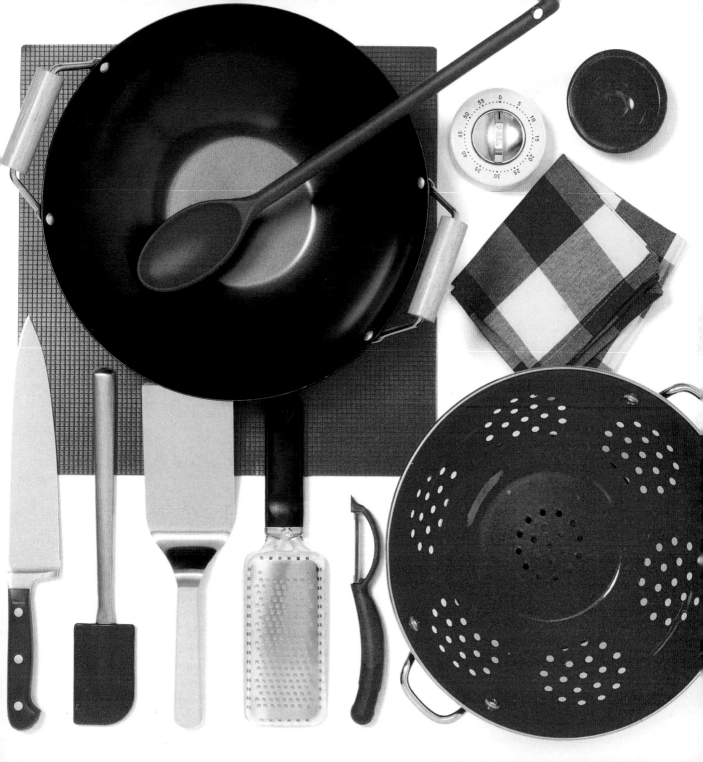

To cook the 400-calorie way, you need the right equipment. Don't worry, you don't have to go out and buy special pots and pans or lots of expensive ingredients. In fact, you probably already have cupboards and drawers full of the utensils and appliances required to make almost any recipe in this book. But now's the time to learn how to use them the 400-calorie way.

The Basics

Any well-stocked kitchen should have good-quality tools that make cooking faster and easier, and the 400-calorie kitchen is no different. First, you'll want to invest in tools to help you measure portions. Keep in mind that measuring will be more accurate if you use tools that are specifically designed for liquids or solids. Here's what you need:

- Nested measuring cups for dry foods and ingredients
- 2-cup liquid measuring cup
- Set of measuring spoons
- Inexpensive digital kitchen scale for weighing food
- ½-cup, 1-cup, 2-cup, and 4-cup sealable plastic containers for storage

Next, make sure you have the right tools for cooking. Here's a list of essentials for your 400-calorie recipes:

- Set of knives, including a small paring knife for peeling and cutting, a chef's knife for cutting and chopping, and a serrated knife for slicing bread and meat
- Two washable cutting boards, one just for raw meat, poultry, and fish
- Instant-read meat thermometer
- Metal colander and/or medium strainer
- Several saucepans with lids
- Large soup pot
- Regular and nonstick skillets, with lids if available
- Regular or nonstick wok with a rack or bamboo basket for steaming
- 8" x 8" baking pan
- 8" or 9" springform pan
- 13" x 9" lasagna or roasting pan
- 10" or 11" tart pan
- Baking sheets
- Muffin pan
- Loaf pan
- Stovetop grill pan
- 8-ounce ovenproof ramekins or custard dishes

400-Calorie Cooking Techniques

Cooking the 400-calorie way has become second nature for me, but it was not always that way. I made sure that the main parts of my meal were healthy—I cooked with plenty of vegetables and fruit, fish or lean meat, and whole grains—but I did not pay a lot of attention to the amount of extra fat I was adding from foods such as olive oil and nuts. While these are nutrition-packed foods that should be a part of everyone's diet, they do have a lot of calories. No wonder I had gained weight eating healthy foods!

Instead, try cooking methods that do not require a lot of added fat so that most of your 400 calories go toward generous portions of food. You will feel more satisfied after eating while knowing that your plate is filled with healthy foods. These are our favorite 400-calorie cooking methods:

COOKING METHOD	BEST FOR	EQUIPMENT
STEAMING	✦ Vegetables ✦ Fish	✦ Double boiler ✦ Rice cooker ✦ Wok with a rack ✦ Microwave ✦ Parchment or foil packet ✦ Pot or skillet with a lid
SLOW COOKING, BRAISING	✦ Soups ✦ Stews ✦ Casseroles ✦ Lower-fat or tough meats	✦ Slow cooker ✦ Large covered skillet or Dutch oven
STIR-FRYING	✦ Meat ✦ Chicken ✦ Tofu ✦ Vegetables	✦ Cooking spray ✦ Regular and/or nonstick wok ✦ Regular and/or nonstick skillet
GRILLING	✦ Meat ✦ Chicken ✦ Fish ✦ Vegetables	✦ Outdoor or indoor grill ✦ Stovetop grill pan
BROILING	✦ Meat	✦ Oven

400-Calorie Kitchen Gadgets

Using our 400 Calorie Lens, let's look at several common kitchen items and see how they can do double duty, performing their original function and supporting your new 400-calorie lifestyle. You'll never look at a cheese grater the same way again!

For Measuring

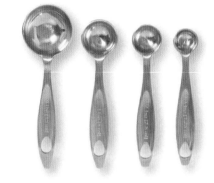

MEASURING SPOON SET
New Use: Sprinkle on just the right amount of sugar (8 calories per ½ teaspoon), nuts (15 to 20 calories per teaspoon), or mini chocolate chips (20 calories per teaspoon).

DIGITAL KITCHEN SCALE
New Use: Double-check the weights of whole fruits and vegetables and visually compare different portion sizes to avoid calorie creep. For example, a small (6-ounce) potato has 130 calories and a medium (7½-ounce) potato has 160 calories. A 1-ounce slice of Italian bread has 70 calories and a 2-ounce slice has 140 calories.

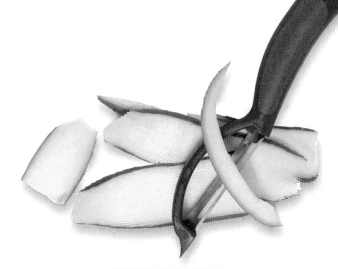

VEGETABLE PEELER

New Use: Slice cheese or chocolate into ultrathin 10-calorie curls, or make zucchini or eggplant ribbons to cook and serve like spaghetti or linguine, but with less than half the calories!

CHEESE GRATER

New Use: Use the extra-fine grate for a 20-calorie, 1-tablespoon dusting of cheese on steamed vegetables, or shave medium ribbons of chocolate (25 calories per tablespoon) to liven up a bowl of berries.

PLASTIC STORAGE CONTAINERS, SERVING SPOONS, UTENSILS

New Use: Once you determine which container can hold your 400-calorie serving of pasta, you'll never have to measure it out again. Same for a soup ladle. At ½ cup per ladle, dishing out an 80-calorie serving of tomato sauce is a breeze. Or serve yourself 1 cup, or 2 ladles, of split pea soup for an easy 180-calorie appetizer.

12-CUP, NONSTICK MUFFIN PAN

New Use: Bake quiche, cake, quick bread, and hors d'oeuvres in right-size portions.

COFFEE GRINDER

New Use: Chop 1 tablespoon of nuts for a quick 50-calorie garnish.

For Cooking

NESTED, HEAVY-GAUGE, STAINLESS STEEL MEASURING CUPS

New Use: Use directly on the stove to heat or reduce small amounts of liquid for sauces and salad dressings.

2-CUP GLASS LIQUID MEASURING CUP

New Use: For melting and warming: Measure soft butter or margarine, chocolate chips, milk, and so on directly in the cup, then microwave. For salad dressing: Layer oil, vinegar, and other ingredients using the measurement markings, and combine with a small whisk or immersion blender.

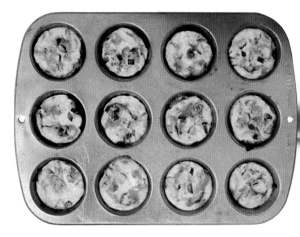

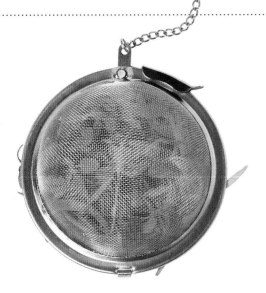

METAL TEA BALL
New Use: For calorie-free flavor, fill with herbs or spices and add to the pot when cooking soups and desserts.

COLLAPSIBLE METAL VEGETABLE STEAMER
New Use: You can steam much more than broccoli! Cook Asian dumplings without adding calories or prepare cubes of delicate silken tofu that still hold their shape.

COFFEE DRIP CONE
New Use: Line with a paper or gold filter, fill with plain yogurt, and place over a bowl in the fridge; as the whey drains off, you get Greek-style yogurt. Because it's thicker than regular yogurt, some folks find it more of an indulgence.

PARCHMENT PAPER
New Use: Wrap fish or chicken fillets, or thinly sliced meat, along with vegetables in a parchment packet and bake for a flavorful, low-calorie meal.

MINI FOOD PROCESSOR
New Use: Make bread and cracker crumbs for a quick, 10-calorie-per-tablespoon crunchy topping.

RICE COOKER
New Use: It's not just for rice anymore. Steam vegetables perfectly al dente. Bonus: Steamed vegetables retain more of their vitamins than when they are boiled.

SLOW COOKER
New Use: Soak dry beans for a couple hours and then cook overnight; they hold their shape and are cooked just right.

DON'T FORGET THE DISHES

What does your china have to do with eating the 400-calorie way? Plenty. I got a set of humongous Pottery Barn dishes after I got married. I loved them, but I didn't realize that using oversize plates could lead me to eat bigger portions. It's true. Brian Wansink, PhD, of Cornell University found that even nutrition experts served themselves bigger portions—and ate more—when they had bigger bowls. That is why we recommend using smaller plates and bowls on the 400 Calorie Fix. Your meals will look larger, and you'll feel like you're eating a larger portion. So make sure to have small plates on which to serve your 400-calorie meals:

✦ 8" salad plates

✦ 8- to 12-ounce soup/salad bowls

✦ Tall, skinny drinking glasses

✦ Small serving bowls and spoons

✦ 8- to 10-ounce mugs for lattes, hot cocoa

3

400 CALORIES AT THE GROCERY STORE

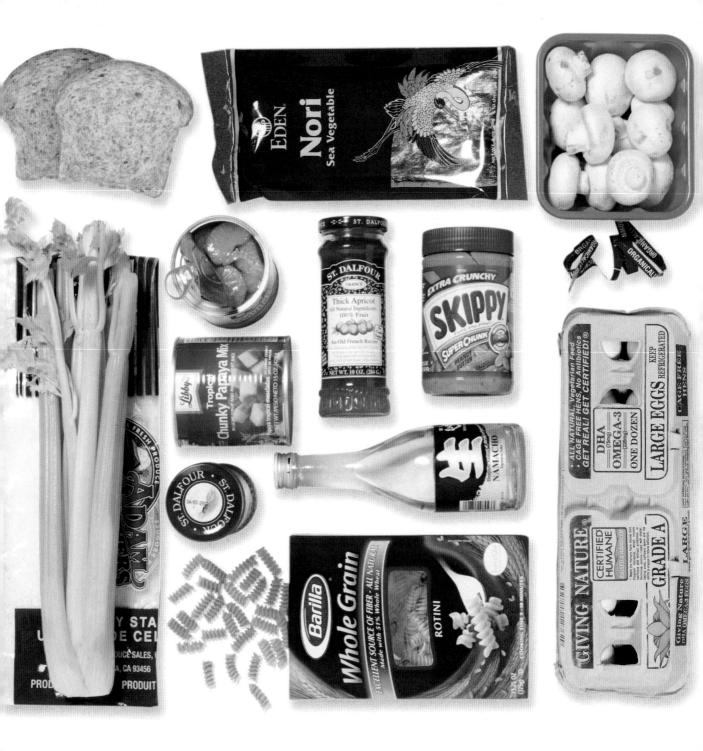

Before I started eating the 400-calorie way, I did not give much thought to grocery shopping (except that I'd do anything to get out of doing it!). I went to the market once a week—usually, but not always, with a grocery list—and filled up my cart with a combination of foods my family ate every week (frozen wild salmon fillets, sweet potatoes, and lots of romaine lettuce) and items that were on sale. I knew which foods were healthiest and those were the ones I bought, save for the occasional package of Oreos.

Now, I've learned to embrace the process and leverage the list. My strategy is twofold: First, I check my inventory of eggs, whole grain pasta, and so on—the 400-calorie staples listed on pages 28–31. It's important to have a combination of long-lasting items in your pantry or cupboard—dry foods such as pasta, rice, other grains, cereals, and baking supplies, plus foods in cans, such as tuna and salmon, beans, and fruit. Freezer foods include meats and poultry, wrapped in 1-pound packages for easy portion control, plus breads, well-marked leftovers, and a selection of frozen vegetables and fruits, which are particularly good during the off-season. Refrigerator foods—fresh fruits and vegetables, meats and proteins, eggs, and dairy products—need to be restocked most often because they're highly perishable.

Second, I review the specific foods I'll need to make meals during the week, whether they're school lunches or a few recipes from this book. I also use the 4 Star Nutrition System as a guide to make sure I'm filling up my cart—and my kitchen—with a nutritionally balanced assortment of foods. I write down the four categories—protein, fiber, good fats, fruits and vegetables—at the top of my grocery list. I scan the list after it's complete just to be sure I see good representation in each of the categories. And when I'm shopping I make a mental note to visit each of those sections of the store. I certainly don't have time to create anything more complicated (spreadsheets with color-coordinated stars?), but just writing down those words and making a list keep me focused on the 400-calorie lifestyle.

Loving the Label

It used to be really tough to know what was in a packaged food—how many calories or fat grams—before the government mandated standardized food package labels about 25 years ago. Today, packaged goods manufacturers are required to display nutrition information, so it is quick work to look up calories and nutrients.

SPOT THE SUGAR

Foods that you might not think of as overly sweet, such as ketchup, barbecue sauce, salad dressing, and breakfast cereals, often have added sweeteners (which give you unnecessary, nutrition-free calories). To spot the sugar, look for one of these listed in the top three ingredients:

- sugar
- corn syrup
- evaporated cane juice
- fruit juice
- fruit juice concentrate
- honey
- glucose
- sucrose
- fructose
- maltodextrin
- dextrose

FIND THE FAT

Almost every dairy product comes in a regular version plus at least one lower-fat version. (Our recipes specify exactly which to use.) The wording on the label can help guide you. Reduced-fat means at least 25 percent less fat than the traditional version. Low-fat foods have no more than 3 grams of fat per serving and fat-free have less than $\frac{1}{2}$ gram. A "light" food has one-third fewer calories and at least 50 percent less fat.

REGULAR VERSION	LOWER-FAT ALTERNATIVE	FAT-FREE ALTERNATIVE
CHEDDAR CHEESE SHREDS 1 tablespoon **30 calories**	REDUCED-FAT CHEDDAR CHEESE SHREDS 1 tablespoon **20 calories**	FAT-FREE CHEDDAR CHEESE SHREDS 1 tablespoon **10 calories**
SOUR CREAM 1 tablespoon **25 calories**	LIGHT SOUR CREAM 1 tablespoon **20 calories**	FAT-FREE (0%) PLAIN GREEK YOGURT 1 tablespoon **10 calories**
WHOLE MILK 1 cup **150 calories**	LOW-FAT MILK 1 cup **100 calories**	FAT-FREE MILK 1 cup **80 calories**
PLAIN YOGURT 6 ounces **140 calories**	LOW-FAT PLAIN 6 ounces **110 calories**	FAT-FREE PLAIN YOGURT 6 ounces **100 calories**
BUTTER 1 teaspoon **30 calories**	WHIPPED BUTTER 1 teaspoon **20 calories**	FAT-FREE BUTTER GRANULES 1 teaspoon **5 calories**
HALF-AND-HALF 1 tablespoon **20 calories**	LOW-FAT NONDAIRY CREAMER 1 tablespoon **10 calories**	FAT-FREE HALF-AND-HALF 1 tablespoon **10 calories**

SEASONINGS AROUND THE WORLD

Stock up on seasonings and spices that add flavor without calories. The *400 Calorie Fix Cookbook* features recipes from many international cuisines. A well-stocked spice drawer is essential. It also is handy for creating your own dishes or modifying ours with seasonings from other regions. We put together this list of typical seasonings to help you get started:

CUISINE	TYPICAL SEASONINGS
Greek	Dill, lemon, marjoram, oregano
French	Bay leaf, tarragon, thyme
Italian	Basil, oregano, marjoram
Spanish	Paprika, saffron, smoked paprika
German and Northern European	Salt, pepper, mustard, rye, cardamom
Eastern European	Salt, pepper, paprika
North African	Cinnamon, cardamom, chile pepper, cumin, turmeric, ginger, nutmeg, za'atar
Caribbean	Allspice, nutmeg, chile pepper, cinnamon, curry powder, ginger
Mexican	Chile pepper, cinnamon, oregano, allspice, cumin
Indian	Curry powder, cardamom, cinnamon, coriander seeds, cumin, fennel seeds, mustard, turmeric
Thai	Chile pepper, basil, cumin, curry paste, star anise, sriracha sauce, turmeric
Chinese	Chile pepper, cinnamon, five-spice powder, star anise

When you're shopping, focus on the top section of the Nutrition Facts panel. Here you can find information on suggested serving size, number of servings per package, and calories per serving. This information might differ from what you see in the book. We are using standard amounts such as $1/4$ cup and $1/2$ cup to make portion control easy; manufacturers can set their own portion sizes within certain limits.

FREEBIES

Although freebies are not entirely calorie-free, they are low enough that most people would find it difficult to overdo. The free veggies and condiments are particularly well suited to sandwiches, burgers, and salads.

RAW VEGGIES

- Alfalfa sprouts
- Bean sprouts
- Bell peppers
- Broccoli
- Cabbage
- Celery
- Cucumber
- Dill pickles
- Fennel
- Jalapeño chile peppers
- Lettuce
- Mushrooms
- Onions
- Sauerkraut
- Spinach
- Tomato

CONDIMENTS

- Capers
- Hot-pepper sauce
- Ketchup*
- Lemon juice
- Mustard
- Prepared horse-radish
- Tomato salsas
- Soy sauce*
- Vinegars
- Worcestershire sauce

Reduced- or low-sodium

BEVERAGES

- Black coffee or tea with no or noncaloric sweeteners
- Diet colas or diet sports drinks
- Sparkling water

3 SPECTACULAR SALAD DRESSINGS

Salads are an easy way to add low-calorie, good-for-you vegetables to your meals, but prepared salad dressings can sabotage your weight loss with hidden fats and sugar that can add more calories than are in the salad. Instead, try whipping up your own simple salad dressings. This trio is bursting with flavor, not calories.

CARROT-GINGER DRESSING

TOTAL TIME: 10 minutes /
Makes 16 servings (2 Tbsp each)

- ¼ cup red miso paste
- ¼ cup rice vinegar
- ¼ cup canola or peanut oil
- ¼ cup water
- 1 piece (1") fresh ginger, peeled
- 2 tablespoons sugar
- 1 teaspoon toasted sesame oil
- 3 medium carrots, cut into ½" pieces

1. **PLACE** the miso, vinegar, oil, water, ginger, sugar, and sesame oil in a blender, and process to puree.

2. **WITH** the blender running, add the carrots, a few pieces at a time, and blend until smooth before adding the next couple of pieces. If the dressing seems too thick, add up to ¼ cup of additional water.

CALORIES PER SERVING = 50

> **SAVE AT LEAST 65 CALORIES!**

HONEY-MUSTARD BALSAMIC VINAIGRETTE

TOTAL TIME: 20 minutes /
Makes 10 servings
(2 Tbsp each)

- 1 cup balsamic vinegar
- 2 tablespoons olive oil
- 1 tablespoon Dijon mustard
- 1 tablespoon honey
- ½ teaspoon coarse sea salt
- ½ teaspoon freshly ground black pepper

1. **SIMMER** the balsamic vinegar in a small nonstick saucepan until reduced by half and syruplike, at least 10 minutes. Let cool to room temperature.

2. **PLACE** the balsamic syrup in a small jar or sealable plastic container. Add the oil, mustard, honey, salt, and pepper, and shake until well blended.

CALORIES PER SERVING = 50

> **SAVE 50 CALORIES!**

BLUE CHEESE DRESSING

TOTAL TIME: 5 minutes /
Makes 8 servings (2 Tbsp each)

- ⅓ cup buttermilk
- ⅓ cup low-fat or fat-free plain yogurt
- ⅓ cup crumbled blue cheese
- ½ teaspoon salt-free garlic-and-herb seasoning

COMBINE the buttermilk, yogurt, blue cheese, and seasoning in a small jar or sealable plastic container. Shake until well blended.

CALORIES PER SERVING = 30

> **SAVE 110 CALORIES!**

400-Calorie STAPLES

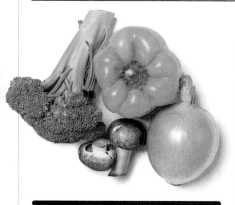

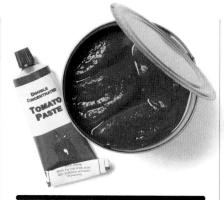

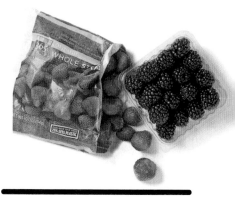

STAPLE:

Freebie vegetables

Most veggies that can be eaten raw are so low in calories that you can eat as much as you'd like without worrying about calories. See the full list of freebie vegetables in the box on page 26.

USES:

FOR DUNKING INTO DIP

RAW BROCCOLI FLORETS
1 cup (baseball)
20 calories

ON A SANDWICH

LETTUCE + TOMATO
2 leaves + 2 slices (tennis ball)
20 calories

IN A SALAD

SALAD GREENS +
SALAD DRESSING SPRAY
1 cup + 10 sprays (baseball)
30 calories

STAPLE:

Canned tomato products (no-salt-added)

Canned tomatoes come in many forms for use in soups, stews, casseroles, and sauces. Buy no-salt-added varieties whenever possible so that you can control the salt content.

USES:

FOR A SAUCE

TOMATO PASTE
1 tablespoon (large marble)
15 calories

IN A STEW

DICED TOMATOES
½ cup (tennis ball)
20 calories

FOR A SOUP

TOMATO PUREE
¼ cup (golf ball)
25 calories

STAPLE:

Frozen and fresh berries

Packed with vitamin C and fiber and relatively low in calories, berries brighten up breakfast, dessert, or a smoothie. Frozen berries are a perfect alternative when fresh are not available.

USES:

ON CEREAL

SLICED FRESH
STRAWBERRIES
½ cup (tennis ball)
30 calories

IN A SMOOTHIE

FROZEN MIXED BERRIES
1 cup (baseball)
60 calories

ON ICE CREAM

THAWED BLUEBERRIES
1 cup (baseball)
80 calories

WHEN YOUR KITCHEN IS STOCKED WITH THE RIGHT INGREDIENTS—IN THE PANTRY, FREEZER, AND REFRIGERATOR—WHIPPING UP A DELICIOUS 400-CALORIE MEAL IS A BREEZE.

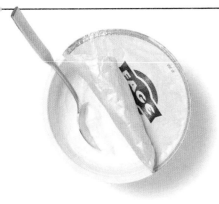

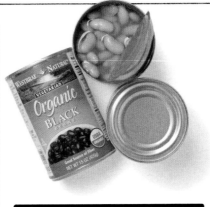

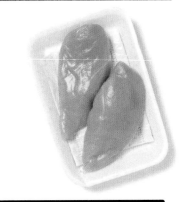

STAPLE:

Fat-free (0%) plain Greek yogurt

Greek yogurt has less moisture, so it's thicker than American- or European-style yogurt, and it gives you the texture and creaminess of sour cream while saving about 15 calories per tablespoon.

USES:

AS A DESSERT TOPPING

FAT-FREE (0%) PLAIN GREEK YOGURT
2 tablespoons (2 large marbles)
15 calories

IN A BREAKFAST PARFAIT

FAT-FREE (0%) PLAIN GREEK YOGURT
½ cup (tennis ball)
60 calories

IN A SMOOTHIE

FAT-FREE (0%) PLAIN GREEK YOGURT
1 cup (baseball)
120 calories

STAPLE:

Canned beans

Keep an assortment of black, kidney, cannellini, and pinto beans, and chickpeas handy in the cupboard to add to salads or soups, and to puree into dips and spreads. They're high in fiber and protein and reasonable in calories.

USES:

IN A SALAD

KIDNEY BEANS
¼ cup (golf ball)
50 calories

IN A SOUP

BLACK BEANS
½ cup (tennis ball)
70 calories

AS A DIP

CHICKPEA HUMMUS
⅓ cup (5 large marbles)
140 calories

STAPLE:

Boneless, skinless chicken

Freeze boneless, skinless breasts and thighs in individual 4-ounce (hockey puck) portions and in recipe-ready 1-pound (4 hockey pucks) packages.

USES:

IN A SALAD

DICED CHICKEN BREAST
¼ cup (golf ball)
60 calories

IN A SANDWICH

GRILLED CHICKEN BREAST CUTLET
3-ounce (hockey puck)
140 calories

IN A STEW

CUBED CHICKEN THIGH
½ cup (tennis ball)
180 CALORIES

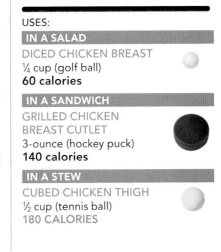

400-Calorie STAPLES

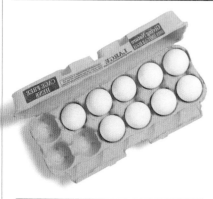

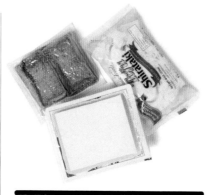

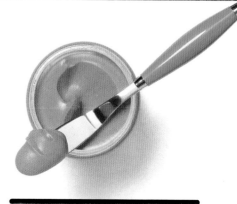

STAPLE:
Eggs

Eggs are among the least expensive and fastest cooking sources of protein. All the fat, but also most of the nutrients, are in the yolk.

USES:

FOR AN EGG WHITE OMELETTE

EGG WHITES
2 egg whites (golf ball)
30 calories

IN A SALAD

CHOPPED EGG
¼ cup (golf ball)
50 calories

AS A SNACK

EGG, HARD-COOKED
1 large (golf ball)
80 calories

STAPLE:
Tofu

Made from soybeans, tofu comes in a wide range of forms—extra-firm for stir-frying, soft silken, seasoned and ready-to-use, and even firm (Chinese) and soft (Japanese) noodles.

USES:

IN A SOUP

SHIRATAKI TOFU NOODLES
½ cup (tennis ball)
20 calories

IN A SMOOTHIE

SILKEN TOFU
½ cup (tennis ball)
60 calories

IN A STIR-FRY

EXTRA-FIRM TOFU
½ cup (tennis ball)
100 calories

STAPLE:
Peanut butter

This American classic supplies protein and good fats, plus B vitamins, vitamin E, and a slew of minerals. It's perfect as a snack, in a main dish, or as a condiment. Peanut butter in moderate amounts is filling, helps stave off hunger, and feels like an indulgence.

USES:

ON AN ENGLISH MUFFIN

PEANUT BUTTER
2 teaspoons (2 small marbles)
60 calories

IN A PEANUT SAUCE

PEANUT BUTTER
1 tablespoon (large marble)
90 calories

ON A RIB OF CELERY

PEANUT BUTTER
2 tablespoons (2 large marbles)
190 calories

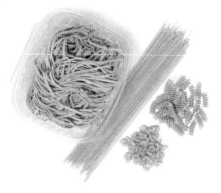

STAPLE:

Whole grain pasta

Whole grain pasta is relatively quick to prepare, with even the longest-cooking shapes taking less than 20 minutes. Although many people think couscous is a type of grain, it actually is very fine nuggets of pasta.

USES:

IN ASIAN SOUP

COOKED BUCKWHEAT
SOBA NOODLES
½ cup (tennis ball)
60 calories

WITH TOMATO SAUCE

COOKED WHOLE WHEAT SPAGHETTI
½ cup (tennis ball)
90 calories

AS A SIDE DISH

COOKED COUSCOUS
⅔ cup (a little less
than 3 golf balls)
120 calories

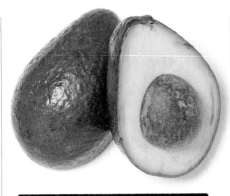

STAPLE:

Avocado

Avocado is worth every calorie for its flavor, creamy texture, and vitamin-packed flesh. Its versatility as a spread, a dip (plain or mixed with tomato and seasonings for guaca-mole), and a topper for salads and sandwiches is hard to match.

USES:

ON A SANDWICH

MASHED AVOCADO
2 tablespoons (2 large marbles)
50 calories

IN A SALAD

DICED AVOCADO
⅓ cup (5 large marbles)
80 calories

AS A DIP

GUACAMOLE
¼ cup (golf ball)
110 calories

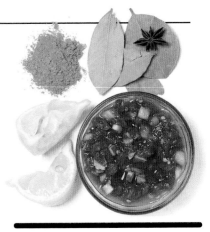

STAPLE:

Freebie condiments

You're home free with these virtually calorie-free condiments. Just keep in mind that some are high in sodium. See the full list of freebie condiments in the box on page 26.

USES:

IN A SALAD

RED WINE VINEGAR
1 teaspoon (small marble)
1 calorie

ON A FISH ENTRÉE

LEMON JUICE
1 teaspoon (small marble)
1 calorie

ON A QUESADILLA

TOMATO SALSA
1 tablespoon (1 large marble)
5 calories

BE A 4-STAR SHOPPER

Cooking the 400-calorie way starts with ingredients that provide maximum taste and nutrition without extra fat, sugar, or calories. Here are a few things to look for as you're cruising the aisles.

CHOOSE PROTEIN

Each *400 Calorie Fix Cookbook* meal specifies exactly which type of protein to use in a recipe, as well as in the dishes that accompany the recipe. Recipes with meat, poultry, or fish usually call for 1 pound, enough for 4 hockey puck–size servings. Larger packages may be a better value. Just divide the contents into suitable portions when you get home and freeze the rest. Cut beef, pork, and lamb into 1-pound (4 hockey pucks) or 4-ounce (1 hockey puck) pieces. For a large fish fillet, use a scale or visual cues to divide it into 1-pound or 4-ounce portions, or cut it up based on the weight of the fish; for example, you might split a 3-pound fish into 3 fairly equal pieces that each weighs about 1 pound.

GO LEAN

These leanest cuts of meat and poultry are lowest in calories (per 3-ounce cooked portion):

- TURKEY BREAST 110 calories
- PORK TENDERLOIN 120 calories
- DUCK BREAST, SKINLESS 120 calories
- 95% EXTRA-LEAN GROUND BEEF 130 calories

Tip

Eating a chicken breast with the skin on adds more than 20 percent more calories. But leaving the skin on during cooking—and removing it before serving—helps keep the meat moist without adding extra calories.

- CHICKEN BREAST, BONELESS, SKINLESS 140 calories
- BEEF TOP ROUND 140 calories
- BEEF EYE ROUND 140 calories
- BEEF ROUND TIP ROAST 150 calories
- TURKEY DARK MEAT 160 calories
- BEEF SIRLOIN TIP 160 calories
- BEEF TOP SIRLOIN 160 calories
- CHICKEN THIGH, BONELESS, SKINLESS 180 calories
- 90% LEAN GROUND BEEF 180 calories
- BEEF BOTTOM ROUND 190 calories
- BEEF ROUND STEAK 190 calories
- PORK BLADE LOIN 200 calories
- PORK SHOULDER BUTT 200 calories

FIND FIBER

The top foods for fiber are canned and dried beans, along with fruits and vegetables, whole grains, and cereals and breads that list a whole grain as the first ingredient. A standard portion of beans is about $1/2$ cup cooked, the size of a tennis ball. Our portions of cooked pasta, rice, and other grains range from $1/3$ cup (5 large marbles) to $2/3$ cup (a little less than 3 golf balls), depending on the number of calories in the other foods in the meal. When you are buying dry pasta, figure on at least 8 servings in a pound.

BEWARE CEREAL SUGAR

High-fiber cereals are proven hunger busters, so read labels to help you pick brands that fit into your 400-calorie framework. Some high-fiber kids' cereals have a fair amount of sugar. Here, we list calories and grams of sugar per 1 cup (baseball) of cereal.

CEREAL	CALORIES	GRAMS OF SUGARS
Puffed wheat	100	0
Shredded wheat, small size	170	0
Fiber cereal, twig shape	120	0
Crispy rice	100	3
Oat bran flakes	140	8
Bran flakes	130	8
Bran cereal, twig shape	160	10
Sugar-dusted shredded wheat, small	180	12
Sugar-coated cornflakes	150	15
Raisin bran	130	18
Granola	530	23

COOK THE RIGHT AMOUNT

Some of our recipes and meals call for cooked pasta, rice, grains, or beans. Unfortunately, food packages may not provide information on the amount of uncooked grain or beans that you need for a cooked portion. We put together this short guide to help you figure out how much is required to make 1 cup cooked.

FOOD	DRY AMOUNT (VOLUME) WEIGHT
Pasta	$1/2$ cup (tennis ball) 2 ounces
Rice	$1/3$ cup (5 large marbles) $2 2/3$ ounces
Couscous	Scant $1/2$ cup (tennis ball) $2 1/2$ ounces
Barley	Heaping $1/4$ cup (golf ball) 2 ounces
Dried beans	Scant $1/2$ cup (tennis ball) $2 2/3$ ounces

Tip

A 16-ounce box of pasta contains at least 8 servings of about 200 calories each. It's easy to make too much, so use a scale to measure accurately. To serve 4, use 6 ounces, a bit less than half a box.

SEEK OUT GOOD FATS

Shop for "good fats" foods in the smallest packages possible since most of our recipes and meals call for no more than $\frac{1}{4}$ cup, or about 1 tablespoon (large marble) per serving. Also, nuts and chocolate can be trigger foods for some people (I'm not mentioning any names!). They're hard to resist and can lead to overeating. Chocolate chips are particularly easy to measure for recipes and easy to eat in small amounts for a quick chocolate fix. Other good fats such as olives, avocados, and fish are perishable, so buy only what you need. At the same time, watch out for extra "bad" fats (like saturated and trans fats) in rice and pasta mixes, frozen vegetable blends, granola-type cereals, crackers, and dairy foods.

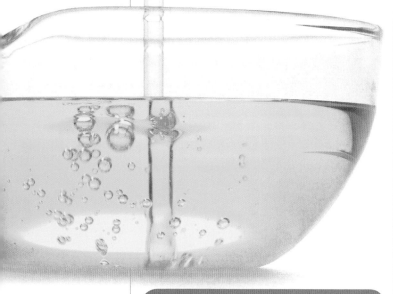

THE GOOD

Most "good fats" foods, with the exception of pure oils, are not 100 percent fat, so their calories per tablespoon vary.

- OLIVES 10 calories
- AVOCADO 15 calories
- SLICED ALMONDS 30 calories
- SUNFLOWER SEEDS 50 calories
- CHOCOLATE CHIPS 50 calories
- PEANUTS 50 calories
- CASHEWS 50 calories
- CHOPPED PECANS 50 calories
- CHOPPED WALNUTS 50 calories
- PESTO SAUCE 80 calories
- TAHINI 90 calories
- PEANUT BUTTER 90 calories
- ALMOND BUTTER 100 calories
- OLIVE OIL 120 calories
- CANOLA OIL 120 calories
- SESAME OIL 120 calories
- PEANUT OIL 120 calories

Tip

Olives and avocados, both high-fat fruits, are packed with nutrients, but also calories. Keep portions down to 5 olives (about 50 calories) or $\frac{1}{4}$ cup (golf ball) of cubed avocado (about 60 calories).

LOAD UP ON FRUITS AND VEGGIES

Most of the *400 Calorie Fix Cookbook* meals call for fruits and vegetables by size rather than weight or volume, for example, a small apple or medium carrot. If you're chopping or slicing them, a serving portion would be $\frac{1}{2}$ to 1 cup. It's hard to beat the flavor and texture of fresh fruits and vegetables when they are in season and reasonably priced. But frozen vegetables and fruits are just as nutritious and are a great substitute when fresh ones will blow your budget. If you use canned vegetables, choose those without added salt and canned fruit without added sugar.

CANNING CALORIES

Canned fruit is okay, but watch out for the sugar! The different types of canning liquids pack different amounts of calories (per ½-cup portion).

- PEACH SLICES (IN WATER)
  30 calories

- PEACH SLICES (IN JUICE)
  50 calories

- PEACH SLICES (IN LIGHT SYRUP)
  70 calories

- PEACH SLICES (IN HEAVY SYRUP)
  90 calories

- PEACH SLICES
  (IN EXTRA-HEAVY SYRUP)
  130 calories

PERFECT PRODUCE PORTIONS

Produce department scales can be hard to find and often are inaccurate, so use your 400 Calorie Lens when picking out common fruits and veggies.

SIZE	APPROXIMATE WEIGHT OR VOLUME	VISUAL CUE
SMALL		
Apple	5¼ ounces	10 large marbles
Potato	4 ounces	Tennis ball
MEDIUM		
Banana	6½ ounces	Pencil length, diameter of a quarter
Beet	2 ounces	Golf ball
Carrot	2½ ounces	Pencil length, diameter of a nickel
Onion	4¼ ounces	Tennis ball
Orange	6¼ ounces	3 golf balls
Sweet potato	6½ ounces	3 golf balls
Tomato	4¾ ounces	Tennis ball
ASSORTED		
Head of broccoli	1 pound	4 baseballs
Head of romaine	1 pound	6 wiffle balls
Bag of lettuce	8 ounces	3 wiffle balls
Half pint of berries	1 cup	1 baseball
Pint of berries	2 cups	2 baseballs

4

BREAKFAST & BRUNCH

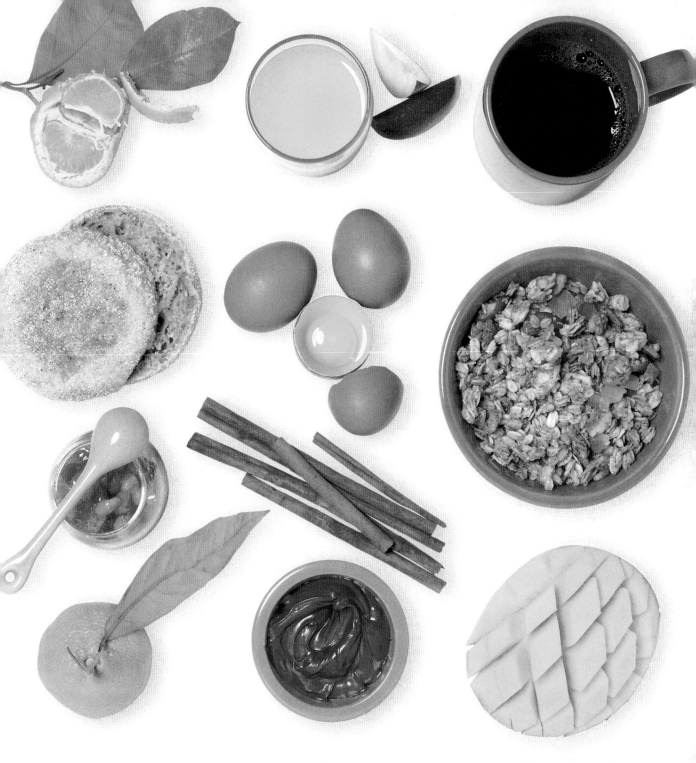

MEXICAN EGGS BENEDICT

PREP TIME: 20 MINUTES / **COOK TIME:** 12 MINUTES / **MAKES** 4 SERVINGS

This recipe features a fresh tomato-avocado salsa in place of high-fat hollandaise sauce. If tomatoes are not in season, substitute a bottled tomato-based salsa or use canned diced tomatoes, preferably no-salt-added.

- 3 plum tomatoes, seeded and chopped
- ⅓ cup chopped Hass avocado (¼ avocado)
- 2 tablespoons finely chopped red onion
- 1 tablespoon chopped fresh cilantro
- 2 teaspoons fresh lime juice
- ½ teaspoon salt
- ⅛ teaspoon freshly ground black pepper
- 2 teaspoons white vinegar
- 8 large eggs
- 8 cups baby spinach
- 4 light (100-calorie) multigrain English muffins, split and toasted
- 4 tablespoons low-fat plain yogurt

1. **COMBINE** the tomatoes, avocado, onion, cilantro, lime juice, ¼ teaspoon of the salt, and the pepper in a bowl. Set the salsa aside.

2. **BRING** 2" of water to a very gentle simmer in a large skillet. Add the vinegar. Carefully break the eggs into the skillet, holding them just above the water level so they slide in without breaking the yolks. Simmer for 5 to 6 minutes, or until the egg whites are firm and the yolks have barely started to set. One at a time, lift the eggs out with a slotted spoon and place on a plate lined with paper towels to absorb the excess water.

3. **MEANWHILE,** coat a large nonstick skillet with cooking spray and heat over medium-high heat. Add the spinach and cook for 1½ to 2 minutes, tossing often, until wilted. Sprinkle with the remaining ¼ teaspoon salt.

4. **ARRANGE** 2 English muffin halves on each of 4 plates. Top each half with ½ cup spinach. Place 1 egg on top of each muffin half. Spoon ½ cup salsa over the eggs and serve with 1 tablespoon yogurt. Serve hot.

MAKE IT A MEAL

Mexican Hot Chocolate: Combine 2½ cups fat-free milk, ¼ cup packed light brown sugar, 3 tablespoons unsweetened cocoa powder, and ⅛ teaspoon ground cinnamon in a medium saucepan over medium heat. Cook, stirring, until the sugar dissolves and the mixture is hot. Divide among 4 cups.
110 CALORIES

410 CALORIES PER MEAL
★ ★ ★ ★

MAKE IT A MEAL

3 broiled pineapple rings drizzled with lime juice
80 CALORIES

380 CALORIES PER MEAL
★ ★ ★ ★

PER SERVING (1 serving = 2 muffin halves, 2 eggs, ½ cup spinach, ½ cup salsa, 1 tablespoon yogurt)

Calories	Total Fat	Saturated Fat	Sodium	Carbohydrate	Dietary Fiber	Protein	Calcium
300	14 g	3.5 g	690 mg	35 g	12 g	21 g	20%

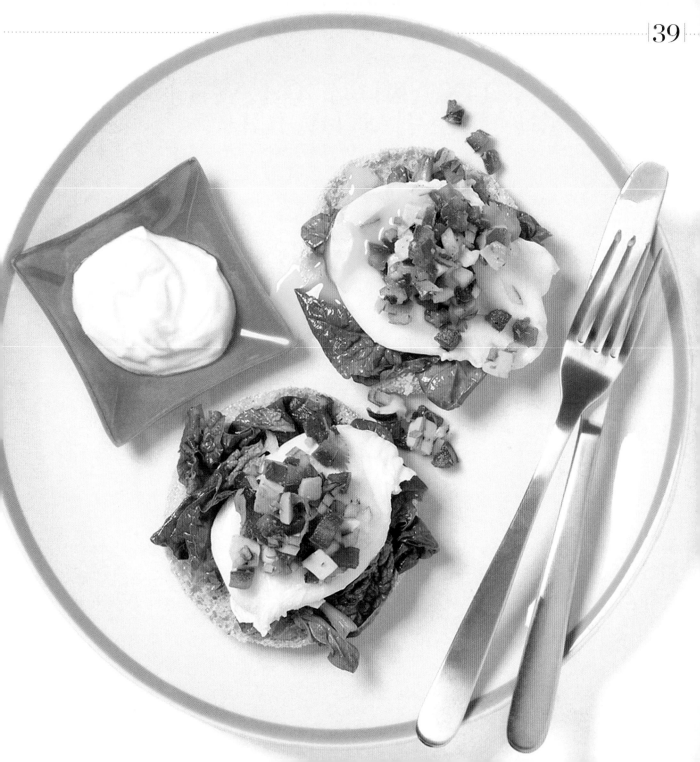

BACON AND EGG ENGLISH MUFFIN SANDWICH

PREP TIME: 5 MINUTES / **COOK TIME:** 9 MINUTES / **MAKES** 1 SERVING

Our version of the classic egg breakfast sandwich trims calories by using a light English muffin—which has plenty of fiber—along with lower-fat versions of bacon and cheese. We've substituted tomato slices for ketchup to add juiciness.

MAKE IT A MEAL

1 small pear
90 CALORIES

Cappuccino made with 1 cup fat-free milk
80 CALORIES

410
CALORIES PER MEAL
★ ★ ★

MAKE IT A MEAL

1 cup fresh fruit salad
100 CALORIES

Cappuccino made with 1 cup fat-free milk
80 CALORIES

420
CALORIES PER MEAL
★ ★ ★

1　light (100-calorie) multigrain English muffin, split

1　slice center-cut, 30%-less-fat bacon, halved crosswise

1　large egg
　 Pinch of freshly ground black pepper

2　tablespoons shredded reduced-fat Cheddar cheese

2　slices tomato

1. **TOAST** the English muffin.

2. **COOK** the bacon in a small nonstick skillet over medium heat for 3 minutes per side, or until crisp. Transfer to a plate lined with paper towels to drain.

3. **RETURN** the skillet to the heat. Add the egg, breaking the yolk, and sprinkle with the pepper. Cook for 1½ minutes, or until starting to set. Flip the egg over, sprinkle with the cheese, cover, and cook for 1 minute, or until the cheese melts and the egg is cooked through.

4. **PLACE** one English muffin half on a plate. Top with the bacon, egg, tomato slices, and the second half of the muffin.

PER SERVING (1 serving = 1 sandwich)

Calories	Total Fat	Saturated Fat	Sodium	Carbohydrate	Dietary Fiber	Protein	Calcium
240	11 g	4 g	440 mg	27 g	9 g	18 g	30%

RINA'S SHAKSHOUKA

PREP TIME: 10 MINUTES / **COOK TIME:** 43 MINUTES / **MAKES** 4 SERVINGS

Sometimes described as Israeli "huevos rancheros," this Middle Eastern favorite with Moroccan roots is so popular that some restaurants in Israel are dedicated to shakshouka in its numerous variations. In our classic version, modified from a recipe from Mindy's Israeli cousin Rina, eggs are cooked on top of a bubbling tomato–bell pepper sauce.

1	tablespoon olive oil
1	medium onion, chopped
6	cloves garlic, finely chopped
3	medium bell peppers (any combination of colors), diced
1	can (14.5 ounces) diced or crushed tomatoes
1	chipotle pepper in adobo sauce, diced
2	tablespoons light brown sugar
1	tablespoon ground cumin
1	teaspoon smoked paprika
½	teaspoon freshly ground black pepper
4	large eggs

1. HEAT the oil in a large saucepan over medium heat. Add the onion and garlic, and cook for 3 minutes. Add the bell peppers and cook for 10 minutes. Add the tomatoes, chipotle pepper, brown sugar, cumin, paprika, and black pepper. Partially cover and cook over medium heat for 20 minutes, until the sauce has thickened.

2. BREAK the eggs one at a time into the sauce, keeping them separate so they don't touch. Cover the pan, reduce the heat to medium-low, and simmer for 10 minutes, until the eggs are fully cooked.

MAKE
IT A
MEAL

Whole wheat
pita (6")
170 CALORIES

½ cup orange juice
50 CALORIES

420
CALORIES
PER MEAL
★ ★

MAKE
IT A
MEAL

1 small
(3¼ ounces)
100% whole
wheat bagel
210 CALORIES

410
CALORIES
PER MEAL
★ ★ ★

PER SERVING (1 serving = 1 egg, 1 cup sauce)

Calories	Total Fat	Saturated Fat	Sodium	Carbohydrate	Dietary Fiber	Protein	Calcium
200	9 g	2 g	230 mg	23 g	4 g	10 g	10%

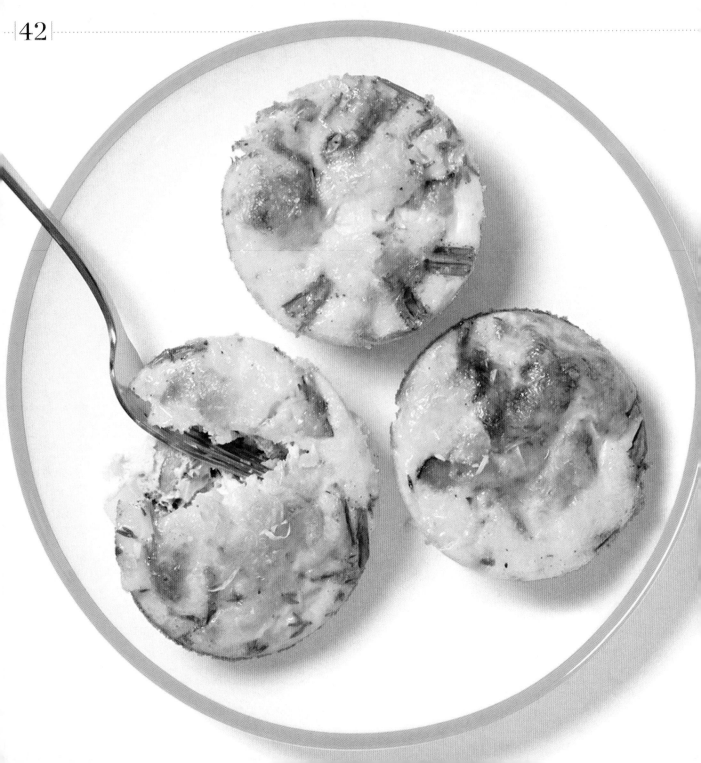

MINI HAM-AND-CHEESE QUICHES

PREP TIME: 15 MINUTES / **COOK TIME:** 34 MINUTES / **MAKES** 4 SERVINGS

You may prefer to use an egg substitute, which works equally well in this recipe. If you can't find reduced-sodium ham in the packaged luncheon meat case, ask for it at the deli counter.

1 large russet (baking) potato (12 ounces), peeled and cut into ¼" dice

1 teaspoon olive oil

¼ cup finely chopped shallots

½ teaspoon dried thyme

6 ounces reduced-sodium deli-sliced ham, chopped

4 large eggs

¾ cup low-fat milk

1 tablespoon chopped fresh chives

⅛ teaspoon ground nutmeg

¼ teaspoon freshly ground black pepper

½ cup shredded reduced-fat Swiss cheese

1. **PREHEAT** the oven to 350°F. Coat 8 large (3-ounce) muffin cups or 12 smaller (2-ounce) muffin cups with cooking spray.

2. **PLACE** the potato in a medium saucepan with enough cold water to cover by 2". Bring to a boil and cook for 10 minutes, or until the potato dice are tender but still hold their shape. Drain.

3. **MEANWHILE,** heat the oil in a medium nonstick skillet over medium-high heat. Add the shallots and thyme, and cook for 1 minute, stirring often. Add the ham and cook for 4 minutes, or until lightly browned. Remove from the heat and set aside to cool for 5 minutes. Stir in the potato.

4. **COMBINE** the eggs, milk, chives, nutmeg, and pepper in a medium bowl. Fill each muffin cup with one-eighth of the ham mixture for the larger cups or one-twelfth for the smaller cups, filling each cup about halfway. Divide the egg mixture among the muffin cups and sprinkle each with some of the cheese.

5. **BAKE** for 22 to 24 minutes for the large muffin cups or 18 to 20 minutes for the smaller muffin cups, until the eggs are set and slightly puffed. Remove from the muffin cups and serve.

MAKE IT A MEAL

1 slice (1 ounce) multigrain toast with 1 teaspoon all-fruit jam
90 CALORIES

½ cup strawberries
30 CALORIES

410 CALORIES PER MEAL
★ ★

MAKE IT A MEAL

Mimosa: Mix 3 ounces orange juice with 3 ounces Champagne
100 CALORIES

½ cup strawberries
30 CALORIES

420 CALORIES PER MEAL
★ ★

PER SERVING (1 serving = 2 large or 3 smaller quiches)

Calories	Total Fat	Saturated Fat	Sodium	Carbohydrate	Dietary Fiber	Protein	Calcium
290	11 g	3.5 g	550 mg	23 g	2 g	24 g	25%

BREAKFAST FRIJOLES TOSTADAS

PREP TIME: 5 MINUTES / **COOK TIME:** 10 MINUTES / **MAKES** 4 SERVINGS

Perfect for brunch or even a weekday breakfast, these tostadas are quick to make if you have all the ingredients on hand. Vary the type of salsa—we used traditional tomato salsa—and reduced-fat cheese to your liking.

4	(6") corn tortillas
1	tablespoon olive oil
½	medium onion, diced
1	cup cooked or rinsed and drained canned pinto beans
½	cup water
½	teaspoon ground cumin
¼	teaspoon salt
½	cup shredded reduced-fat Mexican 4-cheese blend
½	cup salsa
½	cup guacamole
½	cup diced tomato
4	tablespoons low-fat plain yogurt

1. **WRAP** the tortillas in foil and place in a warm oven.

2. **HEAT** the oil in a medium skillet over medium heat. Add the onion and cook, stirring often, for 5 minutes, until softened. Add the beans, water, cumin, and salt. Mash the beans with a potato masher or fork to a slightly chunky consistency. Cook this mixture, which makes the frijoles, for 5 minutes, stirring occasionally.

3. **PLACE** a warmed tortilla on each of 4 plates. Top each tortilla with ¼ cup frijoles, 2 tablespoons each of cheese, salsa, guacamole, and tomato, and 1 tablespoon of yogurt.

BREAKFAST HUEVOS TOSTADAS
(variation)

SCRAMBLE 4 large eggs in a nonstick skillet. Use in place of the frijoles.

MAKE IT A MEAL

¾ cup orange juice
80 CALORIES

Latte made with ¾ cup low-fat milk
80 CALORIES

410
CALORIES PER MEAL
★ ★

MAKE the variation A MEAL

¾ cup orange juice
80 CALORIES

Latte made with 1 cup low-fat milk
100 CALORIES

410
CALORIES PER MEAL
★ ★ ★

PER SERVING (1 serving = 1 tostada) Breakfast Huevos Tostadas (1 serving = 1 tostada)

Calories	Total Fat	Saturated Fat	Sodium	Carbohydrate	Dietary Fiber	Protein	Calcium
250	11 g	3 g	800 mg	30 g	6 g	10 g	25%
230	12 g	4 g	550 mg	20 g	3 g	13 g	25%

PERSIAN HERB OMELET

PREP TIME: 20 MINUTES / **COOK TIME:** 2 HOURS 25 MINUTES / **MAKES** 4 SERVINGS

The combination of herbs gives this dish a unique fresh flavor. The sweetness of the roasted tomatoes provides nice flavor notes.

1	cup halved cherry tomatoes
1	tablespoon olive oil
⅛	teaspoon salt
1	teaspoon balsamic vinegar
6	large eggs
1	tablespoon all-purpose flour
½	teaspoon baking powder
¾	cup chopped fresh parsley
¾	cup chopped chives or scallion greens
¾	cup chopped fresh cilantro
¾	cup chopped fresh dill
¼	cup finely chopped red onion
¼	cup chopped walnuts
2	teaspoons finely grated lemon zest
½	teaspoon salt
¼	teaspoon turmeric
¼	teaspoon freshly ground black pepper
½	lemon

1. **PREHEAT** the oven to 250°F. Toss the tomatoes with the oil and salt. Place in a small baking pan and bake for 2 hours, or until browned and caramelized. Remove from the oven and drizzle with the vinegar.

2. **INCREASE** the oven temperature to 350°F. Coat a 9" pie plate with cooking spray.

3. **BEAT** the eggs, flour, and baking powder in a large bowl for 2 minutes. Add the parsley, chives, cilantro, dill, onion, walnuts, lemon zest, salt, turmeric, and pepper.

4. **SCRAPE** the mixture into the pie plate and bake for 20 minutes, or until lightly browned and firm to the touch. Remove from oven. Squeeze the lemon juice over the omelet.

5. **CUT** into 8 wedges and top with the roasted tomatoes.

MAKE
IT A
MEAL

1 medium (6")
whole wheat pita
170 CALORIES

½ cup cantaloupe
cubes
25 CALORIES

415
CALORIES
PER MEAL
★ ★ ★

MAKE
IT A
MEAL

1 cup fresh
fruit salad
100 CALORIES

6 ounces light
yogurt
80 CALORIES

400
CALORIES
PER MEAL
★ ★

PER SERVING (1 serving = 2 wedges omelet, 2 tablespoons tomatoes)

Calories	Total Fat	Saturated Fat	Sodium	Carbohydrate	Dietary Fiber	Protein	Calcium
220	16 g	3.5 g	540 mg	9 g	2 g	12 g	10%

RICOTTA SOUFFLÉS

PREP TIME: 30 MINUTES / **COOK TIME:** 35 MINUTES / MAKE 4 SERVINGS

Perfect for brunch or dinner, these savory soufflés—accented with bright lemon and delicate chives—are a little more forgiving than a traditional soufflé because the ricotta adds a fair amount of stability.

1	tablespoon butter
2	tablespoons all-purpose flour
1	cup low-fat (2%) evaporated milk
4	large eggs, separated, at room temperature
½	teaspoon cream of tartar
⅓	cup part-skim ricotta cheese
¼	cup grated Parmesan cheese
3	tablespoons finely chopped fresh chives
1½	teaspoons grated lemon zest
½	teaspoon coarse salt
⅛	teaspoon freshly ground black pepper

1. **PREHEAT** the oven to 400°F. Coat four 1-cup ramekins or baking dishes with cooking spray and place on a baking sheet.

2. **MELT** the butter in a small saucepan over medium heat. Add the flour, and cook, stirring, until evenly blended. Slowly whisk in the evaporated milk and bring to a simmer (the mixture will thicken quickly). Remove the white sauce from the heat and let it cool.

3. **COMBINE** the egg whites and cream of tartar in a medium bowl. Beat with an electric mixer on medium speed until frothy. Increase to high speed and beat until soft peaks form. Set aside.

4. **IN** a separate bowl, stir together the cooled white sauce, ricotta, Parmesan, chives, lemon zest, salt, and pepper until evenly blended. Add the egg yolks and stir well to incorporate.

5. **STIR** one-third of the beaten egg whites into the ricotta mixture, gently mixing until evenly blended. Add the remaining egg whites and gently fold in until just combined—do not overmix.

6. **DIVIDE** the soufflé mixture among the ramekins. Place the soufflés in the oven and immediately reduce the oven temperature to 350°F. Bake for 25 minutes, or until puffed and slightly golden.

PER SERVING (1 serving = 1 cup)

Calories	Total Fat	Saturated Fat	Sodium	Carbohydrate	Dietary Fiber	Protein	Calcium
240	14 g	7 g	530 mg	12 g	0 g	17 g	35%

LEMON AND WILD BLUEBERRY MUFFINS

PREP TIME: 10 MINUTES+ 20 MINUTES COOLING / **COOK TIME:** 18 MINUTES / **MAKES** 12 SERVINGS

A light lemon muffin with wild blueberries thrown in for flavor and color, these are nice for breakfast or coffee break/snack time.

1¼	cups all-purpose flour
½	cup white whole wheat flour
½	cup sugar
2	teaspoons baking powder
1	teaspoon baking soda
¼	teaspoon salt
1	container (6 ounces) fat-free lemon yogurt
¼	cup canola oil
1	large egg
2	teaspoons lemon zest
2	tablespoons fresh lemon juice
½	cup frozen wild blueberries

1. **PREHEAT** the oven to 375°F. Line a 12-cup muffin tin with paper liners or coat with cooking spray.

2. **WHISK** together the flours, sugar, baking powder, baking soda, and salt in a medium bowl. Combine the yogurt, oil, egg, lemon zest, and lemon juice in a small bowl. Pour the yogurt mixture into the flour mixture and mix until just blended—do not overmix. Fold in the frozen blueberries, taking care not to smash them.

3. **DIVIDE** the batter among the muffin cups. Bake for 16 to 18 minutes, or until a toothpick inserted in the center of a muffin comes out clean. Let the muffins cool in the pan for 5 minutes before transferring to a rack to cool completely.

MAKE IT A MEAL

Omelet made in a nonstick pan with 1 whole egg, 1 egg white, ½ cup chopped onion, ½ cup sliced mushrooms
135 CALORIES

1 cup low-fat milk
100 CALORIES

385
CALORIES PER MEAL
★ ★

MAKE IT A MEAL

½ cantaloupe filled with ½ cup 1% cottage cheese
240 CALORIES

390
CALORIES PER MEAL
★ ★

PER SERVING (1 serving = 1 muffin)

Calories	Total Fat	Saturated Fat	Sodium	Carbohydrate	Dietary Fiber	Protein	Calcium
150	5 g	0.5 g	250 mg	24 g	1 g	3 g	8%

CRUMBLE-TOP COFFEE CAKE MUFFINS

PREP TIME: 20 MINUTES + 5 MINUTES COOLING / **COOK TIME:** 15 MINUTES / **MAKES** 12 MUFFINS

These cinnamon- and vanilla-kissed muffins can be frozen and thawed as needed, making them perfect for breakfast or snack time.

TOPPING

- ⅓ cup all-purpose flour
- ⅓ cup chopped pecans
- ¼ cup packed light brown sugar
- ½ teaspoon ground cinnamon
- 2 tablespoons butter, melted
- 1 tablespoon water

MUFFINS

- 1½ cups all-purpose flour
- ⅔ cup white whole wheat flour
- ½ cup sugar
- 2 teaspoons baking soda
- 1 teaspoon baking powder
- ¼ teaspoon ground cinnamon
- ¼ teaspoon salt
- 1 cup low-fat buttermilk
- 3 tablespoons canola oil
- 3 tablespoons unsweetened applesauce

1. **PREHEAT** the oven to 375°F. Coat a 12-cup muffin tin with cooking spray or use paper liners.

2. **TO MAKE THE TOPPING:** Combine the flour, pecans, brown sugar, and cinnamon in a small bowl. Stir in the butter and water until crumbly and blended. Set aside.

3. **TO MAKE THE MUFFINS:** Whisk together the flours, sugar, baking soda, baking powder, cinnamon, and salt in a medium bowl. Combine the buttermilk, oil, and applesauce in a small bowl. Pour the buttermilk mixture over the flour mixture and mix until just blended—do not overmix.

4. **SPOON** about ¼ cup batter into each muffin cup. Top each muffin with a scant tablespoon of crumb topping, sprinkling it over the center. Bake for 13 to 15 minutes, or until a toothpick inserted in a muffin comes out clean. Let cool for 5 minutes in the pan before removing.

MAKE IT A MEAL

Parfait made with ¾ cup low-fat plain yogurt and 1 cup thawed frozen berries **180 CALORIES**

400 CALORIES PER MEAL ★

MAKE IT A MEAL

Smoothie made with ½ cup low-fat plain yogurt, ½ cup low-fat milk, and 1 cup frozen peaches **180 CALORIES**

400 CALORIES PER MEAL ★

PER SERVING (1 serving = 1 muffin)

Calories	Total Fat	Saturated Fat	Sodium	Carbohydrate	Dietary Fiber	Protein	Calcium
220	8 g	2 g	340 mg	34 g	2 g	4 g	6%

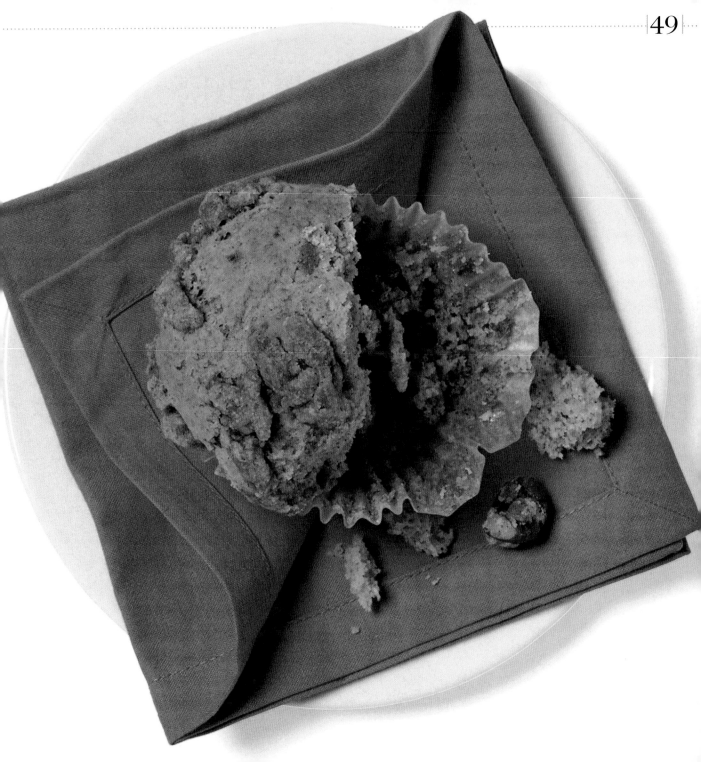

BREAKFAST CUPCAKES

PREP TIME: 20 MINUTES + 10 MINUTES COOLING / **COOK TIME:** 24 MINUTES / **MAKES** 12 SERVINGS

Who wouldn't want to start the day with a treat? Pear and cardamom muffins with a brown sugar–sweetened cranberry-almond topping fit the bill perfectly.

1	teaspoon butter
⅓	cup sliced almonds
2	tablespoons light brown sugar
½	cup dried cranberries or chopped dried cherries
1½	cups all-purpose flour
½	cup white whole wheat flour
½	cup sugar
1	tablespoon ground flaxseeds
2	teaspoons baking soda
1	teaspoon baking powder
¼	teaspoon salt
¼	teaspoon ground cardamom
2	large eggs
¾	cup low-fat buttermilk
¼	cup canola oil
½	teaspoon vanilla extract
1	cup peeled, finely chopped fresh pear (about 1 large)

1. **PREHEAT** the oven to 400°F. Line a 12-cup muffin tin with paper liners or coat with cooking spray.

2. **COAT** a small nonstick skillet with cooking spray and heat over medium heat. Add the butter and almonds, and cook for 2 minutes, stirring, until the almonds are toasted. Sprinkle the brown sugar over the almonds and stir to coat. Remove from the heat and mix in the cranberries. Set aside to cool slightly.

3. **WHISK** together the flours, sugar, ground flaxseeds, baking soda, baking powder, salt, and cardamom in a large bowl. Then whisk together the eggs, buttermilk, oil, and vanilla in a separate bowl. Add the pear to the flour mixture and stir to coat the pear pieces. Add the buttermilk mixture to the flour mixture and stir just until evenly blended—do not overmix.

4. **DIVIDE** the batter among the muffin cups. Top each muffin with 1 tablespoon of the almond-cranberry topping. Bake for 20 to 22 minutes, or until a toothpick inserted in the center of a muffin comes out clean. Let the muffins cool in the pan for 10 minutes before transferring to a rack to cool completely.

PER SERVING (1 serving = 1 breakfast cupcake)

Calories	Total Fat	Saturated Fat	Sodium	Carbohydrate	Dietary Fiber	Protein	Calcium
220	8 g	1 g	330 mg	34 g	2 g	5 g	6%

CURRANT-ALMOND SCONES

PREP TIME: 10 MINUTES / **COOK TIME:** 15 MINUTES / **MAKES** 8 SERVINGS

You can find currants in the same section of the market as raisins. For a different flavor, substitute diced dried apricots or dried tart cherries for the currants.

⅔ cup whole wheat flour

⅓ cup all-purpose flour

½ cup old-fashioned rolled oats

2 tablespoons granulated sugar

1 teaspoon baking powder

¼ teaspoon baking soda

¼ teaspoon ground nutmeg

2 tablespoons unsalted butter, cut into small cubes

2 tablespoons marzipan (we used Solo)

¼ cup buttermilk

1 large egg

½ teaspoon vanilla extract

¼ cup currants

¼ cup slivered almonds

1 egg white whisked with 1 teaspoon water

2 tablespoons white decorating sugar

1. **PREHEAT** the oven to 400°F. Coat a baking sheet with cooking spray or use a nonstick baking sheet.

2. **COMBINE** the flours, oats, granulated sugar, baking powder, baking soda, and nutmeg in a food processor. With the processor running, add the butter 1 cube at a time. Then add the marzipan 1 teaspoon at a time. Process until the mixture looks crumbly. Add the buttermilk, whole egg, and vanilla, and process just until well mixed. Stir in the currants and almonds.

3. **PLACE** the dough on a lightly floured cutting board. Knead lightly to finish distributing all the ingredients. Form into a ball, flatten into an 8" circle (½" thick) with your hands or a floured rolling pin, and cut into 8 wedges. Place the wedges on the baking sheet. Brush with the egg white mixture and sprinkle with the decorating sugar.

4. **BAKE** for 12 to 15 minutes, or until lightly browned.

MAKE IT A MEAL

1 cup orange juice
110 CALORIES

2 tablespoons light cream cheese
60 CALORIES

380 CALORIES PER MEAL
★

MAKE IT A MEAL

1 cup low-fat milk
100 CALORIES

1 medium banana
110 CALORIES

420 CALORIES PER MEAL
★

PER SERVING (1 serving = 1 scone)

Calories	Total Fat	Saturated Fat	Sodium	Carbohydrate	Dietary Fiber	Protein	Calcium
210	7 g	2.5 g	125 mg	32 g	3 g	6 g	8%

MAPLE, DATE, AND NUT BREAD

PREP TIME: 15 MINUTES + 1 HOUR COOLING / **COOK TIME:** 55 MINUTES / **MAKES** 10 SERVINGS

A maple syrup–sweetened loaf packed with sweet dates and chopped walnuts, this bread freezes nicely in a freezer bag and keeps for 3 days at room temperature (wrap well).

1	cup chopped dates
1	cup very hot water
1¾	cups all-purpose flour
1	teaspoon baking soda
¼	teaspoon salt
3	tablespoons Smart Balance spread
¼	cup packed light brown sugar
½	cup maple syrup
1	large egg
½	teaspoon vanilla or maple extract
½	cup chopped walnuts

1. **PREHEAT** the oven to 350°F. Coat a 9" x 5" loaf pan with cooking spray.

2. **STIR** together the dates and hot water in a small bowl. Set aside to soak while preparing the rest of the recipe.

3. **STIR** together the flour, baking soda, and salt in a small bowl.

4. **COMBINE** the spread, brown sugar, and maple syrup in a medium bowl. Beat with an electric mixer on medium speed until smooth. Beat in the egg and vanilla until smooth.

5. **ADD** the dates and soaking water to the bowl and mix on low speed until blended. Stir in the walnuts. Scrape the batter into the loaf pan.

6. **BAKE** for 45 to 55 minutes, or until a toothpick inserted in the center of the loaf comes out clean. Let cool in the pan for 10 minutes before transferring to a rack to cool completely. Cut the loaf into 10 slices.

PER SERVING (1 serving = 1 slice)

Calories	Total Fat	Saturated Fat	Sodium	Carbohydrate	Dietary Fiber	Protein	Calcium
260	7 g	1.5 g	220 mg	45 g	2 g	4 g	4%

NUTTY BREAKFAST BARS

PREP TIME: 10 MINUTES + 1 HOUR COOLING / **COOK TIME:** 5 MINUTES / **MAKES** 8 SERVINGS

When sticking to a healthy eating plan, nothing beats the grab-and-go breakfast. These granola bars are packed with sliced almonds and dried blueberries. If the blueberries are hard to find, substitute dried currants, found near the raisins at the market.

2½	cups crispy brown rice cereal
½	cup sliced almonds
1	tablespoon ground flaxseeds
1	tablespoon toasted wheat germ
3	tablespoons dried blueberries
3	tablespoons natural creamy peanut butter
3	tablespoons honey
2	tablespoons apricot preserves
½	teaspoon vanilla extract
¼	teaspoon almond extract

1. **COAT** an 8" x 8" baking pan with cooking spray.

2. **STIR** together the cereal, almonds, ground flaxseeds, wheat germ, and blueberries in a medium bowl.

3. **COMBINE** the peanut butter, honey, and preserves in a large saucepan. Stir over medium heat until smooth. When the mixture comes to a simmer, reduce the heat to medium-low and simmer for 3 minutes, stirring constantly. Stir in the vanilla and almond extracts.

4. **REMOVE** the pan from the heat and, working quickly, mix in the cereal mixture, stirring until evenly coated. Transfer the mixture to the baking dish. Coat a silicone spatula with cooking spray and press the mixture evenly and firmly into the baking pan.

5. **ALLOW** the mixture to cool for at least 1 hour before cutting it into 8 bars. Bars can be individually wrapped and kept at room temperature for up to 5 days, or frozen until needed.

MAKE IT A MEAL

¼ cup chopped dried fruit
120 CALORIES

1 container (6 ounces) fat-free (0%) plain Greek yogurt
90 CALORIES

Coffee with 2 tablespoons low-fat milk
15 CALORIES

385 CALORIES PER MEAL
★ ★ ★

MAKE IT A MEAL

½ cup 1% cottage cheese mixed with 1 tablespoon sliced almonds and 1 medium sliced banana
220 CALORIES

380 CALORIES PER MEAL
★ ★ ★

PER SERVING (1 serving = one 2" x 4" bar)

Calories	Total Fat	Saturated Fat	Sodium	Carbohydrate	Dietary Fiber	Protein	Calcium
160	7 g	0.5 g	65 mg	24 g	2 g	4 g	2%

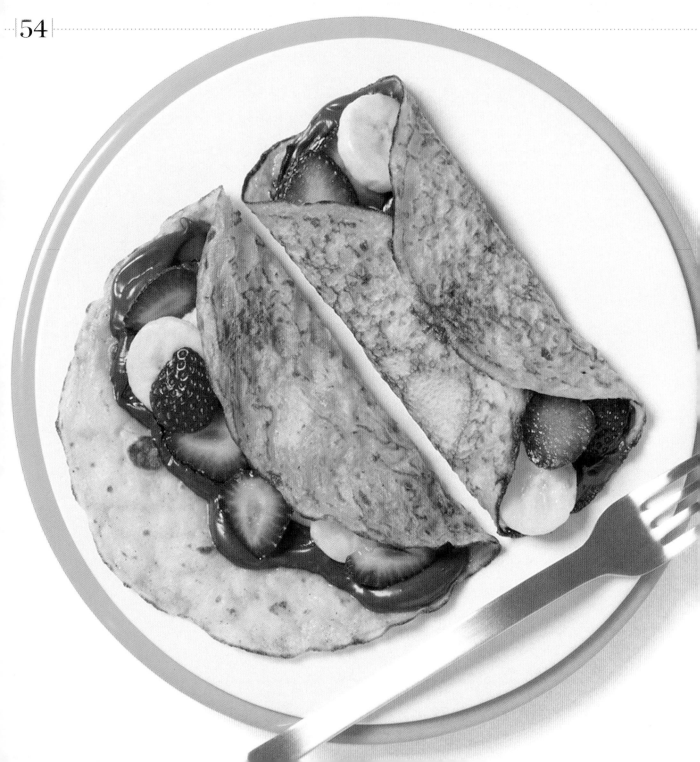

CRÊPES WITH STRAWBERRIES, BANANAS, AND NUTELLA

PREP TIME: 25 MINUTES + 1 HOUR RESTING / **COOK TIME:** 35 MINUTES / **MAKES** 4 SERVINGS

The key to successful crêpes is a pan that allows the crêpes to release easily without sticking. Crêpes can be made ahead of time, separated with foil, parchment, or waxed paper, then wrapped and refrigerated until ready to use.

CRÊPES

- ½ cup all-purpose flour
- 1 tablespoon sugar
- ⅛ teaspoon ground cinnamon
- ⅛ teaspoon salt
- 2 large eggs
- 1 cup fat-free milk

FILLING

- 2 cups strawberries, sliced
- 1 banana, sliced
- 2 teaspoons sugar
- ½ teaspoon vanilla extract
- 4 tablespoons chocolate-hazelnut spread, such as Nutella, warmed

1. TO MAKE THE CRÊPES: Combine the flour, sugar, cinnamon, and salt in a bowl. Whisk together the eggs and milk in a separate bowl. Whisk the egg mixture into the flour mixture until well combined. Cover and let rest in the refrigerator for at least 1 hour or overnight.

2. PREHEAT the oven to 275°F. Coat a large baking sheet with cooking spray.

3. COAT a nonstick crêpe pan or 8" skillet with cooking spray and heat over medium heat. Pour 3 tablespoons of crêpe batter into the pan, tipping to coat the bottom evenly. Cook for 1 to 1½ minutes per side, until lightly browned. Repeat 7 more times with the remaining batter. Stack the crêpes as you work and cover to keep warm.

4. TO MAKE THE FILLING: Combine the strawberries, banana, sugar, and vanilla in a medium bowl.

5. ARRANGE the crêpes on a work surface. Spread each with 1½ teaspoons chocolate-hazelnut spread in a straight line across the center. Top the spread with 6 tablespoons of the strawberry mixture, then roll up jelly-roll style. Transfer the crêpes to the baking sheet, seam-side up. Bake for 9 to 10 minutes, until the filling is warm.

MAKE IT A MEAL

¾ cup low-fat or fat-free plain yogurt as a topping
120 CALORIES

400 CALORIES PER MEAL
★

MAKE IT A MEAL

1 cup low-fat milk
100 CALORIES

380 CALORIES PER MEAL
★

PER SERVING (1 serving = 2 filled crêpes)

Calories	Total Fat	Saturated Fat	Sodium	Carbohydrate	Dietary Fiber	Protein	Calcium
280	9 g	2.5 g	135 mg	44 g	3 g	9 g	10%

CHALLAH BREAD PUDDING WITH APPLE SYRUP

PREP TIME: 10 MINUTES / **COOK TIME:** 35 MINUTES / **MAKES** 4 SERVINGS

Granny Smith and Golden Delicious apples hold their shape well during cooking. In the summer months, try this recipe with peaches and use peach nectar in place of the apple cider.

3	large eggs
1	cup low-fat or fat-free milk
1	tablespoon sugar
½	teaspoon vanilla extract
6	ounces (about 6 standard slices) challah bread, cut into 1" cubes
1¼	cups apple cider
1	tablespoon maple syrup
2	medium Granny Smith or Golden Delicious apples
1	teaspoon unsalted butter
1	tablespoon light brown sugar
½	teaspoon ground cinnamon

1. **PREHEAT** the oven to 350°F. Coat a 13" x 9" baking pan with cooking spray.

2. **WHISK** together the eggs, milk, sugar, and vanilla in a medium bowl. Put the challah cubes into the baking pan. Pour the egg mixture over the bread cubes and mix gently to combine. Cover with foil and bake for 30 minutes. Remove the foil. Bake for 5 minutes, or until the top is lightly browned.

3. **MEANWHILE,** combine 1 cup of the apple cider and the maple syrup in a small saucepan. Simmer over low heat for at least 20 minutes, until reduced to ¼ cup. The syrup should lightly coat the back of a spoon. Set aside.

4. **NEXT,** core the apples and cut into ¼" slices. Melt the butter in a large skillet over medium heat. Add the apples, ¼ cup apple cider, brown sugar, and cinnamon. Cook over medium heat for 10 minutes, or until the apples are soft.

5. **SERVE** the bread pudding topped with one-fourth of the apple mixture and 1 tablespoon of apple syrup.

PER SERVING (1 serving = 1 cup bread pudding, ½ cup apples, 1 tablespoon syrup)

Calories	Total Fat	Saturated Fat	Sodium	Carbohydrate	Dietary Fiber	Protein	Calcium
330	8 g	3 g	300 mg	56 g	3 g	11 g	15%

BANANA PANCAKES WITH MAPLE SYRUP

PREP TIME: 10 MINUTES / **COOK TIME:** 15 MINUTES / **MAKES** 4 SERVINGS

The bananas add sweetness and texture to this traditional breakfast dish. For extra fiber, use white whole wheat flour for some of the all-purpose flour.

1½	cups all-purpose flour
1	tablespoon sugar
1¾	teaspoons baking powder
⅛	teaspoon salt
1	cup fat-free milk
1	large egg, lightly beaten
1	tablespoon canola oil
½	teaspoon vanilla extract
1	large banana, sliced
16	teaspoons maple syrup

1. **COMBINE** the flour, sugar, baking powder, and salt in a large bowl. Combine the milk, egg, oil, and vanilla in a separate bowl. Stir the milk mixture into the flour mixture until smooth. Gently fold in the banana slices.

2. **COAT** a large nonstick skillet with cooking spray and heat over medium heat. Spoon 4 scant ¼ cups of batter into the skillet and cook for 2 to 3 minutes, or until the tops are covered with bubbles and the edges look cooked. Flip and cook for 2 minutes, or until browned on the second side. Transfer to a plate and keep warm. Repeat with the remaining batter and cooking spray as needed. Serve 3 pancakes per person, drizzled with 4 teaspoons maple syrup.

MAKE
IT A
MEAL

3 slices cooked
turkey bacon
60 CALORIES

390
**CALORIES
PER MEAL**

MAKE
IT A
MEAL

¾ cup grapefruit
juice
70 CALORIES

400
**CALORIES
PER MEAL**
★

PER SERVING (1 serving = 3 pancakes, 4 teaspoons maple syrup)

Calories	Total Fat	Saturated Fat	Sodium	Carbohydrate	Dietary Fiber	Protein	Calcium
330	5 g	0.5 g	330 mg	66 g	2 g	9 g	20%

BREAKFAST FRUIT PIZZA

PREP TIME: 15 MINUTES + 5 MINUTES COOLING / **COOK TIME:** 15 MINUTES / **MAKES** 4 SERVINGS

Fresh fruit arranged artfully on a pizza crust with sweetened cheese topping makes for a satisfying breakfast. Vary the fruit according to season or your taste—bananas, grapes, cherries, and peaches would all be delicious.

MAKE
IT A
MEAL

1 tablespoon
sliced almonds
30 CALORIES

400
CALORIES
PER MEAL
★

MAKE
IT A
MEAL

½ cup low-fat milk
50 CALORIES

420
CALORIES
PER MEAL

1   tube (11 ounces) refrigerated thin-crust pizza dough

⅔   cup part-skim ricotta cheese

3   ounces Neufchâtel cheese, at room temperature

2   tablespoons sugar

¼   teaspoon vanilla extract

2   medium plums, sliced

½   cup fresh blueberries

½   teaspoon ground cinnamon

1. PREHEAT the oven to 425°F. Coat a 12" pizza pan or baking sheet with cooking spray.

2. REMOVE the pizza dough from the tube. Spread the dough onto the pizza pan or baking sheet, pressing it lightly with your fingers (the dough will not spread all the way to the edge of the pan). Bake for 10 to 12 minutes. Remove the crust from the oven but leave the oven on.

3. MEANWHILE, combine the ricotta, Neufchâtel, sugar, and vanilla in a small bowl and stir to blend. Spread the cheese mixture over the crust, leaving approximately a ½" border all around.

4. ARRANGE the plums and blueberries decoratively on top of the cheese layer. Sprinkle the cinnamon over the fruit. Bake for 13 to 15 minutes, or until the crust is nicely browned and the fruit appears barely cooked. Let the pizza cool for 5 minutes before cutting into 4 wedges.

PER SERVING (1 serving = one 7" wedge)

Calories	Total Fat	Saturated Fat	Sodium	Carbohydrate	Dietary Fiber	Protein	Calcium
370	11 g	5 g	700 mg	53 g	2 g	14 g	15%

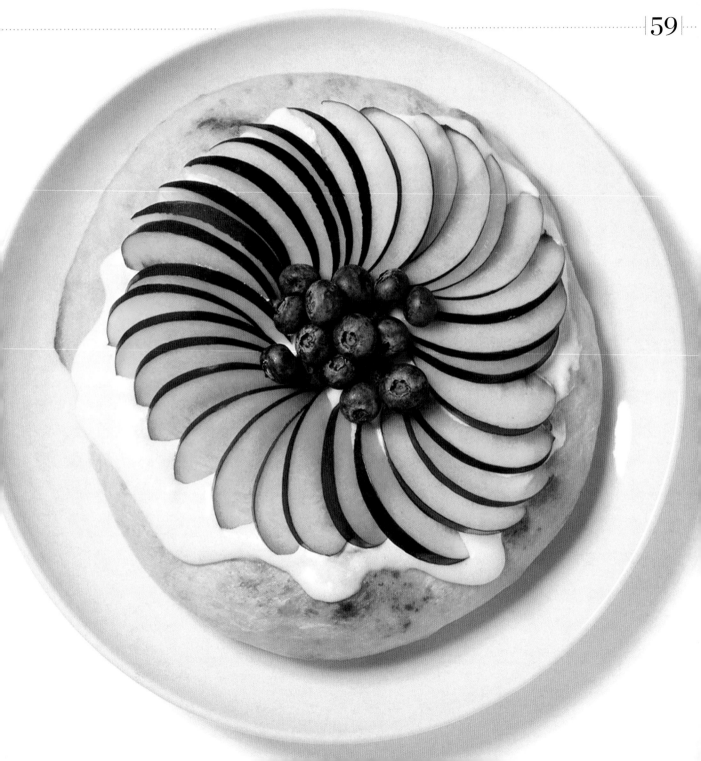

BERRY BREAKFAST COBBLER

PREP TIME: 20 MINUTES + 15 MINUTES COOLING / **COOK TIME:** 35 MINUTES / **MAKES** 4 SERVINGS

Sweet, juicy berries topped with an oat biscuit and sliced almonds—what a way to start the day! The dough can be made a day ahead of time and refrigerated until baking. For apple-cranberry cobbler topped with cinnamon biscuits, use the variation that follows.

BISCUIT DOUGH

- ⅓ cup all-purpose flour
- ⅓ cup white whole wheat flour
- ½ cup old-fashioned rolled oats
- 2 tablespoons sugar
- 1 teaspoon baking powder
- ⅛ teaspoon salt
- 3 tablespoons cold unsalted butter, cut into small cubes
- ½ teaspoon vanilla extract
- ½ cup low-fat buttermilk

BERRY FILLING

- 2 cups fresh or thawed frozen blueberries
- 1 cup fresh or thawed frozen raspberries
- 2 tablespoons sugar
- 1 tablespoon all-purpose flour
- ½ teaspoon fresh lemon juice
- ¼ cup sliced almonds

1. PREHEAT the oven to 375°F. Coat four 1-cup baking dishes, such as custard cups or ramekins, with cooking spray and place them on a baking sheet.

2. TO MAKE THE BISCUIT DOUGH: Whisk together the flours, oats, sugar, baking powder, and salt in a medium bowl. Cut the butter into the flour mixture, using a pastry blender or 2 knives used scissor fashion, until the butter pieces are smaller than peas and the mixture is crumbly.

3. STIR the vanilla into the buttermilk in a separate bowl. Add the buttermilk mixture to the flour mixture, stirring just until the dough comes together—do not overmix.

4. TO MAKE THE BERRY FILLING: Stir together the berries, sugar, flour, and lemon juice in a medium bowl. Divide the berries among the baking dishes. Divide the biscuit dough into 4 even pieces and pat into a round shape that will fit the top of the dish. Gently place over the berries. Sprinkle each cobbler with 1 tablespoon of the almonds.

5. BAKE for 30 to 35 minutes, until the fruit is bubbling and the biscuits are golden. Let cool for 15 minutes before serving. Cobbler is best served warm, but it may also be served at room temperature.

PER SERVING (1 serving = 1 cup) Apple-Cranberry Breakfast Cobbler (1 serving = 1 cup)

Calories	Total Fat	Saturated Fat	Sodium	Carbohydrate	Dietary Fiber	Protein	Calcium
350	13 g	6 g	290 mg	54 g	7 g	8 g	15%
390	13 g	6 g	290 mg	67 g	6 g	7 g	15%

APPLE-CRANBERRY BREAKFAST
COBBLER *(variation)*

OMIT the vanilla extract in the dough and substitute ½ teaspoon ground cinnamon.

OMIT the berries and substitute 4 medium apples, thinly sliced (about 3 cups) and ½ cup fresh or frozen cranberries.

SUBSTITUTE an equal amount of light brown sugar for the granulated sugar in the berry mixture.

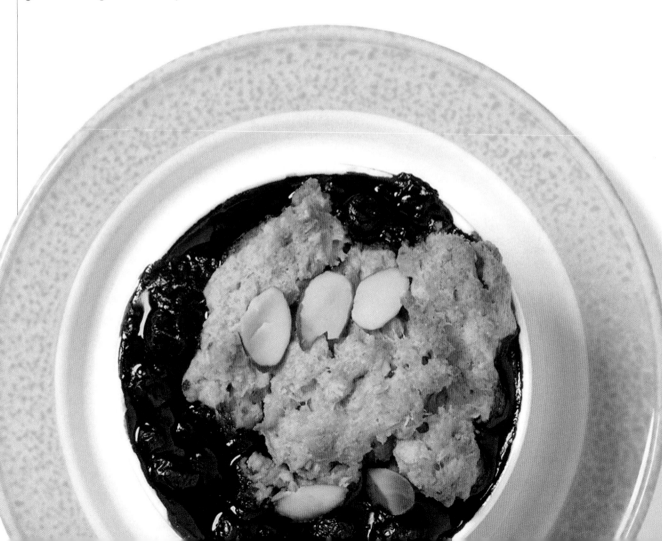

GREEK YOGURT BREAKFAST FOOL

PREP TIME: 5 MINUTES + 5 MINUTES COOLING / **COOK TIME:** 5 MINUTES / **MAKES** 1 SERVING

Traditional fool is made with fruit puree folded into whipped cream. This recipe lightens it up with fat-free vanilla yogurt and fresh fruit, with honey and walnuts added for interest.

2	tablespoons walnuts
12	blueberries
9	raspberries
¼	medium peach, sliced
1	container (6 ounces) fat-free (0%) vanilla Greek yogurt
1	tablespoon honey

1. **PLACE** the walnuts in a small nonstick skillet and cook over medium heat, shaking the pan often, until lightly toasted, 3 to 5 minutes. Transfer the nuts to a cutting board and let cool 5 minutes, then coarsely chop.

2. **COMBINE** 8 of the blueberries, 6 of the raspberries, the peach slices, and yogurt in a medium bowl and gently fold together. Place half of the mixture in a parfait glass. Top with half of the walnuts and 1½ teaspoons of the honey. Top with the remaining yogurt-fruit mixture. Top with the remaining walnuts, 4 blueberries, 3 raspberries, and 1½ teaspoons honey.

MAKE IT A MEAL

¼ cup low-fat granola
90 CALORIES

390
CALORIES
PER MEAL
★ ★

MAKE IT A MEAL

1 slice (1 ounce) whole wheat toast spread with 2 teaspoons all-fruit jam
90 CALORIES

390
CALORIES
PER MEAL
★ ★

PER SERVING (1 serving = 1½ cups)

Calories	Total Fat	Saturated Fat	Sodium	Carbohydrate	Dietary Fiber	Protein	Calcium
300	8 g	1 g	70 mg	41 g	3 g	20 g	25%

TROPICAL FRUIT SMOOTHIE

PREP TIME: 5 MINUTES / **MAKES** 2 SERVINGS

For an extra-slushy and refreshing smoothie on a hot summer day, freeze the mango and pineapple the day before and add frozen to the blender. You may prefer a flavored light yogurt like piña colada to enhance the tropical flavors.

1	mango, cubed
1	cup fresh pineapple chunks
¾	cup orange juice
1	container (6 ounces) fat-free plain yogurt
3	tablespoons sugar
1	tablespoon fresh lime juice
8	ice cubes

COMBINE the mango, pineapple, orange juice, yogurt, sugar, lime juice, and ice cubes in a blender. Puree and serve.

MAKE IT A MEAL

1 small (2-ounce) bran muffin
150 CALORIES

410
CALORIES
PER MEAL
★ ★

MAKE IT A MEAL

20 almonds
140 CALORIES

400
CALORIES
PER MEAL
★ ★

PER SERVING (1 serving = 2 cups)

Calories	Total Fat	Saturated Fat	Sodium	Carbohydrate	Dietary Fiber	Protein	Calcium
260	0.5 g	0 g	55 mg	65 g	3 g	5 g	15%

5

SOUPS & SANDWICHES

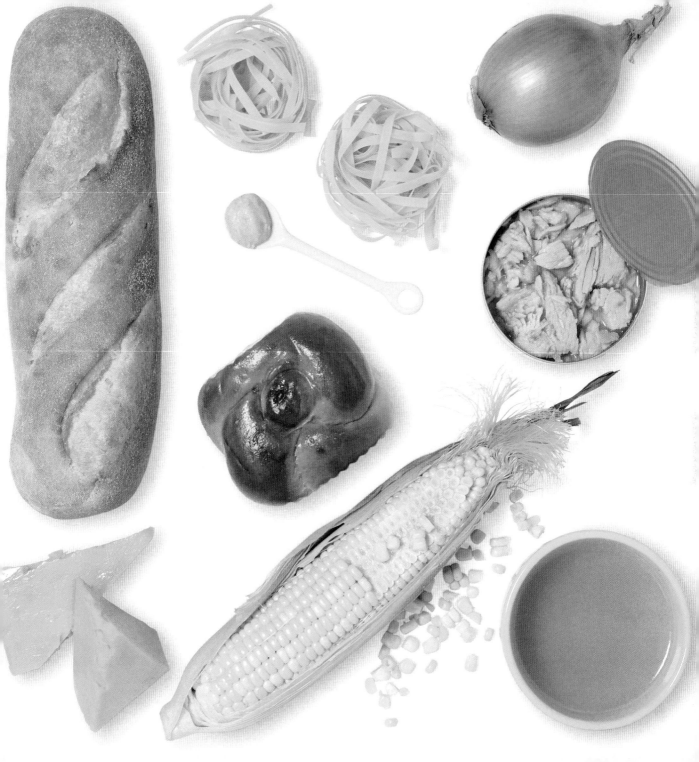

FRENCH ONION SOUP

PREP TIME: 10 MINUTES / **COOK TIME:** 1 HOUR 20 MINUTES / **MAKES** 4 SERVINGS

In this recipe we control calories by using just modest amounts of two high-calorie ingredients, olive oil and cheese. Switch to vegetable broth to make this soup vegetarian.

1	tablespoon olive oil
2½	pounds medium onions, thinly sliced
2	teaspoons sugar
5	cups fat-free, reduced-sodium beef broth
1	teaspoon chopped fresh thyme
1	bay leaf
¼	teaspoon freshly ground black pepper
4	slices (1 ounce each) French bread, toasted
4	slices (⅔ ounce each) reduced-fat Swiss cheese

1. **HEAT** the oil in a large saucepan over medium heat. Add the onions and sugar, and cook, stirring occasionally, for 48 to 50 minutes, or until very soft and golden.

2. **STIR** in the broth, thyme, bay leaf, and pepper. Bring to a boil over medium-high heat. Reduce to a simmer and cook, uncovered, for 30 minutes. Remove the bay leaf.

3. **PREHEAT** the broiler. Place the bread slices on a baking sheet and top each with 1 slice of cheese. Broil for 1½ minutes, or until the cheese melts and browns slightly.

4. **DIVIDE** the soup among 4 bowls and top each with 1 cheese toast.

PER SERVING (1 serving = 1¾ cups soup, 1 cheese toast)

Calories	Total Fat	Saturated Fat	Sodium	Carbohydrate	Dietary Fiber	Protein	Calcium
320	8 g	2.5 g	810 mg	47 g	6 g	18 g	30%

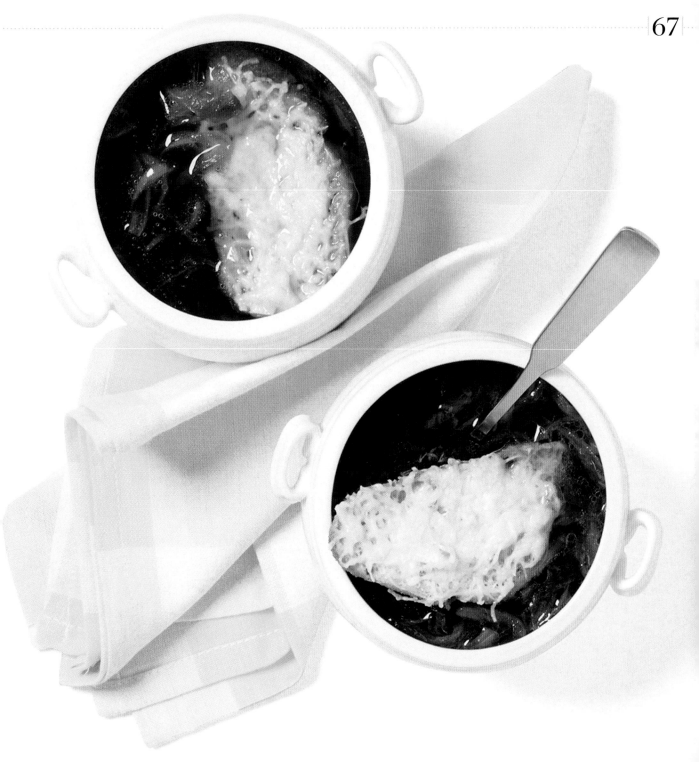

SLOW-COOKER TORTILLA SOUP

PREP TIME: 10 MINUTES / **COOK TIME:** 3 TO 6 HOURS / **MAKES** 4 SERVINGS

Chicken thighs hold up better to slow cooking than chicken breast, which tends to overcook and dry out. This recipe calls for no-salt-added tomatoes, reduced-sodium chicken broth, and homemade tortilla chips so that you can better control the sodium levels.

MAKE IT A MEAL

½ medium sliced mango
70 CALORIES

380 CALORIES PER MEAL
★ ★ ★ ★

MAKE IT A MEAL

1 frozen fruit bar (2¾ ounces)
80 CALORIES

390 CALORIES PER MEAL
★ ★ ★ ★

1   can (28 ounces) no-salt-added crushed tomatoes
1   can (14.5 ounces) fat-free, reduced-sodium chicken broth
1   cup water
¾   pound boneless, skinless chicken thighs, trimmed of visible fat and cut into 1" cubes
1   medium onion, finely chopped
1   chipotle pepper in adobo sauce, finely chopped
1   clove garlic, minced
1   tablespoon chili powder or no-salt chili seasoning blend
¾   teaspoon salt
4   (6") corn tortillas
½   Hass avocado, diced
¼   cup finely chopped fresh cilantro
1   lime, cut into 8 wedges

1. **PLACE** the tomatoes, broth, water, chicken, onion, chipotle, garlic, chili powder, and salt in a slow cooker. Cook for 3 hours on high or 6 hours on low.

2. **MEANWHILE,** preheat the oven to 350°F. Spray the tortillas on one side with cooking spray. Cut the tortillas into eighths. Place on a baking sheet and bake for 20 minutes, or until crisp.

3. **LADLE** the soup into 4 bowls. Top each bowl with 8 tortilla wedges, about 1 tablespoon avocado, and 1 tablespoon cilantro. Serve with 2 lime wedges.

PER SERVING (1 serving = 1½ cups)

Calories	Total Fat	Saturated Fat	Sodium	Carbohydrate	Dietary Fiber	Protein	Calcium
310	11 g	2.5 g	790 mg	32 g	8 g	22 g	8%

TURKEY NOODLE SOUP

PREP TIME: 10 MINUTES / **COOK TIME:** 1 HOUR 21 MINUTES / **MAKES** 6 SERVINGS

If turkey necks are not readily available at your local market, ask the butcher to set them aside for you. Make this soup even heartier by adding more vegetables and chunks of leftover turkey.

1	tablespoon olive oil
1	medium onion, chopped
2	large carrots, sliced
2	ribs celery, sliced
1	parsnip, sliced
1	teaspoon fresh thyme leaves
6	cups fat-free, reduced-sodium chicken broth
1	pound skinless turkey necks
4	sprigs of parsley
1	bay leaf
4	ounces wide yolk-free noodles
¼	teaspoon freshly ground black pepper

1. HEAT the oil in a Dutch oven over medium heat. Add the onion, carrots, celery, parsnip, and thyme. Cook, stirring occasionally, for 9 to 10 minutes, or until the vegetables are softened.

2. INCREASE the heat to medium-high and stir in the broth, turkey necks, parsley, and bay leaf. Bring to a boil, reduce to a simmer, cover, and cook for 1 hour. Remove the turkey necks and transfer to cutting board. When cool enough to handle, remove the turkey meat from the bones with 2 forks or your fingers and shred.

3. MEANWHILE, add the noodles to the Dutch oven, cover, and return to a simmer. Cook for 10 minutes, or until the noodles are tender.

4. STIR the turkey and pepper into the soup and cook for 1 minute to heat through. Remove the bay leaf before serving.

PER SERVING (1 serving = 1½ cups)

Calories	Total Fat	Saturated Fat	Sodium	Carbohydrate	Dietary Fiber	Protein	Calcium
230	7 g	1.5 g	560 mg	21 g	3 g	19 g	6%

MAKE IT A MEAL

Salad made with 1½ cups baby spinach, 1 medium diced tomato, 1 teaspoon olive oil, 1½ teaspoons balsamic vinegar **85 CALORIES**

1 cup orange sections **80 CALORIES**

395

CALORIES PER MEAL

★ ★ ★

MAKE IT A MEAL

Sandwich made with 1 whole wheat English muffin, 1 wedge Laughing Cow Light cheese, 2 tomato slices **175 CALORIES**

405

CALORIES PER MEAL

★ ★ ★

TURKEY CHILI VERDE

PREP TIME: 30 MINUTES / **COOK TIME:** 15 MINUTES / **MAKES** 6 SERVINGS

Lean ground turkey is cooked with aromatic chile peppers and seasoned with cumin and cilantro. If you want a spicier chili, substitute 3 poblano peppers for the cubanelles (also called Italian frying peppers). Leftovers freeze and reheat well.

CHIPOTLE SOUR CREAM
- ⅓ cup light sour cream
- ¼ teaspoon chipotle pepper powder
- 1 tablespoon finely chopped fresh cilantro or parsley
- ½ teaspoon grated lime zest

1. TO MAKE THE CHIPOTLE SOUR CREAM: Combine the sour cream, chipotle powder, cilantro or parsley, and lime zest in a small bowl. Refrigerate until serving time.

2. TO MAKE THE CHILI: Heat the oil in a large soup pot over medium heat. When hot, add the onion, cubanelle peppers, garlic, jalapeño chile pepper, cumin, oregano, salt, and black pepper. Cook for 5 minutes, stirring, until the onions and peppers begin to soften.

PER SERVING (1 serving = 2 cups chili, 1 tablespoon chipotle sour cream)

Calories	Total Fat	Saturated Fat	Sodium	Carbohydrate	Dietary Fiber	Protein	Calcium
280	9 g	2.5 g	370 mg	23 g	7 g	26 g	8%

CHILI

1	teaspoon canola oil
1	medium onion, finely chopped
3	cubanelle peppers, finely chopped (1½ cups)
4	cloves garlic, minced
1	jalapeño chile pepper, seeded and finely chopped (wear plastic gloves when handling)
1	tablespoon ground cumin
2	teaspoons dried oregano
¼	teaspoon coarse salt
¼	teaspoon freshly ground black pepper
1¼	pounds 93% lean ground turkey
1	can (4 ounces) chopped mild green chiles, drained
1	cup water
2	packets (4 grams each) fat-free, salt-free chicken bouillon
2	cans (15.5 ounces each) cannellini beans, rinsed and drained
½	cup tomatillo salsa (salsa verde)
⅓	cup finely chopped fresh cilantro
¼	cup finely chopped fresh flat-leaf parsley

3. ADD the turkey and cook for 5 minutes, breaking up the meat with a spoon, until almost cooked through.

4. ADD the green chilies, water, bouillon, beans, and salsa. Mix until evenly blended. Simmer for 5 minutes, stirring occasionally. Stir in the cilantro and parsley. Top each serving of chili with 1 tablespoon of chipotle sour cream.

GREEK LEMON-CHICKEN SOUP

PREP TIME: 10 MINUTES / **COOK TIME:** 10 MINUTES / **MAKES** 4 SERVINGS

This soup is a refreshing alternative to traditional chicken noodle soup. With 3 ounces of chicken per serving, it makes a hearty main course.

5	cups fat-free, reduced-sodium chicken broth
4	large eggs
¼	cup fresh lemon juice
12	ounces cooked chicken breast, shredded (2 cups)
1	cup cooked brown rice
¼	teaspoon ground white pepper

1. BRING the broth to a boil in a large saucepan over medium-high heat. Reduce the heat to medium.

2. MEANWHILE, whisk together the eggs and lemon juice in a medium bowl. Whisk 1 cup of the hot broth into the egg mixture. Whisk the warmed egg mixture into the saucepan and cook, stirring, for 1 minute. Add the chicken, rice, and pepper, and cook, stirring often, for 1 to 2 minutes to heat through.

MAKE IT A MEAL

1 small (4") whole wheat pita
70 CALORIES

1 cup watermelon cubes
50 CALORIES

400
CALORIES PER MEAL
★ ★

MAKE IT A MEAL

½ cup sliced cucumber
10 CALORIES

1 ounce reduced-fat feta cheese
60 CALORIES

1 cup cantaloupe cubes
50 CALORIES

400
CALORIES PER MEAL
★ ★

PER SERVING (1 serving = 2 cups)

Calories	Total Fat	Saturated Fat	Sodium	Carbohydrate	Dietary Fiber	Protein	Calcium
280	8 g	2.5 g	700 mg	13 g	1 g	35 g	4%

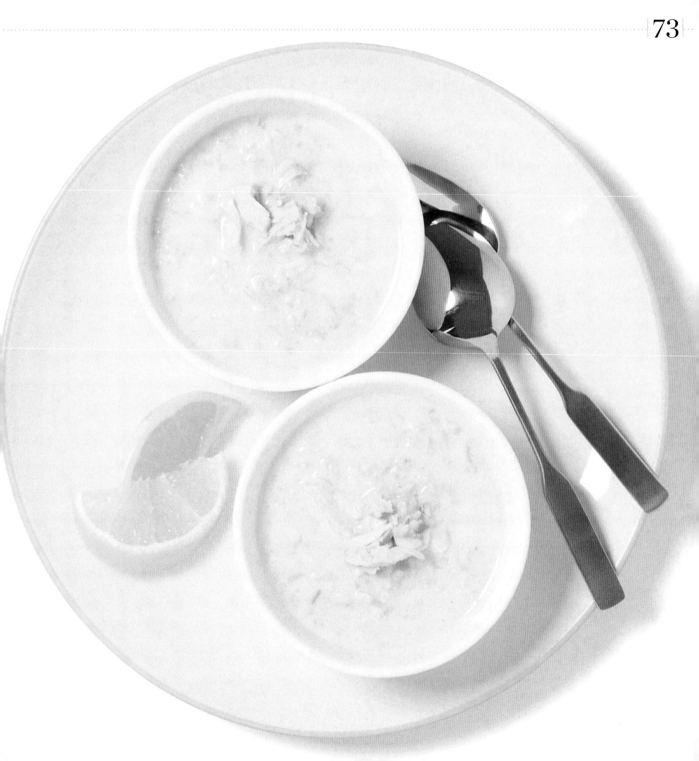

TOMATO AND BEEF SOUP

PREP TIME: 5 MINUTES / **COOK TIME:** 37 MINUTES / **MAKES** 4 SERVINGS

This soup is the perfect winter meal when vegetable choices in the market are limited. During the summer, use fresh vegetables and fresh tomatoes for a light supper.

MAKE IT A MEAL

½ toasted whole wheat English muffin
70 CALORIES

10 baby carrots and 1 medium rib celery
50 CALORIES

390
CALORIES PER MEAL
★ ★ ★

MAKE IT A MEAL

10 low-sodium thin wheat crackers
90 CALORIES

10 baby carrots and 1 medium rib celery
50 CALORIES

410
CALORIES PER MEAL
★ ★ ★

2	teaspoons olive oil
¾	pound well-trimmed bottom round beef roast, cut into ½" cubes
3	cloves garlic, minced
1	teaspoon dried basil
1½	cups frozen mixed vegetables
2	cans (14.5 ounces each) no-salt-added petite diced tomatoes
1	can (14.5 ounces) fat-free, reduced-sodium chicken broth
2	ounces ditalini pasta
½	teaspoon salt
¼	teaspoon freshly ground black pepper

1. HEAT the oil in a nonstick Dutch oven over medium-high heat. Add the beef and cook for 4 to 5 minutes, turning occasionally, until browned. Add the garlic and basil, and cook for 1 minute, stirring occasionally. Add the mixed vegetables and cook for 1 minute. Add the tomatoes and broth, bring to a boil, reduce to a simmer, cover, and cook for 20 minutes, or until the beef is tender.

2. STIR in the pasta, cover, return to a simmer, and cook for 10 minutes, or until the pasta is cooked. Remove from the heat and stir in the salt and pepper.

PER SERVING (1 serving = 1¾ cups)

Calories	Total Fat	Saturated Fat	Sodium	Carbohydrate	Dietary Fiber	Protein	Calcium
270	7 g	2 g	660 mg	25 g	3 g	24 g	2%

SIMPLE LOBSTER STEW

PREP TIME: 10 MINUTES / **COOK TIME:** 20 MINUTES / **MAKES** 4 SERVINGS

Rich, creamy, and full of succulent lobster meat, this stew makes a special dinner. Many supermarkets will cook the lobster for you free of charge—a great time-saver. For a more economical seafood stew, follow the variation and substitute raw haddock or cod for the lobster.

1	pound Yukon gold potatoes, peeled and cut into ½" chunks
2	tablespoons butter
1	cup sliced leeks (white part only)
2	cups coarsely chopped cooked lobster meat (about 10 ounces)
2	tablespoons all-purpose flour
1	bottle (8 ounces) clam juice
1	cup fat-free milk
⅓	cup heavy cream
¼	teaspoon coarse salt
¼	teaspoon freshly ground black pepper
⅛	teaspoon dried thyme

1. **PLACE** the potatoes in a medium saucepan. Add hot water to cover and bring to a boil over high heat. Reduce to a simmer, cover, and cook for 10 minutes, or until tender. Drain and set aside.

2. **MEANWHILE,** melt the butter in a large saucepan or deep skillet over medium heat. Add the leeks and cook for 3 minutes, or until softened. Stir in the lobster and flour. Cook, stirring constantly, for 2 minutes, until the leeks and lobster are well coated with flour and the mixture starts to brown on the bottom of the pan. Slowly stir in the clam juice and bring to a simmer (it will thicken).

3. **ADD** the cooked potatoes, milk, cream, salt, pepper, and thyme. Cook, stirring, until the stew just reaches a simmer. Serve hot.

SIMPLE FISH STEW *(variation)*

SUBSTITUTE ¾ pound raw, bite-sized pieces of haddock or cod for the cooked lobster.

MAKE IT A MEAL

Salad made with 2 cups romaine lettuce, ¼ cup chopped tomato, 1 teaspoon olive oil, 1 teaspoon red wine vinegar **70 CALORIES**

400 CALORIES PER MEAL ★ ★ ★

MAKE the variation A MEAL

Salad made with 2 cups romaine lettuce, ¼ cup chopped tomato, 1 teaspoon olive oil, 1 teaspoon red wine vinegar **70 CALORIES**

390 CALORIES PER MEAL ★ ★ ★

PER SERVING (1 serving = 1½ cups) Simple Fish Stew (1 serving = 1½ cups)

Calories	Total Fat	Saturated Fat	Sodium	Carbohydrate	Dietary Fiber	Protein	Calcium
330	15 g	9 g	600 mg	29 g	2 g	19 g	15%
320	14 g	8 g	380 mg	28 g	2 g	21 g	15%

MANHATTAN SEAFOOD CHOWDER

PREP TIME: 20 MINUTES / **COOK TIME:** 35 MINUTES / **MAKES** 4 SERVINGS

Unlike its cousin, New England chowder, Manhattan seafood chowder uses a light, vitamin C–rich tomato base rather than milk or cream. The fennel and basil add a touch of Italian flavor.

5	slices bacon, chopped
2	ribs celery, chopped
1	onion, chopped
1	russet (baking) potato (8 ounces), peeled and cut into ½" cubes
½	bulb fennel, chopped
4	cloves garlic, minced
1	teaspoon dried basil
1	can (14.5 ounces) no-salt-added diced tomatoes
2	bottles (8 ounces each) clam juice
¾	pound peeled and deveined small shrimp
1	can (6.5 ounces) chopped clams, drained
¼	teaspoon freshly ground black pepper

1. COOK the bacon in a large saucepan over medium-high heat for 4 to 5 minutes, or until just starting to brown. Reduce the heat to medium and add the celery, onion, potato, fennel, garlic, and basil. Cook, stirring occasionally, for 6 to 7 minutes, or until the vegetables are crisp-tender.

2. STIR in the tomatoes and clam juice. Bring to a boil over medium-high heat. Reduce to a simmer, cover, and cook for 18 to 20 minutes, or until the potatoes are tender.

3. ADD the shrimp, clams, and pepper, and cook for 4 to 5 minutes, or until the shrimp are cooked through.

PER SERVING (1 serving = 2 cups)

Calories	Total Fat	Saturated Fat	Sodium	Carbohydrate	Dietary Fiber	Protein	Calcium
340	13 g	4 g	690 mg	23 g	4 g	32 g	15%

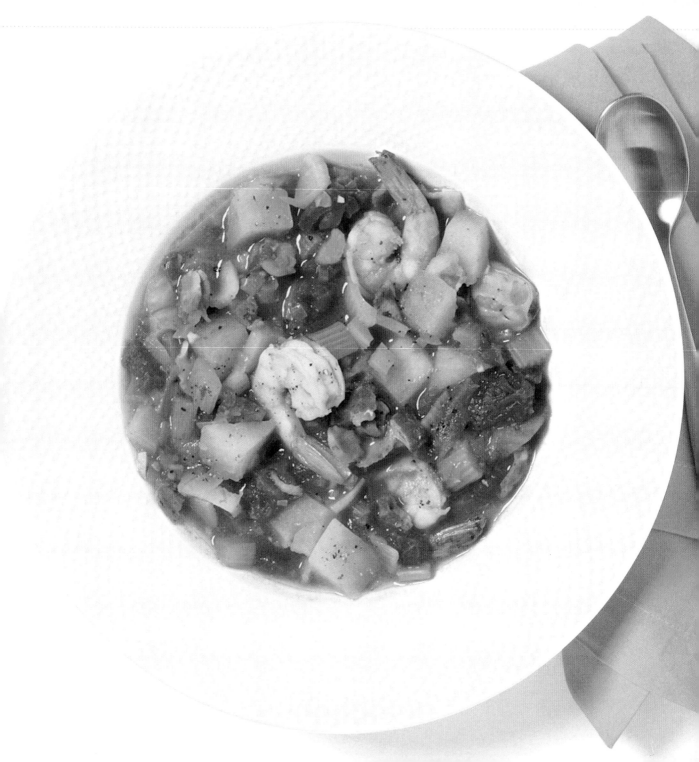

SOUTHWEST CORN AND BEAN CHOWDER

PREP TIME: 5 MINUTES / **COOK TIME:** 12 MINUTES / **MAKES** 4 SERVINGS

Colorful and packed with veggies, this easy chowder comes together quickly for dinner in a hurry.

MAKE IT A MEAL

Small piece (2¼ ounces) cornbread
150 CALORIES

CALORIES PER MEAL
★ ★

MAKE IT A MEAL

1 bottle (12 ounces) beer
150 CALORIES

CALORIES PER MEAL
★ ★

1	tablespoon olive oil
½	small onion, finely chopped
½	medium green bell pepper, chopped
2	cloves garlic, minced
½	teaspoon ground cumin
¼	teaspoon smoked paprika
2	tablespoons all-purpose flour
2½	cups fat-free, reduced-sodium chicken broth
2½	cups frozen corn kernels
1	can (15.5 ounces) black beans, rinsed and drained
¼	pound ham, finely diced (about 1 cup)
½	cup salsa
½	cup fat-free half-and-half
4	tablespoons low-fat plain yogurt

1. **HEAT** the oil in a large saucepan over medium heat. Add the onion, bell pepper, garlic, cumin, and paprika. Cook, stirring, for 2 minutes, or until the onion has softened a bit. Stir in the flour and cook for 2 minutes, stirring. Slowly pour in the broth a little at a time, continuing to stir. The broth will thicken.

2. **STIR** in the corn, beans, ham, and salsa. Bring the mixture to a simmer. Cook, mixing occasionally, for 3 to 5 minutes, until heated through. Stir in the half-and-half.

3. **DIVIDE** the chowder among 4 bowls and top each portion with 1 tablespoon of yogurt.

PER SERVING (1 serving = 2 cups chowder, 1 tablespoon yogurt)

Calories	Total Fat	Saturated Fat	Sodium	Carbohydrate	Dietary Fiber	Protein	Calcium
270	6 g	1 g	1,080 mg	44 g	7 g	15 g	10%

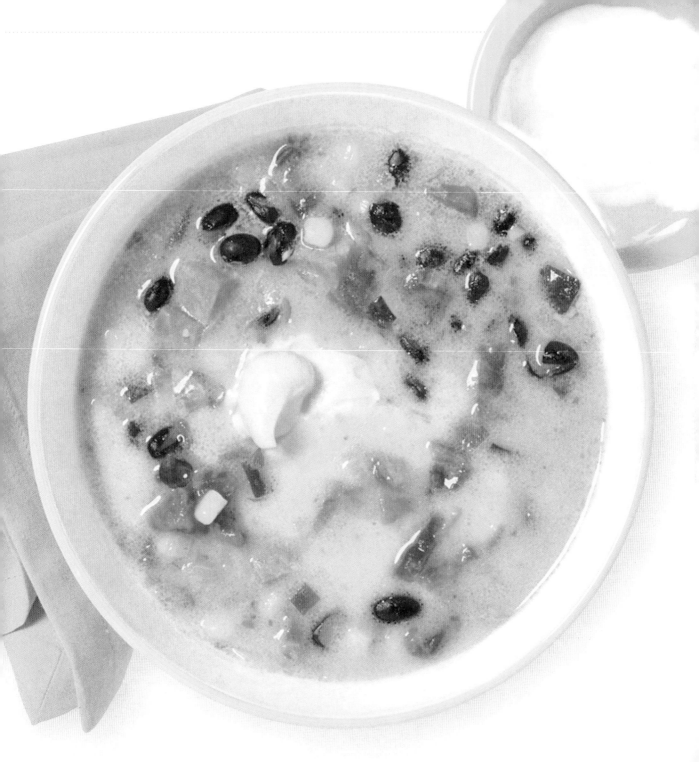

WINTER SQUASH AND APPLE SOUP

PREP TIME: 10 MINUTES / **COOK TIME:** 30 MINUTES / **MAKES** 4 SERVINGS

Beautiful, tasty, and nutritious, this soup makes a simple dinner for four when served with salad and a roll, or serves six as an appetizer.

- 2 tablespoons Smart Balance spread
- 2 medium leeks, well washed and thinly sliced
- 1 medium onion, chopped
- ¾ pound winter squash (butternut or acorn), peeled and cubed
- 2 medium carrots, halved lengthwise and thinly sliced crosswise
- 1½ cups peeled, chopped apple (1 large or 2 small)
- 3 cups fat-free, reduced-sodium chicken broth
- ½ cup fat-free half-and-half
- ¼ teaspoon ground nutmeg
- ⅛ teaspoon ground ginger
- ⅛ teaspoon garlic salt
- ⅛ teaspoon coarse salt
- ⅛ teaspoon freshly ground black pepper
- ½ cup low-fat plain yogurt
- 2 tablespoons chopped fresh chives

1. **MELT** the spread in a large soup pot over medium heat. Add the leeks and onion, and cook, stirring often, for 5 minutes, or until the onion softens. Stir in the squash, carrots, apple, and broth, and bring to a boil. Reduce to a simmer, cover, and cook for 20 minutes, or until the vegetables are soft.

2. **TRANSFER** the soup in batches to a blender, puree until smooth, and return to the pot (or use a hand blender to puree the soup right in the pot). Add the half-and-half, nutmeg, ginger, garlic salt, coarse salt, and pepper. Stir well and bring to a low simmer to reheat.

3. **GARNISH** each serving with 2 tablespoons of yogurt and a sprinkling of the chives.

PER SERVING (1 serving = 1½ cups)

Calories	Total Fat	Saturated Fat	Sodium	Carbohydrate	Dietary Fiber	Protein	Calcium
210	5 g	1.5 g	560 mg	37 g	5 g	6 g	20%

CREAMY MUSHROOM SOUP

PREP TIME: 10 MINUTES / **COOK TIME:** 30 MINUTES / **MAKES** 4 SERVINGS

Dried mushrooms—any combination or single variety, including porcini, morels, and others—impart a rich and earthy flavor to this satisfying soup. Increase the thyme to ¹/₂ teaspoon if you use chicken broth.

½ cup assorted dried mushrooms, crumbled

2 teaspoons unsalted butter

1 medium onion, finely chopped

1 clove garlic, minced

10 ounces sliced cremini (brown) mushrooms

2 tablespoons all-purpose flour

3 cups low-sodium vegetable or chicken broth

2 tablespoons dry sherry

½ teaspoon coarse salt

½ teaspoon freshly ground black pepper

¼ teaspoon dried thyme

1 cup low-fat (2%) evaporated milk

2 tablespoons chopped fresh parsley

1. PLACE the dried mushrooms in a medium heatproof bowl and add boiling water to cover. Let stand for 20 minutes to soften.

2. MEANWHILE, melt the butter in a medium saucepan over medium heat. Add the onion and garlic, and cook for 6 minutes, or until the onion begins to brown.

3. ADD the cremini mushrooms and cook for 8 minutes, until the mushrooms have released their liquid and most of the liquid has evaporated. Sprinkle the flour over the mushrooms and onion and garlic, and cook, stirring, for 1 minute. Add the dried mushrooms and their soaking liquid, the broth, sherry, salt, pepper, and thyme. Cover and simmer over low heat for 15 minutes.

4. WHISK in the evaporated milk and remove from the heat. Serve garnished with parsley.

MAKE
IT A
MEAL

½ grilled cheese sandwich made with 1 slice (1 ounce) whole wheat bread and 1 slice (⅔ ounce) American cheese
140 CALORIES

1 small apple
80 CALORIES

420
CALORIES
PER MEAL
★ ★ ★

MAKE
IT A
MEAL

Salad made with 2 cups mixed baby greens, 10 cherry tomatoes, and 1 tablespoon light Italian dressing, topped with 3 ounces grilled chicken breast
220 CALORIES

420
CALORIES
PER MEAL
★ ★ ★

PER SERVING (1 serving = 1½ cups)

Calories	Total Fat	Saturated Fat	Sodium	Carbohydrate	Dietary Fiber	Protein	Calcium
200	4 g	2 g	430 mg	27 g	5 g	13 g	20%

VEGETABLE STEW WITH QUINOA

PREP TIME: 25 MINUTES / **COOK TIME:** 32 MINUTES / **MAKES** 4 SERVINGS

Vibrant sweet potatoes and tender mushrooms create a hearty vegetarian stew. For a dish with Mediterranean flair, follow the instructions in the variation.

MAKE IT A MEAL

1 medium (1¼ ounces) whole wheat roll
100 CALORIES

390 CALORIES PER MEAL
★ ★

MAKE the variation A MEAL

1 medium (1¼ ounces) whole wheat roll
100 CALORIES

400 CALORIES PER MEAL
★ ★ ★

1	teaspoon olive oil
1	small onion, finely chopped
2	cloves garlic, minced
16	ounces mushrooms, quartered
1	large (about 14 ounces) sweet potato, peeled and cut into ½"chunks
2½	cups low-sodium vegetable broth
1	tablespoon fresh lemon juice
1	teaspoon Dijon mustard
¼	teaspoon dried thyme
¼	teaspoon coarse salt
⅛	teaspoon freshly ground black pepper
¾	cup quinoa, rinsed
8	tablespoons crumbled reduced-fat feta cheese

1. **HEAT** the oil in a large saucepan over medium heat. Add the onion, garlic, mushrooms, and sweet potato, and stir well. Add ½ cup of the broth, the lemon juice, mustard, thyme, salt, and pepper. Stir to coat the vegetables. Simmer, uncovered, for 8 to 10 minutes, stirring occasionally. Increase the heat to medium-high and add the remaining 2 cups broth. Simmer for 8 to 10 minutes, or until the sweet potato is nearly cooked through.

2. **STIR** in the quinoa. Cover the pan, reduce the heat to a simmer, and cook for 10 to 12 minutes, until the quinoa is tender but still a bit chewy.

3. **DIVIDE** the stew among 4 bowls and garnish each portion with 2 tablespoons of the cheese.

MEDITERRANEAN STEW WITH QUINOA
(variation)

OMIT the mushrooms and sweet potato.

ADD 1 medium zucchini, halved lengthwise and thinly sliced, when you cook the onion and garlic. Add 2 cans (14.5 ounces each) no-salt-added diced tomatoes when you add the broth, and decrease the broth to 2 cups. Simmer for 2 minutes after adding the broth. Omit the dried thyme and substitute ½ teaspoon dried basil.

INCREASE the quinoa to 1 cup.

ADD 4 cups coarsely chopped arugula and 12 pitted kalamata olives, halved, to the stew in Step 2, after the quinoa has cooked.

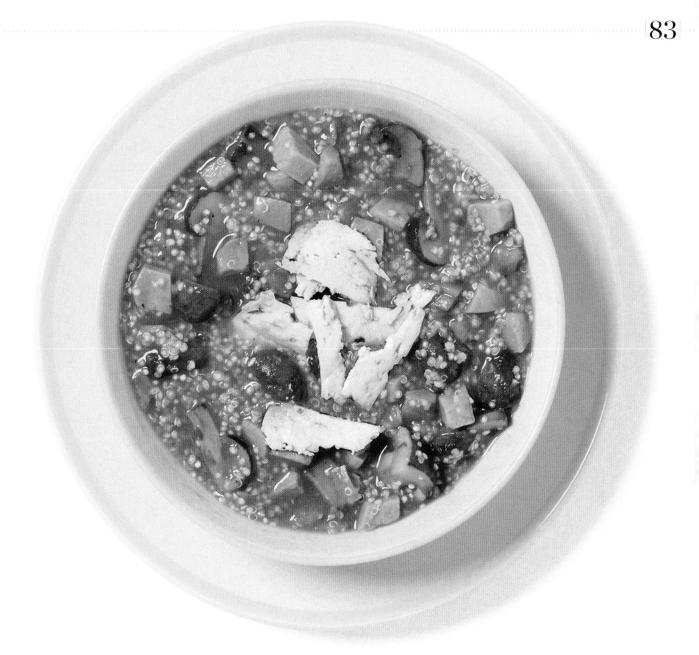

PER SERVING (1 serving = 1¼ cups stew, 2 tablespoons feta cheese)
Mediterranean Stew with Quinoa (1 serving = 1¼ cups)

Calories	Total Fat	Saturated Fat	Sodium	Carbohydrate	Dietary Fiber	Protein	Calcium
290	6 g	2 g	520 mg	49 g	8 g	13 g	10%
300	9 g	2.5 g	720 mg	45 g	8 g	13 g	15%

AFRICAN PEANUT SOUP

PREP TIME: 10 MINUTES / **COOK TIME:** 30 MINUTES / **MAKES** 4 SERVINGS

This hearty soup is extremely filling, much more than you would expect for the calories. We added an assortment of vegetables for color, flavor, and even greater satisfaction.

1 teaspoon peanut oil
1 medium onion, chopped
1 medium yellow or red bell pepper, chopped
1 or 2 serrano chile peppers, minced (optional)
1 tablespoon curry powder
3 cups water
1 cup canned crushed tomatoes
1 cup cubed (½") winter squash
1 medium carrot, cut into ½" chunks
1 medium red potato, cut into ½" chunks
¼ cup creamy peanut butter
½ teaspoon salt
¼ cup finely chopped honey-roasted peanuts

1. HEAT the oil in a medium saucepan over medium heat. Add the onion, bell pepper, and serrano chile pepper (if using), and cook for 5 minutes, or until soft. Stir in the curry powder and cook for 1 minute.

2. ADD the water, tomatoes, squash, carrot, potato, peanut butter, and salt. Bring to a boil. Reduce to a simmer, cover, and cook for 25 minutes, or until the vegetables are just tender.

3. GARNISH each serving with 1 tablespoon chopped peanuts.

MAKE
IT A
MEAL

1 slice (2 ounces)
Italian bread
150 CALORIES

410
CALORIES
PER MEAL
★ ★ ★

MAKE
IT A
MEAL

⅔ cup cooked
brown rice stirred
into the soup
150 CALORIES

410
CALORIES
PER MEAL
★ ★ ★

PER SERVING (1 serving = 2 cups)

Calories	Total Fat	Saturated Fat	Sodium	Carbohydrate	Dietary Fiber	Protein	Calcium
260	14 g	3 g	500 mg	28 g	6 g	10 g	6%

CHICKEN, JACK CHEESE, AND TOMATO ON GARLIC BREAD

PREP TIME: 10 MINUTES / **COOK TIME:** 15 MINUTES / **MAKES** 4 SERVINGS

Monitor the temperature of the chicken breast halves carefully so that they stay juicy and are not overcooked. Leftover grilled vegetables make a nice addition if you prefer a bulkier sandwich.

3 boneless, skinless chicken breast halves (4 ounces each)

1 teaspoon extra-virgin olive oil

¼ teaspoon salt

¼ teaspoon freshly ground black pepper

1 baguette (8 ounces), halved lengthwise

1 clove garlic

4 teaspoons Dijon mustard

4 slices reduced-fat Monterey Jack cheese (about 3 ounces)

1 large tomato, cut into 8 slices

8 fresh basil leaves

1. PREHEAT the oven to 400°F.

2. TOSS the chicken with the oil, salt, and pepper. Coat a nonstick grill pan with cooking spray and heat over medium-high heat. Add the chicken to the pan and cook for 5 to 6 minutes per side or until cooked through but still juicy. Transfer the chicken to a cutting board and when cool enough to handle, thinly slice.

3. MEANWHILE, place the baguette on a baking sheet and bake for 8 to 10 minutes, or until toasted. Let cool slightly, then rub the cut sides of the bread with the garlic clove. Spread with the mustard. Arrange the cheese over the bottom half of the baguette and return to the oven for 1 to 2 minutes to melt the cheese. Remove from the oven and top with the tomato, basil, sliced chicken, and the top half of the bread. Cut crosswise into 4 sandwiches.

TURKEY, SWISS, AND TOMATO *(variation)*

SUBSTITUTE ¾ pound turkey breast cutlets for the chicken breasts and reduced-fat Swiss cheese for the Jack cheese

MAKE IT A MEAL

Salad made with 2 cups romaine lettuce, ¼ cup chopped tomato, 1 teaspoon olive oil, 1 teaspoon red wine vinegar
70 CALORIES

400
CALORIES PER MEAL
★ ★

MAKE the variation A MEAL

Salad made with 2 cups romaine lettuce, ¼ cup chopped tomato, 1 teaspoon olive oil, 1 teaspoon red wine vinegar
70 CALORIES

420
CALORIES PER MEAL
★ ★

PER SERVING (1 serving = 1 sandwich) Turkey, Swiss, and Tomato (1 serving = 1 sandwich)

Calories	Total Fat	Saturated Fat	Sodium	Carbohydrate	Dietary Fiber	Protein	Calcium
330	8 g	3.5 g	860 mg	35 g	1 g	28 g	15%
350	6 g	2.5 g	710 mg	35 g	1 g	38 g	20%

FRUITY CHICKEN SALAD FINGER SANDWICHES

PREP TIME: 10 MINUTES / **COOK TIME:** 3 MINUTES / **MAKES** 6 SERVINGS

This cross between Waldorf salad and chicken salad yields a tasty, crunchy concoction that's sandwiched between soft finger rolls. Or, try it paired with wheat crackers for a lighter meal.

MAKE
IT A
MEAL

½ cup sugar-free
gelatin dessert
10 CALORIES

380
CALORIES
PER MEAL
★ ★

MAKE
the variation
A MEAL

6 reduced-fat
Triscuits
100 CALORIES

1 cup fresh
fruit salad
100 CALORIES

410
CALORIES
PER MEAL
★ ★ ★

2	cups (about 10½ ounces) chopped cooked chicken breast
2	ribs celery, finely chopped
1	small apple, finely chopped
¼	cup dried cranberries
¼	cup chopped pecans, walnuts, almonds, or hazelnuts
½	cup light mayonnaise
¼	teaspoon poultry seasoning
⅛	teaspoon celery seeds
⅛	teaspoon poppy seeds
⅛	teaspoon garlic salt
	Freshly ground black pepper
12	finger rolls (1 ounce each), split

1. **STIR** together the chicken, celery, apple, and cranberries in a medium bowl.

2. **PLACE** the nuts in a small skillet and cook over medium heat, shaking the pan often, for 2 to 3 minutes, or until toasted. Add the nuts to the chicken mixture.

3. **STIR** together the mayonnaise, poultry seasoning, celery seeds, poppy seeds, and garlic salt in a small bowl. Add pepper to taste. Combine the mayonnaise mixture with the chicken mixture and stir thoroughly. Refrigerate the chicken salad until ready to serve (it will keep nicely for 2 days).

4. **DIVIDE** the salad mixture evenly among the finger rolls (about ⅓ cup per sandwich).

FRUITY CHICKEN SALAD *(variation)*

OMIT the rolls.

PER SERVING (1 serving = 2 sandwiches)

Calories	Total Fat	Saturated Fat	Sodium	Carbohydrate	Dietary Fiber	Protein	Calcium
370	16 g	3 g	470 mg	37 g	4 g	19 g	2%
210	12 g	2 g	230 mg	11 g	2 g	15 g	2%

GRILLED TURKEY AND ARUGULA SANDWICH WITH BALSAMIC DIJONNAISE

PREP TIME: 5 MINUTES / **COOK TIME:** 8 MINUTES / **MAKES** 4 SERVINGS

Change the flavors in this versatile sandwich by varying the type of mustard and using different vegetables. Try grilling the sandwich on a panini grill or in a skillet for a toasty lunch on a cold day.

3	tablespoons light mayonnaise
2	teaspoons Dijon mustard
2	teaspoons balsamic vinegar
4	turkey breast cutlets (4 ounces each)
1	tablespoon extra-virgin olive oil
½	teaspoon salt
¼	teaspoon freshly ground black pepper
8	slices (1 ounce each) whole wheat bread, toasted
1	cup arugula
2	roasted peppers, rinsed, patted dry, and cut into 4 pieces

1. COMBINE the mayonnaise, mustard, and vinegar in a bowl.

2. COMBINE the turkey, oil, salt, and pepper in a separate bowl. Coat a nonstick grill pan with cooking spray and heat over medium-high heat. Add the turkey to the grill pan and cook for 3 to 4 minutes per side, or until well marked and cooked through.

3. BRUSH one side of each slice of bread with the mayonnaise mixture. Top half the slices with the turkey, arugula, and roasted peppers. Top with the remaining slices of bread and cut each sandwich in half.

MAKE
IT A
MEAL

Lemonade spritzer with ¾ cup lemonade and ¾ cup seltzer **70 CALORIES**

CALORIES
PER MEAL
★

MAKE
IT A
MEAL

1 small apple **80 CALORIES**

CALORIES
PER MEAL
★ ★ ★

PER SERVING (1 serving = 1 sandwich)

Calories	Total Fat	Saturated Fat	Sodium	Carbohydrate	Dietary Fiber	Protein	Calcium
340	10 g	1 g	880 mg	31 g	5 g	34 g	0%

CHICKEN SAUSAGE CALZONES

PREP TIME 20 MINUTES + 15 MINUTES COOLING / COOK TIME: 29 MINUTES / MAKES 4 SERVINGS

Refrigerated pizza dough makes easy work of this crowd-pleasing dish. To bump up the fiber, use whole wheat dough instead.

1   teaspoon extra-virgin olive oil
6   ounces reduced-fat Italian chicken sausage (such as Al Fresco), sliced
1   onion, sliced
3   cloves garlic, minced
1   teaspoon dried oregano
1   green bell pepper, thinly sliced
1   red bell pepper, thinly sliced
⅛   teaspoon salt
½   cup shredded part-skim mozzarella cheese
1   tube (11 ounces) refrigerated thin-crust pizza dough

1. PREHEAT the oven to 400°F. Coat a large baking sheet with cooking spray.

2. HEAT the oil in a large nonstick skillet over medium-high heat. Add the sausage, onion, garlic, and oregano, and cook, stirring occasionally, for 2 to 3 minutes, or until the onion starts to soften. Add the bell peppers and salt. Cook, stirring occasionally, for 7 to 8 minutes, or until the sausage is browned and the vegetables are tender. Remove from the heat and let cool for 10 minutes. Stir in the cheese.

3. DIVIDE the dough into 4 equal pieces. On a lightly floured surface, roll each piece into a 6"-diameter circle. Place one-fourth of the sausage mixture over half of each circle. Fold the dough over the filling to form 4 semicircles. Firmly pinch the edges of the dough to seal. Carefully lift the calzones and transfer them to the baking sheet. Pierce the dough with a fork in four separate places.

4. BAKE the calzones for 16 to 18 minutes, or until the tops are golden brown. Let cool for 5 minutes before serving.

PER SERVING (1 serving = 1 calzone)

Calories	Total Fat	Saturated Fat	Sodium	Carbohydrate	Dietary Fiber	Protein	Calcium
330	11 g	3 g	630 mg	41 g	3 g	19 g	15%

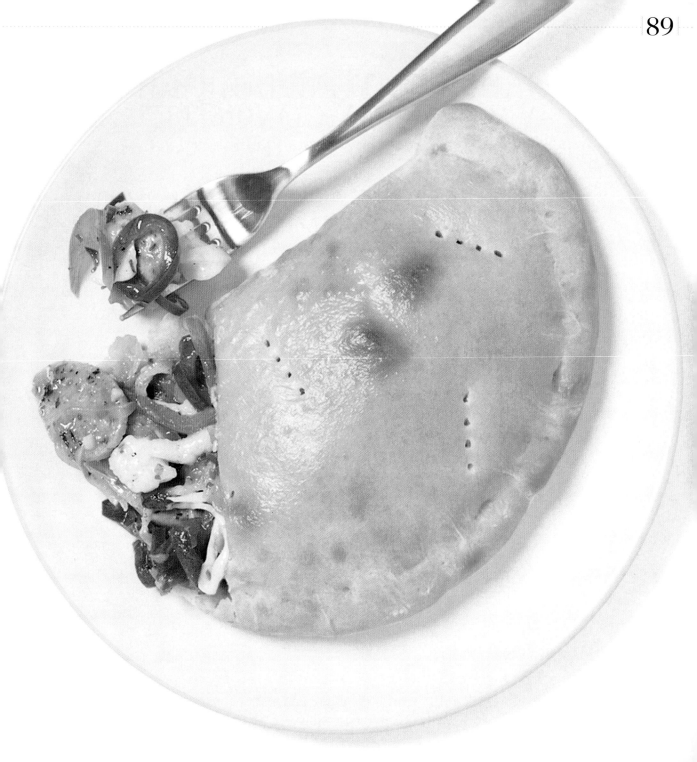

GRILLED STEAK BURGERS WITH ONION COMPOTE

PREP TIME: 15 MINUTES / **COOK TIME:** 20 MINUTES / **MAKES** 4 SERVINGS

Home-ground steak, here skirt steak, is much more flavorful than supermarket ground beef, and you know exactly what is in it. However, you can substitute ready-to-use ground beef or ground turkey if you prefer.

410
CALORIES
PER MEAL
★ ★ ★

(variation)
380
CALORIES
PER MEAL
★ ★ ★

ONION COMPOTE

- 1 teaspoon olive oil
- 2 onions, chopped
- 2 teaspoons light brown sugar
- ⅓ cup red wine
- 1 tablespoon red wine vinegar

STEAK BURGERS

- ¼ cup oil-packed sun-dried tomatoes, well drained
- 1 pound skirt steak, trimmed of visible fat, cut into chunks
- 1 tablespoon chili powder
- ½ teaspoon salt
- ¼ teaspoon freshly ground black pepper
- 4 whole wheat kaiser rolls (2 ounces each), toasted
- 4 slices tomato
- 4 leaves green-leaf lettuce

1. **TO MAKE THE ONION COMPOTE:** Heat the oil in a large regular or nonstick skillet over medium heat. Add the onions and brown sugar. Cook for 8 minutes, or until the onions are soft and lightly browned; stir occasionally to prevent sticking or burning. Add the wine and vinegar. Simmer for 5 minutes, or until the wine is almost completely cooked off. Set aside.

2. **TO MAKE THE STEAK BURGERS:** Puree the sun-dried tomatoes in a mini food processor. Set aside.

3. **COARSELY** chop the steak in a food processor or meat grinder until slightly chunkier than hamburger meat. Mix in the chili powder, salt, and pepper.

4. **FORM** the meat into 4 balls. Make a hole in the center of each ball and fill with 1 tablespoon of the pureed sun-dried tomatoes. Gently form the ball into a patty by bringing up the sides to enclose the tomato puree in the center.

5. **PREHEAT** a grill to medium. Place the patties on a grill rack coated with cooking spray. Grill for 7 minutes per side or until an instant-read thermometer inserted sideways in a burger registers 160°F and the meat is no longer pink.

6. **SERVE** each burger on a toasted roll. Top with tomato, lettuce, and ¼ cup onion compote.

PER SERVING (1 serving = 1 burger, ¼ cup onion compote)
Steak Burgers with Sautéed Mushrooms (1 serving = 1 burger, ½ cup sautéed mushrooms)

Calories	Total Fat	Saturated Fat	Sodium	Carbohydrate	Dietary Fiber	Protein	Calcium
410	14 g	4 g	670 mg	41 g	7 g	30 g	10%
380	15 g	4 g	820 mg	36 g	7 g	31 g	8%

STEAK BURGERS WITH SAUTÉED MUSHROOMS *(variation)*

OMIT the onion compote and make sautéed mushrooms. Heat 1 teaspoon olive oil in a large regular or nonstick skillet over medium heat. Add 2 cloves minced garlic, 10 ounces sliced cremini (brown) mushrooms, 2 tablespoons chopped parsley, ¼ teaspoon salt, and ⅛ teaspoon freshly ground black pepper. Cook, stirring occasionally, for 5 minutes, or until the mushrooms release their liquid and soften. Reduce to a simmer and cook for 10 minutes, until most of liquid has evaporated.

SERVE each burger topped with one-fourth of the mushrooms (plus tomato and lettuce).

MUSHROOM-STUFFED TURKEY BURGERS

PREP TIME: 10 MINUTES + 10 MINUTES COOLING / **COOK TIME:** 22 MINUTES / **MAKES** 4 SERVINGS

In this recipe, sautéed mushrooms are tucked inside turkey burgers to add flavor and moisture.

2	teaspoons olive oil
4	ounces mushrooms, chopped
½	small onion, finely chopped
¼	teaspoon dried thyme
½	teaspoon salt
1	clove garlic, minced
1	pound lean ground turkey
4	whole wheat hamburger buns
4	teaspoons Dijon mustard
1	cup mixed greens
1	medium tomato, cut into 4 slices

1. **HEAT** the oil in a medium nonstick skillet over medium-high heat. Add the mushrooms, onion, thyme, and ¼ teaspoon of the salt, and cook, stirring occasionally, for 4 minutes or until starting to brown. Add the garlic and cook for 2 minutes. Remove from the heat and set aside to cool for 10 minutes.

2. **DIVIDE** the turkey into 4 portions and shape each into a ball. Make a deep indentation in each with your finger and fill with one-fourth of the mushroom mixture. Close the turkey around the mushroom mixture and form each ball into a patty 3½" in diameter. Sprinkle the patties with the remaining ¼ teaspoon salt.

3. **COAT** a nonstick grill pan with cooking spray and heat over medium-high heat. Add the patties and cook for 14 to 16 minutes, turning once, until cooked through.

4. **BRUSH** each hamburger bun bottom with 1 teaspoon mustard. Top with ¼ cup of the greens, 1 tomato slice, a turkey patty, and the bun top.

MAKE IT A MEAL

Potato salad made with ½ cup cooked potato cubes, 2 tablespoons fat-free (0%) Greek yogurt, slivered fresh herbs
85 CALORIES

395 CALORIES PER MEAL
★ ★

MAKE IT A MEAL

Salad made with 2 cups mixed baby greens, 1 tablespoon dried cranberries, 1 tablespoon goat cheese, 1 tablespoon balsamic vinegar
105 CALORIES

415 CALORIES PER MEAL
★ ★

PER SERVING (1 serving = 1 burger)

Calories	Total Fat	Saturated Fat	Sodium	Carbohydrate	Dietary Fiber	Protein	Calcium
310	11 g	2.5 g	700 mg	27 g	4 g	27 g	6%

SMOKED TURKEY BLT

PREP TIME: 5 MINUTES / **MAKES** 1 SERVING

The combination of bacon and smoked turkey gives this sandwich a double dose of smokiness. If you're watching your sodium, ask for lower-sodium sliced turkey at the deli counter.

2   slices (1 ounce each) multigrain bread, toasted

2   teaspoons light mayonnaise

1   Boston lettuce leaf

2   tomato slices

1   slice bacon, cooked

2   ounces sliced smoked turkey

SPREAD one side of one slice of toast with the mayonnaise. Top with the lettuce, tomato, bacon, turkey, and remaining toast. Cut in half.

MAKE
IT A
MEAL

1 cup raw broccoli florets with
2 tablespoons guacamole
60 CALORIES

1 small apple
80 CALORIES

410

CALORIES
PER MEAL

★ ★ ★ ★

MAKE
IT A
MEAL

1 cup reduced-sodium cream of tomato soup with 10 low-sodium oyster crackers
140 CALORIES

410

CALORIES
PER MEAL

★

PER SERVING (1 serving = 1 sandwich)

Calories	Total Fat	Saturated Fat	Sodium	Carbohydrate	Dietary Fiber	Protein	Calcium
270	9 g	2 g	840 mg	25 g	4 g	22 g	6%

PEKING DUCK QUESADILLAS

PREP TIME: 15 MINUTES + UP TO 4 HOURS MARINATING / **COOK TIME:** 48 MINUTES / **MAKES** 4 SERVINGS

Though duck skin is extremely fatty, duck breast meat is extremely lean. Cooking the breast with the skin on helps the meat stay moist.

MAKE IT A MEAL

⅓ cup diced Hass avocado drizzled with lime juice
80 CALORIES

390
CALORIES PER MEAL
★ ★ ★

MAKE IT A MEAL

1 cup cubed tomato and jicama
40 CALORIES

¼ cup frozen yogurt
50 CALORIES

400
CALORIES PER MEAL
★ ★ ★

- 3 tablespoons dry sherry
- ¼ teaspoon salt
- ¼ teaspoon five-spice powder
- 1 pound boneless, skin-on duck breasts
- ¼ cup chopped fresh cilantro
- 3 scallions, thinly sliced
- 1 chipotle pepper in adobo sauce, minced
- 4 (8") whole wheat tortillas
- 2 tablespoons hoisin sauce
- ¼ cup grated queso blanco light or part-skim mozzarella cheese
- ¼ cup low-fat plain yogurt
- 2 tablespoons chopped hulled pumpkin seeds

1. **COMBINE** the sherry, salt, and five-spice powder in a resealable plastic bag or container. Add the duck. Marinate in the refrigerator for 1 to 4 hours.

2. **REMOVE** the duck from the marinade (discard the marinade). Pierce the duck skin all over with a sharp skewer.

3. **FILL** a wok or large pot with about 2" of water. Set a steamer basket or rack above the water. Bring the water to a boil over medium heat. Place the duck skin-side down in the steamer basket or on the rack. Cover and steam for 20 minutes.

4. **MEANWHILE,** preheat the oven to 350°F. Coat a 13" x 9" baking dish with cooking spray.

5. **PLACE** a rack that is large enough to hold the duck in the baking dish. Place the duck skin-side up on the rack. Bake for 15 to 20 minutes, until the skin is sizzling and a thermometer inserted in the thickest part of a breast registers 160°F.

PER SERVING (1 serving = 2 wedges, 1 tablespoon yogurt, 1½ teaspoons pumpkin seeds)

Calories	Total Fat	Saturated Fat	Sodium	Carbohydrate	Dietary Fiber	Protein	Calcium
310	5 g	1.5 g	780 mg	40 g	4 g	33 g	8%

6. MEANWHILE, combine the cilantro, 2 of the scallions, and the chipotle pepper in a small bowl. Spread 2 of the tortillas with the hoisin sauce. Top the hoisin sauce with the cilantro mixture.

7. DISCARD the duck skin and slice the duck into thin slices. Place on top of the cilantro mixture on the tortillas. Sprinkle with the cheese. Top with the 2 remaining tortillas.

8. SPRAY a large skillet with cooking spray. Cook each quesadilla for 2 minutes on each side. Cut each quesadilla into 4 wedges and serve 2 wedges per person. Top each serving with 1 tablespoon yogurt, 1½ teaspoons pumpkin seeds, and a sprinkling of the remaining scallion.

SPICY SHRIMP SALAD PITAS

PREP TIME: 10 MINUTES / **COOK TIME:** 5 MINUTES / **MAKES** 4 SERVINGS

Shrimp are always a calorie-smart pick, as they have almost no fat and plenty of protein. Most people prefer the extra-dense, creamy flesh of the pebbly-skinned Hass, or California, avocado over the larger, smooth-skinned Florida avocado.

¾	pound peeled and deveined large shrimp
1	teaspoon olive oil
¼	teaspoon salt
½	Hass avocado, chopped
1	small red onion, chopped
1	rib celery, chopped
1	cup shredded lettuce
1	tablespoon chopped fresh cilantro
3	tablespoons light mayonnaise
1	jalapeño chile pepper, finely chopped (wear plastic gloves when handling)
4	large (6½") whole wheat pitas

1. **PREHEAT** a grill to medium-high.

2. **COMBINE** the shrimp, oil, and salt in a bowl, and toss well. Set the shrimp on a grill rack (or in a grill basket) that has been coated with cooking spray. Grill for 2½ minutes per side, or until opaque and cooked through. Transfer to a cutting board. When cool enough to handle, coarsely chop and transfer to a bowl.

3. **ADD** the avocado, onion, celery, lettuce, cilantro, mayonnaise, and jalapeño chile pepper to the shrimp, and toss gently to combine.

4. **SLICE** the top one-eighth off each pita and discard. Divide the shrimp mixture among the pitas (about 1 cup salad per sandwich).

MAKE
IT A
MEAL

½ cup deli 3-bean salad
90 CALORIES

1 cup fresh papaya cubes
50 CALORIES

420
CALORIES
PER MEAL
★ ★ ★ ★

MAKE
IT A
MEAL

½ cup lemon sorbet
110 CALORIES

390
CALORIES
PER MEAL
★

PER SERVING (1 serving = 1 sandwich)

Calories	Total Fat	Saturated Fat	Sodium	Carbohydrate	Dietary Fiber	Protein	Calcium
280	9 g	1.5 g	640 mg	30 g	6 g	19 g	4%

TOMATO, ARUGULA, PROSCIUTTO, AND FETA PANINI

PREP TIME: 5 MINUTES / **COOK TIME:** 6 MINUTES / **MAKES** 1 SERVING

This quick grilled sandwich can be a light accompaniment to a hearty salad. Or pair it with a favorite dessert.

1	small piece (2 ounces) baguette, halved horizontally
1	teaspoon balsamic vinegar
¼	cup arugula
3	slices (1 ounce total) prosciutto
2	medium tomato slices
2	teaspoons crumbled reduced-fat feta cheese

1. BRUSH the bottom half of the baguette with the vinegar. Top with the arugula, prosciutto, tomato slices, cheese, and top half of the bread.

2. COAT a nonstick grill pan with cooking spray and heat over medium heat.

3. LIGHTLY coat the outside of the sandwich with cooking spray. Place the sandwich on the grill pan, set a heavy pan on top, and press down slightly to partially flatten. Cook for 3 minutes per side, or until the center is warm and the bread is marked and toasted. Transfer to a cutting board and cut in half before serving.

MAKE IT A MEAL

Salad made with 2 cups romaine lettuce, 1 tablespoon chopped walnuts, ¼ cup rinsed and drained chickpeas, 1 chopped dried fig, 10 sprays salad dressing spray **170 CALORIES**

410 CALORIES PER MEAL
★ ★ ★

MAKE IT A MEAL

2 mini brownie bites (such as Hostess) **110 CALORIES**

¼ cup vanilla ice cream **70 CALORIES**

420 CALORIES PER MEAL

PER SERVING (1 serving = 1 sandwich)

Calories	Total Fat	Saturated Fat	Sodium	Carbohydrate	Dietary Fiber	Protein	Calcium
240	5 g	2 g	960 mg	35 g	1 g	14 g	4%

TUSCAN TUNA SALAD SANDWICH

PREP TIME: 10 MINUTES / **MAKES** 4 SERVINGS

Try this recipe as a light and refreshing change from traditional mayonnaise-laden tuna salad. Use strongly flavored olive oil to enhance the flavor of the other ingredients.

1	can (6 ounces) water-packed light tuna, drained
1	can (15 to 19 ounces) small white beans, rinsed and drained
¼	cup chopped fresh parsley
¼	cup chopped dry-pack sun-dried tomatoes
2	tablespoons chopped fresh basil
2	tablespoons finely chopped shallots
2	tablespoons fresh lemon juice
2	tablespoons olive oil
2	tablespoons low-fat plain yogurt
4	large (6½") whole wheat pitas
1	cup shredded romaine lettuce

1. **COMBINE** the tuna, beans, parsley, sun-dried tomatoes, basil, shallots, lemon juice, oil, and yogurt in a medium bowl.

2. **CUT** each pita crosswise in half. Fill each half with 2 tablespoons lettuce and about ½ cup tuna mixture.

MAKE IT A MEAL

Salad made with 2 cups mixed baby greens, 10 cherry tomatoes, 1 tablespoon light Italian dressing
80 CALORIES

420
CALORIES PER MEAL
★ ★ ★

MAKE IT A MEAL

10 baby carrots
40 CALORIES

1 clementine
30 CALORIES

410
CALORIES PER MEAL
★ ★ ★

PER SERVING (1 serving = 2 pita halves)

Calories	Total Fat	Saturated Fat	Sodium	Carbohydrate	Dietary Fiber	Protein	Calcium
340	10 g	1.5 g	620 mg	43 g	8 g	21 g	15%

HALIBUT SANDWICH WITH EASY TARTAR SAUCE

PREP TIME: 10 MINUTES / **COOK TIME:** 10 MINUTES / **MAKES** 4 SERVINGS

After eating this fresh, light sandwich, you'll never crave greasy fast-food fish sandwiches again. Any type of white, firm-fleshed fish, such as mahi mahi, tilapia, or cod, works well. For a tangier tartar sauce, substitute plain yogurt for the mayo.

¼	cup light mayonnaise
2	tablespoons sweet pickle relish
1	tablespoon finely chopped onion
4	skinless halibut fillets (4 ounces each)
¼	teaspoon salt
¼	teaspoon freshly ground black pepper
4	whole wheat hamburger buns, toasted
1	medium tomato, cut into 4 slices
4	Boston lettuce leaves

1. COMBINE the mayonnaise, relish, and onion to make the tartar sauce in a small bowl, and mix well.

2. COAT a nonstick grill pan with cooking spray and heat over medium-high heat. Sprinkle the halibut with the salt and pepper, and add to the pan. Cook, turning once, for 9 to 10 minues, or until the fish flakes easily with a fork. Remove from the heat.

3. TOP each hamburger bun bottom with 1 tomato slice, 1 lettuce leaf, and 1 halibut fillet. Spread the top half of each bun with the tartar sauce and set over the fillet.

MAKE IT A MEAL

1 medium ear corn
80 CALORIES

380
CALORIES
PER MEAL
★

MAKE IT A MEAL

12 ounces sweetened iced tea
120 CALORIES

420
CALORIES
PER MEAL
★

PER SERVING (1 serving = 1 sandwich)

Calories	Total Fat	Saturated Fat	Sodium	Carbohydrate	Dietary Fiber	Protein	Calcium
300	10 g	1.5 g	590 mg	27 g	4 g	27 g	10%

CURRIED CHICKPEAS WITH CUCUMBER RAITA IN A PITA

PREP TIME: 15 MINUTES + 1 HOUR CHILLING / **COOK TIME:** 30 MINUTES / **MAKES** 4 SERVINGS

This dish is delicious warm, at room temperature, or cold. Prepare at least 1 hour before serving to allow the flavors to blend.

MAKE
IT A
MEAL

½ medium mango,
sliced
70 CALORIES

390
CALORIES
PER MEAL
★ ★

MAKE
IT A
MEAL

1 frozen fruit bar
(2¾ ounces)
80 CALORIES

400
CALORIES
PER MEAL
★ ★

1	tablespoon olive oil
2	medium onions, chopped
2	cloves garlic, minced
1	teaspoon honey
2	cups cooked or rinsed and drained canned chickpeas
1	medium tomato, diced
½	cup finely chopped fresh cilantro
2	tablespoons currants
1	tablespoon curry powder
¾	teaspoon salt
1	medium cucumber
1	cup low-fat plain yogurt
2	tablespoons finely chopped fresh mint
1	tablespoon fresh lemon juice
2	large (6½") whole wheat pitas, halved crosswise

1. **HEAT** the oil in a large skillet over medium heat. Add the onions, half of the garlic, and the honey. Cover and cook for 5 minutes to soften the onions. Uncover and cook for 20 minutes, or until the onions are very soft and light brown. Add the chickpeas, tomato, ¼ cup of the cilantro, the currants, curry powder, and ½ teaspoon of the salt. Simmer for 5 minutes to blend the flavors. Let cool to room temperature, then refrigerate for 1 hour.

2. **MEANWHILE,** grate the cucumber into a colander. Squeeze or press out as much cucumber liquid as possible. Combine the cucumber, yogurt, mint, lemon juice, and the remaining garlic, ¼ teaspoon salt, and ¼ cup cilantro in a medium bowl to make the raita.

3. **WARM** the pitas if desired. Fill each half with the chickpea mixture (about ¾ cup) and top with ⅓ cup of the cucumber raita.

PER SERVING (1 serving = 1 stuffed pita half, ⅓ cup raita)

Calories	Total Fat	Saturated Fat	Sodium	Carbohydrate	Dietary Fiber	Protein	Calcium
320	7 g	1.5 g	610 mg	53 g	11 g	14 g	20%

SWISS AND CHEDDAR GRILLED CHEESE ON THIN WHOLE WHEAT

PREP TIME: 5 MINUTES / **COOK TIME:** 6 MINUTES / **MAKES** 1 SERVING

This recipe calls for Cheddar and Swiss cheeses but you can use any reduced-fat sliced cheese, including varieties with herbs and seasonings. If you have a panini maker, try it out on this recipe.

2	thin slices (about ½ ounce each) whole wheat bread
1	teaspoon Dijon mustard
1	slice (1 ounce) reduced-fat Cheddar cheese
2	medium tomato slices
1	slice (1 ounce) reduced-fat Swiss cheese

1. BRUSH one side of one slice of bread with the mustard. Top with the Cheddar, tomato, Swiss, and remaining slice of bread.

2. HEAT a small nonstick skillet coated with cooking spray over medium heat. Lightly coat the outside of the sandwich with cooking spray and add to the skillet. Cook for 3 minutes per side, or until the cheese has melted and the outside of the bread is golden. Cut in half before serving.

MAKE IT A MEAL

1 small apple
80 CALORIES

390
CALORIES PER MEAL
★ ★ ★

MAKE IT A MEAL

Salad made with 2 cups mixed baby greens, 1 teaspoon olive oil, 1 teaspoon red wine vinegar
60 CALORIES

½ cup blueberries
40 CALORIES

410
CALORIES PER MEAL
★ ★ ★

PER SERVING (1 serving = 1 sandwich)

Calories	Total Fat	Saturated Fat	Sodium	Carbohydrate	Dietary Fiber	Protein	Calcium
310	14 g	6 g	470 mg	26 g	4 g	23 g	50%

NEW ENGLAND LOBSTER ROLL

PREP TIME: 10 MINUTES / **MAKES** 4 SERVINGS

We lightened up this Down East classic by using just enough light mayo to moisten the ingredients while allowing the flavor of the lobster to shine through. The fresh tarragon adds an unexpected flavor twist.

12	ounces cooked lobster meat, chopped (about 3 cups)
¼	cup finely chopped celery
3	tablespoons light mayonnaise
2	tablespoons finely chopped red onion
2	teaspoons chopped fresh tarragon
1	teaspoon fresh lemon juice
⅛	teaspoon freshly ground black pepper
4	top-split New England–style hot dog rolls, toasted (we used Pepperidge Farm)

COMBINE the lobster, celery, mayonnaise, onion, tarragon, lemon juice, and pepper in a medium bowl. Divide the mixture among the 4 hot dog rolls.

Sidebar

MAKE
IT A
MEAL

⅓ cup deli coleslaw
110 CALORIES

½ cup tomato slices
20 CALORIES

390
CALORIES
PER MEAL
★ ★

MAKE
IT A
MEAL

1 bottle (12 ounces) beer
150 CALORIES

410
CALORIES
PER MEAL
★

PER SERVING (1 serving = 1 roll, ¾ cup lobster salad)

Calories	Total Fat	Saturated Fat	Sodium	Carbohydrate	Dietary Fiber	Protein	Calcium
260	8 g	2.5 g	640 mg	24 g	1 g	21 g	10%

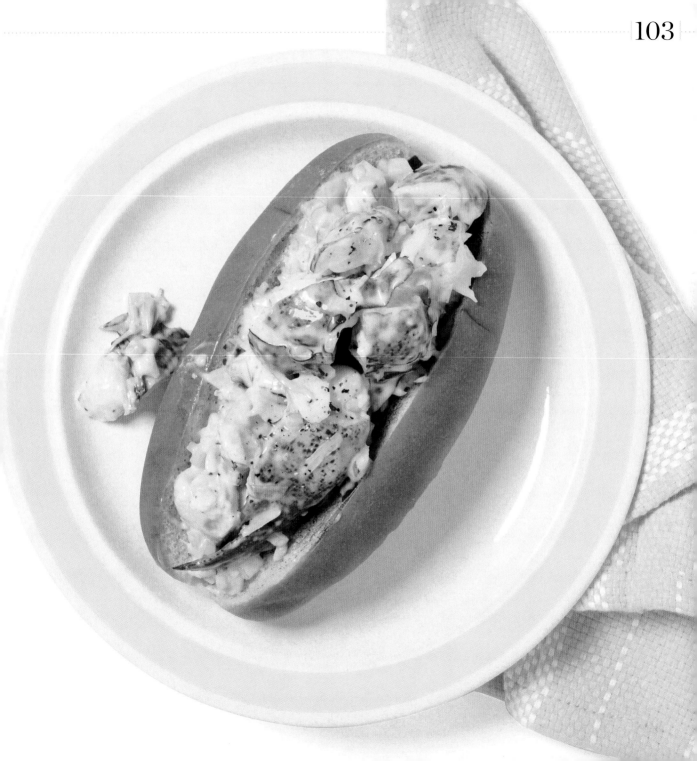

6

SALADS & SIDES

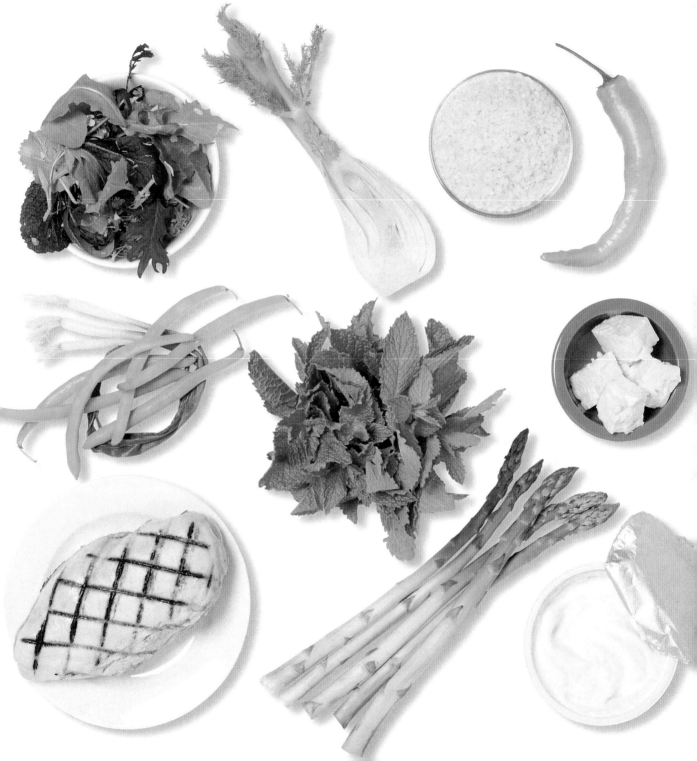

SUMMER CHOPPED SALAD WITH GRILLED SHRIMP

PREP TIME: 35 MINUTES / **COOK TIME:** 12 MINUTES / **MAKES** 4 SERVINGS

This salad is light and refreshing on a hot summer day. The honey and the mustard help keep the salad dressing from separating.

MAKE IT A MEAL

½ cup light vanilla ice cream
100 CALORIES

410
CALORIES PER MEAL
★ ★ ★ ★

MAKE the variation A MEAL

1 medium banana, grilled
110 CALORIES

420
CALORIES PER MEAL
★ ★ ★ ★

3	ounces French bread, cut into ½" cubes
3	cups chopped romaine lettuce
3	tomatoes, seeded and chopped
1	carrot, chopped
1	rib celery, chopped
1	cucumber, seeded and chopped
½	fennel bulb, chopped
4	radishes, chopped
¾	pound peeled and deveined large shrimp
3	tablespoons extra-virgin olive oil
⅜	teaspoon salt
¼	teaspoon freshly ground black pepper
¼	cup finely chopped shallots
1	tablespoon balsamic vinegar
2	teaspoons honey
2	teaspoons Dijon mustard

1. PREHEAT the oven to 425°F. Arrange the bread cubes on a baking sheet in a single layer. Bake for 6 to 8 minutes, or until golden and crisp. Let cool on the baking sheet.

2. MEANWHILE, combine the lettuce, tomatoes, carrot, celery, cucumber, fennel, and radishes in a large bowl.

3. COAT a grill pan with cooking spray and heat over medium-high heat. Toss the shrimp with 2 teaspoons of the oil in a small bowl. Sprinkle with ⅛ teaspoon of the salt and ⅛ teaspoon of the pepper. Set the shrimp on the grill pan and cook for 1½ to 2 minutes per side, or until opaque. Transfer to a plate and set aside.

4. COMBINE the shallots, vinegar, honey, mustard, and the remaining ¼ teaspoon salt and ⅛ teaspoon pepper in a medium bowl. Slowly whisk in the remaining 2 tablespoons + 1 teaspoon oil. Pour the dressing over the lettuce mixture, add the cooled bread cubes, and toss well. Divide the mixture among 4 plates and top with the shrimp.

PER SERVING (1 serving = 2 cups salad, about 10 shrimp, 1½ tablespoons dressing) Summer Chopped Salad with Grilled Chicken (1 serving = 2 cups salad, about 2 ounces chicken, 1½ tablespoons dressing)

Calories	Total Fat	Saturated Fat	Sodium	Carbohydrate	Dietary Fiber	Protein	Calcium
310	13 g	2 g	570 mg	28 g	4 g	22 g	10%
310	13 g	2 g	480 mg	27 g	4 g	22 g	6%

SUMMER CHOPPED SALAD
WITH GRILLED CHICKEN *(variation)*
SUBSTITUTE ¾ pound sliced boneless, skinless chicken
breast for the shrimp and follow the grilling procedure.

ROASTED CORN AND BLACK BEAN SALAD WITH CHICKEN

PREP TIME: 10 MINUTES / **COOK TIME:** 6 MINUTES / **MAKES** 4 SERVINGS

Though this refreshing summer dish just calls for cooked chicken, if you have leftover grilled chicken, all the better. And instead of pan-roasting the corn, you could cook ears of corn on the grill to add a smoky flavor.

MAKE
IT A
MEAL

2 peanut
butter cookies
(½ ounce each)
120 CALORIES

420
CALORIES
PER MEAL
★ ★ ★ ★

MAKE
the variation
A MEAL

1 cup fresh
fruit salad
100 CALORIES

390
CALORIES
PER MEAL
★ ★ ★

2	tablespoons olive oil
2	cups fresh corn kernels
1	can (15 ounces) no-salt-added black beans, rinsed and drained
8	ounces cooked chicken breast, cubed
2	plum tomatoes, chopped
1	small red onion, chopped
3	tablespoons chopped fresh cilantro
2	tablespoons fresh lime juice
1	jalapeño chile pepper, finely chopped (wear plastic gloves when handling)
½	teaspoon salt

1. **HEAT** 1 tablespoon of the oil in a large nonstick skillet over medium-high heat. Add the corn and cook, stirring occasionally, for 5 to 6 minutes, or until the corn starts to brown.

2. **TRANSFER** the corn to a large bowl and stir in the beans, chicken, tomatoes, onion, cilantro, lime juice, jalapeño chile pepper, and salt.

ROASTED CORN AND BLACK BEAN SALAD WITH PORK TENDERLOIN

(variation)

SUBSTITUTE grilled pork tenderloin for chicken breast.

PER SERVING (1 serving = 1½ cups)
Roasted Corn and Black Bean Salad with Pork Tenderloin (1 serving = 1½ cups)

Calories	Total Fat	Saturated Fat	Sodium	Carbohydrate	Dietary Fiber	Protein	Calcium
300	10 g	1.5 g	360 mg	30 g	7 g	25 g	6%
290	10 g	2 g	350 mg	30 g	7 g	22 g	6%

CHICKEN CAESAR SALAD

PREP TIME: 10 MINUTES / **MAKES** 4 SERVINGS

You will love the lightened-up dressing (we cut way down on the oil) so much that you may want to use it every day. Any greens work in this salad, including baby spinach, field greens, and arugula.

3	tablespoons light mayonnaise
2	tablespoons grated Parmesan cheese
1½	tablespoons fresh lemon juice
1	tablespoon extra-virgin olive oil
2	teaspoons Dijon mustard
1	teaspoon grated lemon zest
¾	teaspoon Worcestershire sauce
½	teaspoon anchovy paste
⅛	teaspoon freshly ground black pepper
6	cups torn romaine lettuce
12	ounces cooked chicken breast, cubed
24	fat-free Italian seasoned croutons

1. **WHISK** together the mayonnaise, Parmesan, lemon juice, oil, mustard, lemon zest, Worcestershire sauce, anchovy paste, and pepper in a small bowl.

2. **COMBINE** the lettuce, chicken, and croutons in a large bowl. Pour the dressing over the lettuce mixture and toss well to coat.

SHRIMP CAESAR SALAD *(variation)*

SUBSTITUTE 1 pound of cooked shrimp for the chicken breast.

MAKE IT A MEAL

Bruschetta made with 2 thin slices (½ ounce each) toasted Italian bread topped with ¼ cup diced tomato and slivered fresh basil **90 CALORIES**

390 CALORIES PER MEAL
★ ★

MAKE the variation A MEAL

Bruschetta made with 2 thin slices (½ ounce each) toasted Italian bread topped with ¼ cup diced tomato and slivered fresh basil **90 CALORIES**

1 slice (2") angel food cake **70 CALORIES**

400 CALORIES PER MEAL
★ ★

PER SERVING (1 serving = 2 cups) Shrimp Caesar Salad (1 serving = 2 cups)

Calories	Total Fat	Saturated Fat	Sodium	Carbohydrate	Dietary Fiber	Protein	Calcium
300	12 g	3 g	400 mg	9 g	2 g	36 g	8%
240	10 g	2 g	580 mg	9 g	2 g	27 g	10%

TARRAGON CHICKEN SALAD

PREP TIME: 10 MINUTES / **MAKES** 4 SERVINGS

A perfect use for leftover chicken, this salad works as a light lunch on a warm summer day. The recipe calls for cooked chicken, a combination of light and dark meat, but you may prefer to use only chicken breast. Try poaching or steaming boneless, skinless breasts to help keep them juicy.

MAKE IT A MEAL

1 small (1 ounce) whole wheat roll
80 CALORIES

½ cup strawberries
30 CALORIES

410
CALORIES PER MEAL
★ ★ ★

MAKE IT A MEAL

1 small (4") pita
70 CALORIES

½ cup blueberries
40 CALORIES

410
CALORIES PER MEAL
★ ★ ★

¼   cup walnut pieces

2   cups cubed (½") cooked chicken

¼   cup light mayonnaise

1   tablespoon Dijon mustard

1   tablespoon dried tarragon, crumbled

¼   teaspoon freshly ground black pepper

1   cup seedless red grapes, halved

12   Belgian endive leaves from 1 or 2 heads

1. **PLACE** the walnut pieces in a small microwaveable bowl and microwave for 30 seconds, until the nuts smell lightly toasted. Set aside.

2. **COMBINE** the chicken, mayonnaise, mustard, tarragon, and pepper in a medium bowl. Fold in the walnuts and gently fold in the grapes.

3. **PLACE** about ¼ cup of chicken salad on each endive leaf.

PER SERVING (1 serving = 3 endive leaves, ¾ cup chicken salad)

Calories	Total Fat	Saturated Fat	Sodium	Carbohydrate	Dietary Fiber	Protein	Calcium
300	18 g	3.5 g	240 mg	12 g	2 g	23 g	4%

SWEET AND SOUR CABBAGE SALAD

PREP TIME: 10 MINUTES + 30 MINUTES STANDING / **COOK TIME:** 3 MINUTES / **MAKES** 6 SERVINGS

Toasting the almonds gives them a touch of sweetness that helps balance the acidity of the vinegar. Shredding the cabbage in a food processor makes quick work of the preparation for this recipe.

½ cup sliced almonds

½ medium head green cabbage, very thinly sliced

½ medium head red cabbage, very thinly sliced

2 medium carrots, grated

1 Gala apple, peeled and cut into matchsticks

½ cup cider vinegar

¼ cup sugar

1 tablespoon olive oil

1 teaspoon salt

¼ teaspoon freshly ground black pepper

1. **PLACE** the almonds in a small nonstick skillet and cook over medium heat, shaking the pan often, for 1 to 3 minutes, or until the almonds are toasted. Transfer to a large bowl.

2. **ADD** the cabbages, carrots, apple, vinegar, sugar, oil, salt, and pepper. Toss well and let stand for 30 minutes, tossing occasionally, before serving.

MAKE IT A MEAL

3 ounces turkey kielbasa
140 CALORIES

⅔ cup mashed potatoes
80 CALORIES

380
CALORIES
PER MEAL
★ ★

MAKE IT A MEAL

3 ounces chicken-apple sausage
110 CALORIES

⅔ cup cooked barley
130 CALORIES

400
CALORIES
PER MEAL
★ ★ ★

PER SERVING (1 serving = 1⅓ cups)

Calories	Total Fat	Saturated Fat	Sodium	Carbohydrate	Dietary Fiber	Protein	Calcium
160	6 g	0.5 g	440 mg	25 g	5 g	4 g	10%

THAI BEEF SALAD

PREP TIME: 20 MINUTES / **COOK TIME:** 20 MINUTES / **MAKES** 4 SERVINGS

For extra flavor, marinate the cooked beef in the dressing for up to 1 hour in the refrigerator before slicing. Green papaya, which is underripe, is very firm, which is why you can shred it; ripe papaya is too soft and should not be substituted.

MAKE
IT A
MEAL

⅔ cup cooked
medium-grain
white rice
160 CALORIES

410
CALORIES
PER MEAL
★ ★

MAKE
IT A
MEAL

1 medium (7"–8")
flour tortilla
140 CALORIES

390
CALORIES
PER MEAL
★ ★

1	pound London broil
2	tablespoons finely chopped shallots
1	clove garlic, minced
	Juice of 1 lime
2	tablespoons rice vinegar
2	tablespoons sugar
1	tablespoon fish sauce
1	teaspoon Thai chili-garlic sauce (sriracha)
1	teaspoon toasted sesame oil
6	cups torn romaine or green leaf lettuce
2	cups shredded green papaya
¼	cup fresh basil leaves (Thai basil if available), coarsely chopped
¼	cup fresh cilantro, coarsely chopped
¼	cup fresh mint leaves, coarsely chopped
1	small cucumber, peeled and thinly sliced
2	scallions, thinly sliced

1. PREHEAT the broiler or grill. Broil or grill the meat for 7 to 10 minutes per side, depending on thickness, or until a thermometer inserted in the center registers 145°F for medium-rare or 160°F for medium. Let rest for 10 minutes before slicing across the grain into 12 slices.

2. MEANWHILE, whisk together the shallots, garlic, lime juice, vinegar, sugar, fish sauce, chili-garlic sauce, and sesame oil in a small bowl. Set the dressing aside.

3. TOSS together the lettuce, papaya, basil, cilantro, mint, cucumber, and scallions in a large bowl. Place the salad on a large platter.

4. ARRANGE the sliced meat over the salad. Drizzle with the dressing.

PER SERVING (1 serving = 3 slices beef, 2 cups salad, 2 tablespoons dressing)

Calories	Total Fat	Saturated Fat	Sodium	Carbohydrate	Dietary Fiber	Protein	Calcium
250	8 g	2.5 g	450 mg	20 g	4 g	27 g	10%

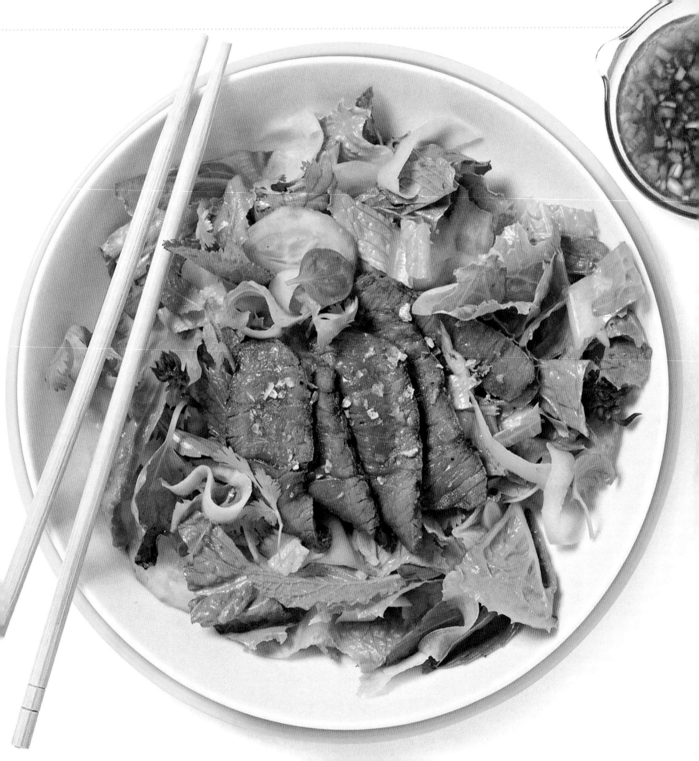

COBB SALAD WITH BLUE CHEESE VINAIGRETTE

PREP TIME: 20 MINUTES / **MAKES** 4 SERVINGS

Cobb salad is a restaurant classic easy to duplicate at home. Ours varies from the traditional in that we put just a small amount of blue cheese in the dressing, not several spoonfuls directly on the salad, which helps keep calories and fat under control. Either serve the salad on individual plates as we've done or, if you're entertaining, present it in a pretty serving bowl as a large, layered salad. (This can be done a few hours in advance and the salad can be refrigerated until needed. Dress the salad just before serving.)

BLUE CHEESE VINAIGRETTE

- 2 tablespoons extra-virgin olive oil
- 2 tablespoons fresh lemon juice
- 1 tablespoon water
- 1 tablespoon red wine vinegar
- 1 teaspoon Worcestershire sauce
- ½ teaspoon Dijon mustard
- ¼ teaspoon coarse salt
- ⅛ teaspoon freshly ground black pepper
- ¼ cup crumbled reduced-fat blue cheese

1. TO MAKE THE BLUE CHEESE VINAIGRETTE: Combine the oil, lemon juice, water, vinegar, Worcestershire sauce, mustard, salt, pepper, and blue cheese in a small bowl and whisk.

MAKE IT A MEAL

Garlic bread made with 1 slice (1 ounce) bread brushed with ½ teaspoon olive oil and sprinkled lightly with garlic powder
100 CALORIES

400
CALORIES PER MEAL
★ ★ ★

MAKE IT A MEAL

2 medium (7½") breadsticks
80 CALORIES

380
CALORIES PER MEAL
★ ★ ★

PER SERVING (1 serving = 2½ cups)

Calories	Total Fat	Saturated Fat	Sodium	Carbohydrate	Dietary Fiber	Protein	Calcium
300	21 g	4.5 g	420 mg	10 g	5 g	19 g	8%

SALAD

- 1 package (5 ounces) baby romaine lettuce
- 1 pint grape tomatoes, halved
- 1 Hass avocado, chopped
- 2 large hard-cooked eggs, peeled and coarsely chopped
- 1 cup diced cooked chicken breast (about 6 ounces)
- 2 tablespoons jarred real bacon bits

   Freshly ground black pepper (optional)

2. **TO ASSEMBLE THE SALAD:** Divide the lettuce and tomatoes among 4 plates. Layer one-fourth of the avocado over each salad and top with one-fourth of the chopped egg and ¼ cup of the chicken.

3. **WHISK** the dressing again and drizzle a generous 2 tablespoons of dressing over each serving. Top each with 1 tablespoon of bacon bits. Serve with black pepper if desired.

GREEK POTATO-BEAN SALAD

PREP TIME: 15 MINUTES / **COOK TIME:** 15 MINUTES / **MAKES** 4 SERVINGS

Potatoes have as much, if not more, fiber and vitamin C as other vegetables, along with about the same amount of carbohydrate as grains. To change the "nationality" of this dish, use a salt-free Italian or French seasoning blend in place of the dill. Asparagus works well in place of the beans.

MAKE
IT A
MEAL

3 ounces grilled
beef kebab made
with London broil
170 CALORIES

¼ cup grapes
30 CALORIES

420
CALORIES
PER MEAL
★ ★ ★

MAKE
IT A
MEAL

3 ounces grilled
lamb kebab
made with lean
leg of lamb
110 CALORIES

1 small (4")
whole wheat pita
70 CALORIES

400
CALORIES
PER MEAL
★ ★ ★ ★

1¼	pounds red potatoes, cut into 1" cubes
¾	pound green beans
¼	medium red onion, thinly sliced
1	rib celery, thinly sliced
3	tablespoons extra-virgin olive oil
1	teaspoon grated lemon zest
1	tablespoon fresh lemon juice
1	tablespoon chopped fresh dill
1	small clove garlic, minced
¾	teaspoon salt
¼	teaspoon freshly ground black pepper

1. **PLACE** the potatoes in a large saucepan with enough cold water to cover by 2". Bring to a boil over medium-high heat and cook for 10 to 12 minutes, or until the potatoes are tender but still hold their shape. Drain and transfer to a large bowl.

2. **MEANWHILE,** bring a large saucepan of lightly salted water to a boil. Add the green beans, return to a boil, and cook for 3 minutes. Drain and rinse under cold water, then drain again. Transfer to the bowl with the potatoes.

3. **ADD** the onion, celery, oil, lemon zest, lemon juice, dill, garlic, salt, and pepper. Toss well and serve warm or at room temperature.

PER SERVING (1 serving = 1½ cups)

Calories	Total Fat	Saturated Fat	Sodium	Carbohydrate	Dietary Fiber	Protein	Calcium
220	11 g	1.5 g	460 mg	30 g	5 g	4 g	6%

TABBOULEH SALAD WITH EXTRA VEGGIES

PREP TIME: 15 MINUTES + 1 HOUR CHILLING / **COOK TIME:** 5 MINUTES + 15 MINUTES STANDING / **MAKES** 4 SERVINGS

This recipe features the traditional refreshing flavors of tabbouleh, but with more vegetables for a more substantial salad. The salad benefits from being made ahead of time so the flavors develop. It can even be prepared a day ahead of serving.

¾ cup bulgur

1¼ cups boiling water

½ pint grape tomatoes, halved

1 small cucumber, cut into ¼" dice

½ yellow bell pepper, chopped

¾ cup shredded carrot

½ cup chopped fresh flat-leaf parsley

2 tablespoons chopped fresh mint

2 cloves garlic, minced

¼ cup crumbled reduced-fat feta cheese

¼ cup fresh lemon juice

3 tablespoons extra-virgin olive oil

¼ teaspoon coarse salt

⅛ teaspoon freshly ground black pepper

1. COMBINE the bulgur and boiling water in a medium heatproof bowl. Stir and set aside to absorb the liquid (about 15 minutes) while you prep the rest of the ingredients.

2. ADD the tomatoes, cucumber, bell pepper, carrot, parsley, mint, garlic, cheese, lemon juice, oil, salt, and black pepper to the bulgur. Stir thoroughly, cover, and refrigerate until chilled, at least 1 hour and up to 1 day ahead of serving. Stir thoroughly before serving.

MAKE IT A MEAL

3 ounces grilled swordfish
130 CALORIES

½ cup blueberries
40 CALORIES

410
CALORIES PER MEAL
★ ★ ★ ★

MAKE IT A MEAL

3 ounces grilled chicken thigh kebabs
180 CALORIES

420
CALORIES PER MEAL
★ ★ ★ ★

PER SERVING (1 serving = 1½ cups)

Calories	Total Fat	Saturated Fat	Sodium	Carbohydrate	Dietary Fiber	Protein	Calcium
240	12 g	2.5 g	260 mg	28 g	7 g	6 g	6%

SCALLOP SALAD WITH HERBED GOAT CHEESE

PREP TIME: 15 MINUTES / **COOK TIME:** 11 MINUTES / **MAKES** 4 SERVINGS

This entrée salad features sautéed scallops in a lemony dressing and tangy chèvre (fresh goat cheese) coated with fresh dill, parsley, and mint.

2	tablespoons finely chopped fresh dill
2	tablespoons finely chopped fresh flat-leaf parsley
1	tablespoon finely chopped fresh mint
½	log (2 ounces) fresh goat cheese
3	tablespoons light mayonnaise
2	tablespoons + 1 teaspoon extra-virgin olive oil
2	tablespoons fresh lemon juice
1	tablespoon red wine vinegar
1	tablespoon water
1	teaspoon Dijon mustard
½	teaspoon coarse salt
¼	teaspoon freshly ground black pepper

1. **COMBINE** the dill, parsley, and mint on a plate. Roll the goat cheese in the herbs, pressing the herbs into the cheese. Transfer the herb-coated goat cheese to a separate plate and refrigerate while you make the rest of the salad.

2. **ADD** the remaining herbs (what didn't stick to the cheese) to a medium bowl. Mix in the mayonnaise, 2 tablespoons of the oil, the lemon juice, vinegar, water, mustard, salt, and pepper. Whisk until smooth.

3. **MICROWAVE** the corn in a microwaveable bowl, covered, for 4 minutes. Rinse the corn under cold water until cool. Drain well.

4. **MEANWHILE,** divide the arugula among 4 plates. Top with the carrots and cucumber. Sprinkle the cooled corn over the salads.

MAKE IT A MEAL

2 small slices (½ ounce each) toasted baguette
80 CALORIES

410
CALORIES PER MEAL
★ ★

MAKE IT A MEAL

10 low-sodium thin wheat crackers
90 CALORIES

420
CALORIES PER MEAL
★ ★

PER SERVING (1 serving = 3 cups salad, 1 slice cheese, about 6 scallops)

Calories	Total Fat	Saturated Fat	Sodium	Carbohydrate	Dietary Fiber	Protein	Calcium
330	18 g	5 g	650 mg	19 g	3 g	25 g	15%

1 cup frozen corn kernels

1 package (5 ounces) baby arugula

1 cup pre-cut matchstick carrots

1 cucumber, peeled, seeded, and chopped

1 pound sea scallops (20/30 count)

2 tablespoons thinly sliced chives

Freshly ground black pepper (optional)

5. REMOVE the cheese from the refrigerator and cut it into 4 equal slices. Set aside.

6. HEAT the remaining 1 teaspoon oil in a large nonstick skillet over medium heat. Add the scallops and cook, without turning, for 4 minutes. Turn over and cook for 2 to 3 minutes, or until just cooked through.

7. ADD the scallops to the dressing and toss well to coat. Divide the scallops among the salad plates. Drizzle any remaining dressing over the salads. Place 1 goat cheese slice on each salad just to the side of the scallops. Garnish each salad with 1½ teaspoons of chives and freshly ground black pepper if desired.

WARM POTATO, PEA, AND PESTO SALAD

PREP TIME: 30 MINUTES / **COOK TIME:** 20 MINUTES / **MAKES** 4 SERVINGS

This warm potato salad skips the heavy dressing and instead is flavored with a "deconstructed" pesto sauce—basil, toasted pine nuts, and freshly shaved Parmesan cheese are sprinkled over the vegetables. A lemony dressing adds zing.

MAKE IT A MEAL

3 ounces grilled tuna
120 CALORIES

400 CALORIES PER MEAL
★ ★ ★

MAKE IT A MEAL

5 ounces white wine
120 CALORIES

400 CALORIES PER MEAL
★ ★

1	pound tiny red potatoes, halved
2	tablespoons fresh lemon juice
2	tablespoons extra-virgin olive oil
1	tablespoon light mayonnaise
1	tablespoon water
1	clove garlic, minced
¼	teaspoon coarse salt
⅛	teaspoon freshly ground black pepper
¼	cup pine nuts
½	pound sugar snap peas
⅓	cup thinly sliced red onion
½	cup thinly sliced fresh basil leaves
¼	cup freshly shaved or shredded Parmesan cheese

1. **PLACE** the potatoes in a medium saucepan. Add cold water to cover potatoes by 2" and bring to a boil over high heat. Cook, uncovered, for 8 to 10 minutes, or until tender.

2. **MEANWHILE,** whisk together the lemon juice, oil, mayonnaise, water, garlic, salt, and pepper in a small bowl or cup.

3. **PLACE** the pine nuts in a small nonstick skillet and cook over medium heat, shaking the pan often, for 2 to 3 minutes, or until fragrant and lightly browned. Transfer the pine nuts to a plate.

4. **PLACE** the snap peas and onion slices in a medium bowl. Drain the cooked potatoes and place on top of the snap peas and onion. Pour the dressing over the vegetables and stir with a wooden spoon to coat all the ingredients.

5. **DIVIDE** the potato and snap pea mixture among 4 salad plates. Sprinkle each portion with 1 tablespoon pine nuts, 2 tablespoons basil, and 1 tablespoon Parmesan. Alternatively, combine all ingredients in the bowl, then divide among the plates. Serve warm or at room temperature.

PER SERVING (1 serving = 1½ cups)

Calories	Total Fat	Saturated Fat	Sodium	Carbohydrate	Dietary Fiber	Protein	Calcium
280	15 g	2.5 g	250 mg	28 g	3 g	7 g	10%

SHAVED FENNEL, CUCUMBER, AND RED ONION SALAD

PREP TIME: 10 MINUTES + 15 MINUTES STANDING / **MAKES** 4 SERVINGS

The texture of fennel resembles celery, but the flavor has mild licorice overtones. The combination of rice vinegar and sugar imparts sweet and sour notes to this salad.

2½	cups thinly sliced fennel
1	large cucumber, peeled, halved lengthwise, seeded, and thinly sliced crosswise
1	small red onion, thinly sliced
1	large carrot, cut into long shreds with a vegetable peeler
2	tablespoons natural rice vinegar
2	tablespoons chopped fresh parsley
1	tablespoon olive oil
2	teaspoons sugar
¼	teaspoon salt
¼	teaspoon freshly ground black pepper

COMBINE the fennel, cucumber, onion, and carrot in a large bowl. Mix together the vinegar, parsley, oil, sugar, salt, and pepper in a small bowl. Pour the dressing over the vegetables and toss well. Let stand 15 minutes, tossing occasionally, before serving.

PER SERVING (1 serving = 1½ cups)

Calories	Total Fat	Saturated Fat	Sodium	Carbohydrate	Dietary Fiber	Protein	Calcium
80	3.5 g	0 g	190 mg	11 g	3 g	2 g	4%

MAKE IT A MEAL

3 ounces pan-seared salmon
180 CALORIES

½ cup cooked orzo
100 CALORIES

2 meringue cookies
60 CALORIES

CALORIES PER MEAL
★ ★ ★

MAKE IT A MEAL

3 ounces grilled chicken thighs
180 CALORIES

Garlic bread made with 1 slice (1 ounce) bread brushed with ½ teaspoon olive oil and sprinkled lightly with garlic powder
100 CALORIES

2 meringue cookies
60 CALORIES

CALORIES PER MEAL
★ ★

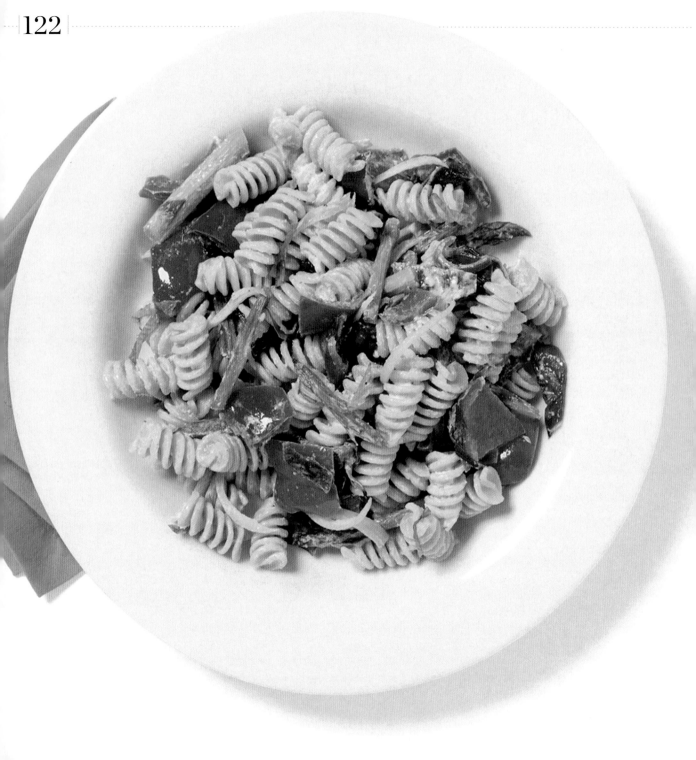

ROASTED-VEGETABLE PASTA SALAD

PREP TIME: 15 MINUTES / **COOK TIME:** 28 MINUTES / **MAKES** 4 SERVINGS

A wonderful side dish for almost any meal: Savory asparagus, red bell pepper, and red onion are roasted, then tossed with a summery basil-lemon vinaigrette and cooked whole grain rotini.

1½	cups whole grain rotini pasta
1	pound asparagus, cut into 1½" pieces
1	red bell pepper, cut into 1" pieces
1	small red onion, cut into 1" pieces
½	cup fresh basil leaves
2	cloves garlic, minced
2	tablespoons fat-free (0%) plain Greek yogurt
2	tablespoons extra-virgin olive oil
½	teaspoon grated lemon zest
2	tablespoons fresh lemon juice
2	tablespoons water
½	teaspoon coarse salt

1. **PREHEAT** the oven to 450°F. Line 2 baking sheets with foil and coat with cooking spray.

2. **BRING** a medium pot of water to a boil over high heat. Add the rotini and cook according to package directions. Drain the pasta and rinse under cold running water. Transfer to a salad bowl.

3. **MEANWHILE,** arrange the asparagus, bell pepper, and onion pieces in a single layer on the baking sheets. Coat the vegetables with cooking spray and bake for 12 minutes, tossing once, until the vegetables are crisp-tender and very lightly browned.

4. **COMBINE** the basil, garlic, yogurt, oil, lemon zest, lemon juice, water, and salt in a blender or food processor, and process until smooth.

5. **ADD** the roasted vegetables and dressing to the pasta and toss well. Serve warm or at room temperature.

MAKE IT A MEAL

3 ounces grilled shrimp
80 CALORIES

2 meringue cookies
60 CALORIES

390
CALORIES PER MEAL
★ ★

MAKE IT A MEAL

3 ounces grilled chicken breast
140 CALORIES

390
CALORIES PER MEAL
★ ★

PER SERVING (1 serving = 1½ cups salad)

Calories	Total Fat	Saturated Fat	Sodium	Carbohydrate	Dietary Fiber	Protein	Calcium
250	8 g	1 g	250 mg	38 g	6 g	9 g	6%

FATTOUSH

PREP TIME: 30 MINUTES / **COOK TIME:** 10 MINUTES / **MAKES** 4 SERVINGS

Fattoush is Lebanese bread salad, made by combining toasted pita bread with lettuce, tomato, assorted vegetables, and, often, cheese. It makes a refreshing meal on a hot summer day. Za'atar is a Middle Eastern seasoning made with thyme, sesame seeds, sumac, and other ingredients, depending on the country of origin.

MAKE IT A MEAL

3 ounces grilled lamb loin kebabs
170 CALORIES

1 slice (2") angel food cake topped with ½ cup frozen, thawed unsweetened berries
100 CALORIES

410
CALORIES PER MEAL
★ ★

MAKE IT A MEAL

3 ounces grilled scallops
100 CALORIES

2 biscotti (⅔ ounce each)
180 CALORIES

420
CALORIES PER MEAL
★ ★

2	tablespoons olive oil
1	teaspoon finely chopped fresh thyme
1	large (6½") whole wheat pita, split horizontally
3	cups shredded romaine lettuce
2	medium tomatoes, cut into ½" cubes
½	medium green bell pepper, cut into ¼" dice
½	medium red bell pepper, cut into ¼" dice
½	cup chopped fresh parsley
½	cup crumbled feta cheese
¼	cup chopped red onion
¼	cup chopped fresh mint
¼	cup chopped fresh chives
2	tablespoons fresh lemon juice
1	clove garlic, minced
2	teaspoons za'atar
½	teaspoon salt
¼	teaspoon freshly ground black pepper

1. **PREHEAT** the oven to 350°F. Combine 1 tablespoon of the oil and the thyme in a small bowl. Brush the cut sides of the pita halves with the oil mixture. Place on a baking sheet and bake for 10 minutes, or until crisp.

2. **MEANWHILE,** combine the lettuce, tomatoes, bell pepper, parsley, cheese, onion, mint, and chives in a large bowl. Whisk together the lemon juice, garlic, za'atar, salt, black pepper, and remaining 1 tablespoon oil in a small bowl. Pour the dressing over the salad and toss to combine.

3. **JUST** before serving, break the pita crisps into small pieces, add to the salad, and toss to combine.

PER SERVING (1 serving = 2 cups)

Calories	Total Fat	Saturated Fat	Sodium	Carbohydrate	Dietary Fiber	Protein	Calcium
140	8 g	1 g	390 mg	17 g	4 g	3 g	6%

ROASTED ASPARAGUS WITH LEMON ZEST

PREP TIME: 5 MINUTES / **COOK TIME:** 10 MINUTES / **MAKES** 4 SERVINGS

Roasting brings out sweet undertones in asparagus, a spring vegetable now available year-round. This recipe also works well with green beans.

1½	pounds asparagus
1	tablespoon extra-virgin olive oil
¼	teaspoon salt
⅛	teaspoon freshly ground black pepper
2	teaspoons grated lemon zest

1. PREHEAT the oven to 425°F. Coat a large baking sheet with cooking spray.

2. COMBINE the asparagus, oil, salt, and pepper in a large bowl and toss well to coat. Arrange on the baking sheet in a single layer and set in the center of the oven. Roast, shaking the pan occasionally, for 8 to 10 minutes, or until crisp-tender. Remove from the oven, sprinkle with the lemon zest, and stir to combine. Serve hot or at room temperature.

MAKE
IT A
MEAL

3 ounces cooked
filet mignon
190 CALORIES

⅔ cup roasted
small red potatoes
cooked with ½
teaspoon olive oil
110 CALORIES

1 cup strawberries
50 CALORIES

420
CALORIES
PER MEAL
★ ★

MAKE
IT A
MEAL

3 ounces
cooked boneless
pork chop
200 CALORIES

½ cup cooked
egg noodles
110 CALORIES

380
CALORIES
PER MEAL
★ ★

PER SERVING (1 serving = 1 cup)

Calories	Total Fat	Saturated Fat	Sodium	Carbohydrate	Dietary Fiber	Protein	Calcium
70	3.5 g	0.5 g	150 mg	7 g	4 g	4 g	4%

EASY TWICE-BAKED POTATOES

PREP TIME: 15 MINUTES + 15 MINUTES COOLING /
COOK TIME: 1 HOUR 25 MINUTES / **MAKES** 4 SERVINGS

A special potato side dish that's not difficult to prepare—and even easier if you're starting with leftover baked potatoes (so bake some extras next time and keep them in the refrigerator ready for this recipe)!

2 medium (7 ounces each) russet (baking) potatoes, well scrubbed
1 tablespoon unsalted butter
⅓ cup low-fat milk
1 scallion, chopped
¼ cup grated Parmesan cheese
¼ teaspoon Italian seasoning
⅛ teaspoon garlic salt

1. **PREHEAT** the oven to 400°F. Prick the potatoes in several places and bake for 1 hour, or until fork-tender. Remove the potatoes from the oven and reduce the oven temperature to 350°F.

2. **LET** the potatoes cool in the refrigerator for 15 minutes. Halve the cooled potatoes lengthwise. Carefully scoop out the potato flesh from each half (a grapefruit spoon works well for this job), leaving enough to form a potato "shell." Set the shells aside on a baking sheet.

3. **COMBINE** the potato flesh, butter, milk, scallion, cheese, Italian seasoning, and garlic salt in a medium bowl and mix to blend. Scoop the mixture into the potato shells. Bake the stuffed potatoes for 25 minutes, or until heated through and golden brown.

PER SERVING (1 serving = 1 potato half)

Calories	Total Fat	Saturated Fat	Sodium	Carbohydrate	Dietary Fiber	Protein	Calcium
150	4.5 g	2.5 g	130 mg	23 g	2 g	5 g	10%

INDIAN-STYLE POTATO PANCAKES

PREP TIME: 15 MINUTES / **COOK TIME:** 1 HOUR / **MAKES** 4 SERVINGS

This recipe was inspired by a friend of Mindy's who brought Indian potato pancakes to a holiday celebration. Precooking and mashing the potatoes gives the inside of the pancakes a creamy texture.

4	medium Yukon gold potatoes (about 1½ pounds), peeled and cut into 1" cubes
1	large egg
1	medium yellow onion, grated
¼	cup chopped fresh cilantro
2	teaspoons curry powder
2	teaspoons mustard seeds
½	teaspoon salt
¼	teaspoon freshly ground black pepper
4	teaspoons olive oil

1. COMBINE the potatoes in a medium saucepan with water to cover. Bring to a gentle boil over medium heat and cook for 20 minutes, or until tender. Drain and place in a large bowl. Mash with a potato masher until mostly smooth but still slightly chunky. (You may prefer to pulse briefly in a food processor; be careful not to overprocess.)

2. ADD the egg, onion, cilantro, curry powder, mustard seeds, salt, and pepper to the potatoes and stir well. Form the potato mixture into 16 patties using a scant ¼ cup for each.

3. SET the oven on warm. Coat a large skillet with cooking spray or use a nonstick skillet. Cooking in batches, heat 1 teaspoon of the oil over medium heat until shimmering. Add 4 pancakes and cook for 5 minutes per side. Place on a baking sheet in the oven to keep warm. Repeat with the remaining oil and pancakes.

PER SERVING (1 serving = 4 pancakes)

Calories	Total Fat	Saturated Fat	Sodium	Carbohydrate	Dietary Fiber	Protein	Calcium
220	7 g	1 g	320 mg	37 g	4 g	5 g	4%

MAKE IT A MEAL

3 ounces lean braised brisket
170 CALORIES

½ cup steamed broccoli
25 CALORIES

415
CALORIES
PER MEAL
★ ★ ★

MAKE IT A MEAL

3 ounces baked trout
110 CALORIES

⅓ cup fat-free (0%) plain Greek yogurt
40 CALORIES

½ cup unsweetened applesauce
50 CALORIES

420
CALORIES
PER MEAL
★ ★

ARUGULA-PARMESAN SALAD WITH ROSEMARY AND KALAMATA FLATBREAD

PREP TIME: 25 MINUTES + 1 HOUR RISING / **COOK TIME:** 15 MINUTES / **MAKES** 4 SERVINGS

Olive-studded flatbread is served alongside a lemony arugula salad—restaurant good, but homemade! For authentic flavor, get Parmigiano Reggiano, the gold standard for Parmesan cheeses. The salad would be equally delicious with baby spinach, watercress, baby lettuce, or a mesclun mix.

DRESSING

2	tablespoons extra-virgin olive oil
½	teaspoon grated lemon zest
2	tablespoons fresh lemon juice
1	tablespoon mild honey
1	tablespoon water
⅛	teaspoon coarse salt

FLATBREAD

1	tablespoon olive oil
1	teaspoon active dry yeast
⅔	cup warm water (about 115°F)
1⅓	cups bread flour
½	teaspoon coarse salt
1	teaspoon fresh rosemary or ½ teaspoon dried
10	pitted kalamata olives (about ⅓ cup), quartered lengthwise

1. TO MAKE THE DRESSING: Combine the oil, lemon zest, lemon juice, honey, water, and salt in a small bowl and whisk until smooth. Set aside.

2. TO MAKE THE FLATBREAD: Place the oil in a small bowl. Use a small amount of the oil to grease a 9" pie plate.

3. SPRINKLE the yeast over the warm water in a medium bowl and let sit until dissolved. Add the flour and ¼ teaspoon of the salt. Stir until the dough comes together. Knead the dough until it forms a ball, about 1 minute. Dip your fingertips into the bowl of oil and press the dough into the pie plate. Set the remaining oil aside. Sprinkle the rosemary over the dough. Press the olives into the dough and sprinkle the remaining ¼ teaspoon salt on top. Cover the dough with a clean linen towel or plastic wrap. Let rise for 1 hour or until doubled in size.

MAKE IT A MEAL

1 cup cantaloupe cubes
50 CALORIES

420
CALORIES PER MEAL
★ ★

MAKE IT A MEAL

1 tablespoon mini chocolate chips
50 CALORIES

420
CALORIES PER MEAL
★ ★

PER SERVING (1 serving = 1¼ cups salad, 2 wedges flatbread)

Calories	Total Fat	Saturated Fat	Sodium	Carbohydrate	Dietary Fiber	Protein	Calcium
370	17 g	4 g	690 mg	41 g	2 g	12 g	20%

SALAD

- 5 cups arugula
- ¼ cup thinly sliced red onion
- 2 ounces Parmesan cheese, cut into shavings with a vegetable peeler

  Freshly ground black pepper (optional)

4. PREHEAT the oven to 400°F. Press your fingers into the dough to make several indentations. Drizzle the remaining oil over the dough. Bake for 15 minutes, or until the bottom crust is crispy. Let cool slightly, then cut into 8 wedges and set aside.

5. TO ASSEMBLE THE SALAD: Toss the arugula and dressing in a medium bowl. Divide the arugula among 4 plates. Top each salad with onion and Parmesan shavings. Garnish each plate with 2 flatbread wedges. Serve with freshly ground pepper, if desired.

FRESH CORN, TOMATO, AND RED ONION SALAD

PREP TIME: 10 MINUTES / **MAKES** 4 SERVINGS

A recipe for the height of the fresh corn season, this scrumptious salad is a nice change of pace from green salads and coleslaw.

2	medium ears corn, husk and silk removed
1	pint grape tomatoes, halved
¼	medium red onion, thinly sliced
⅓	cup fresh basil leaves
1	tablespoon balsamic vinegar
2	teaspoons extra-virgin olive oil
¼	teaspoon coarse salt
⅛	teaspoon freshly ground black pepper

1. HOLDING the tops of the ears of corn over a cutting board, carefully cut the kernels off in strips from top to bottom. Add the tomatoes, onion, and basil, and stir to combine.

2. ADD the vinegar, oil, salt, and pepper to the vegetables and stir again. Serve immediately or refrigerate for up to 4 hours.

MAKE IT A MEAL

3 ounces grilled flank steak
170 CALORIES

½ cup frozen yogurt
100 CALORIES

½ cup fresh fruit salad
50 CALORIES

420 CALORIES PER MEAL
★ ★ ★

MAKE IT A MEAL

3 ounces grilled salmon
180 CALORIES

½ cup frozen yogurt
100 CALORIES

½ cup fresh pineapple chunks
40 CALORIES

420 CALORIES PER MEAL
★ ★ ★

PER SERVING (1 serving = ¾ cup)

Calories	Total Fat	Saturated Fat	Sodium	Carbohydrate	Dietary Fiber	Protein	Calcium
100	3.5 g	0 g	135 mg	17 g	3 g	3g	2%

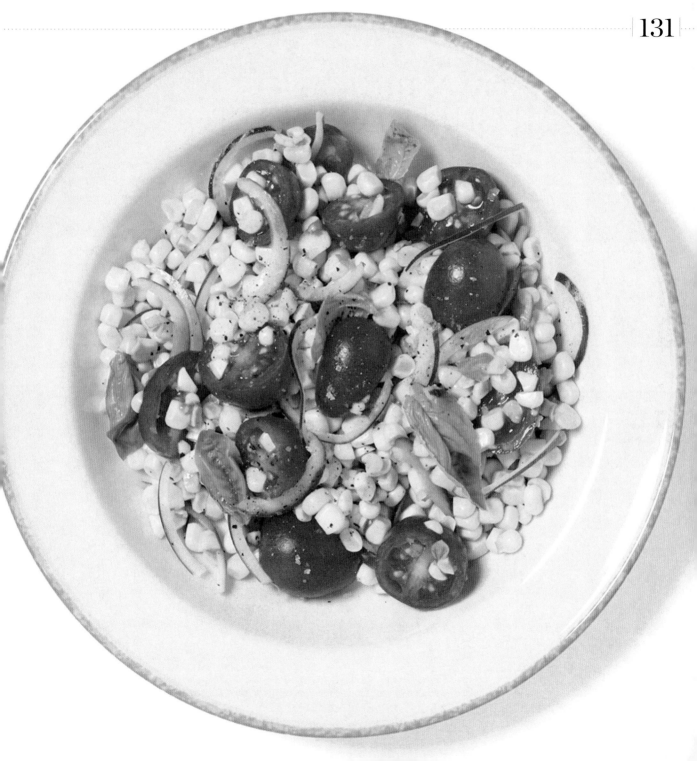

BROWN RICE AND MUSHROOM RISOTTO

PREP TIME: 50 MINUTES / **COOK TIME:** 50 MINUTES / **MAKES** 4 SERVINGS

Creamy rice is blended with a mushroom sauté to deliver a risotto that would please your Italian grandmother. Par-cooking the rice in the microwave saves time stirring at the stove. Yes, risotto requires a lot of stirring, but the end result is so worth it.

MAKE
IT A
MEAL

1 medium (3¾ ounces) chicken drumstick, roasted and skin removed
80 CALORIES

1 cup steamed broccoli
50 CALORIES

400
**CALORIES
PER MEAL**
★ ★ ★

MAKE
IT A
MEAL

3 ounces baked halibut fillet
120 CALORIES

390
**CALORIES
PER MEAL**
★

1	teaspoon olive oil
1	package (8 ounces) sliced white mushrooms
1	package (8 ounces) sliced cremini (brown) mushrooms
½	teaspoon coarse salt
1	cup medium- or short-grain brown rice
1	teaspoon butter
1	shallot, finely chopped
⅛	teaspoon freshly ground black pepper
2	tablespoons dry white wine
3½	cups fat-free, reduced-sodium chicken or vegetable broth
2	tablespoons light cream cheese
2	tablespoons grated Parmesan cheese
2	tablespoons thinly sliced fresh chives

1. HEAT the oil in a large nonstick skillet over medium heat. Add the mushrooms and ¼ teaspoon of the salt. Cook for 15 to 18 minutes, stirring often, until the mushrooms have given off all their liquid and are beginning to brown. Remove from the heat and set aside.

2. MEANWHILE, combine the rice and 2 cups of water in a microwaveable bowl. Microwave on high for 10 minutes. Drain.

3. MELT the butter in a large saucepan over low heat. Add the shallot, pepper, and remaining ¼ teaspoon salt. Cook for 5 minutes, stirring often, until the shallot begins to soften. Add the drained rice and stir well to coat with the seasonings. Increase the heat to medium-high and add the wine. Cook and stir until the wine evaporates.

4. ADD the broth, ½ cup at a time. With each addition of broth, cook and stir until almost all of the broth is absorbed. The rice is done when it becomes tender and the mixture is a bit creamy.

5. STIR in the sautéed mushrooms and cook for 1 minute to heat through. Remove from the heat and stir in the cream cheese and Parmesan until blended. Garnish each serving with a sprinkling of the chives.

PER SERVING (1 serving = ¾ cup)

Calories	Total Fat	Saturated Fat	Sodium	Carbohydrate	Dietary Fiber	Protein	Calcium
270	6 g	2.5 g	720 mg	43 g	3 g	9 g	6%

TRICOLOR RICE PILAF

PREP TIME: 10 MINUTES / **COOK TIME:** 1 HOUR 5 MINUTES / **MAKES** 4 SERVINGS

We used a packaged blend of three different rices—brown, red, and wild—in this hearty side dish. To keep sodium under control and for the best flavor in this recipe, choose brands that do not have added seasonings.

1	cup whole grain rice blend
1½	teaspoons olive oil
1	medium onion, finely chopped
½	small red bell pepper, finely chopped
4	medium cremini (brown) mushrooms, sliced
1	clove garlic, finely chopped
2	cups low-sodium vegetable broth
½	teaspoon dried basil
½	teaspoon salt
½	teaspoon freshly ground black pepper
½	cup frozen peas, thawed

1. **PLACE** the rice blend in a medium saucepan and cook over medium heat for 5 minutes or until lightly toasted. Transfer to a heatproof bowl.

2. **HEAT** the oil in the pan over medium-low heat. Add the onion, bell pepper, mushrooms, and garlic. Cook for 10 minutes, stirring frequently, until the vegetables have released their liquid and begun to brown.

3. **STIR** in the toasted rice, broth, basil, salt, and black pepper. Reduce to a simmer, cover, and cook for 50 minutes, or until the rice is tender.

MAKE IT A MEAL

3 ounces roast pork tenderloin
120 CALORIES

1 cup watermelon cubes
50 CALORIES

380 CALORIES PER MEAL
★ ★

MAKE IT A MEAL

3 ounces pan-roasted catfish
130 CALORIES

1 cup shredded collard greens sautéed in 1 teaspoon olive oil
50 CALORIES

390 CALORIES PER MEAL
★ ★ ★

PER SERVING (1 serving = 1 cup)

Calories	Total Fat	Saturated Fat	Sodium	Carbohydrate	Dietary Fiber	Protein	Calcium
210	3.5 g	0 g	380 mg	43 g	5 g	6 g	2%

OVEN-BAKED FRIES

PREP TIME: 10 MINUTES / **COOK TIME:** 45 MINUTES / **MAKES** 4 SERVINGS

A Yukon gold potato has a creamier texture than a baking potato and its flesh holds its color after cutting. Light mayonnaise gives a crispier crust than low-fat mayo because it is slightly higher in fat.

MAKE IT A MEAL

3 ounces grilled chicken breast brushed with 1 tablespoon barbecue sauce
170 CALORIES

¼ cup sweet-and-sour red cabbage
40 CALORIES

410 CALORIES PER MEAL
★ ★

MAKE IT A MEAL

2 ounces sliced meat loaf served with 1 tablespoon ketchup
135 CALORIES

1 cup steamed carrots
50 CALORIES

385 CALORIES PER MEAL
★ ★

2   tablespoons light mayonnaise

1   teaspoon olive oil

⅔   cup panko bread crumbs

1   tablespoon salt-free fajita seasoning (such as Spice Hunter) or salt-free garlic-and-herb seasoning (such as McCormick's)

½   teaspoon salt

4   medium (6 ounces each) Yukon gold potatoes

1. **PREHEAT** the oven to 400°F. Coat a regular baking sheet with cooking spray or line with a nonstick liner (or use a nonstick baking sheet).

2. **WHISK** together the mayonnaise and oil. Combine the panko crumbs, seasoning, and salt on a small plate.

3. **CUT** each potato into 8 wedges. Brush all sides of the potato wedges with the mayonnaise mixture. Dip the wedges in the crumb mixture to cover each side. Place the wedges on the baking sheet.

4. **BAKE** for 45 minutes, or until the potatoes are crisp and lightly browned.

PER SERVING (1 serving = 8 wedges)

Calories	Total Fat	Saturated Fat	Sodium	Carbohydrate	Dietary Fiber	Protein	Calcium
200	4 g	0.5 g	380 mg	37 g	4 g	5 g	2%

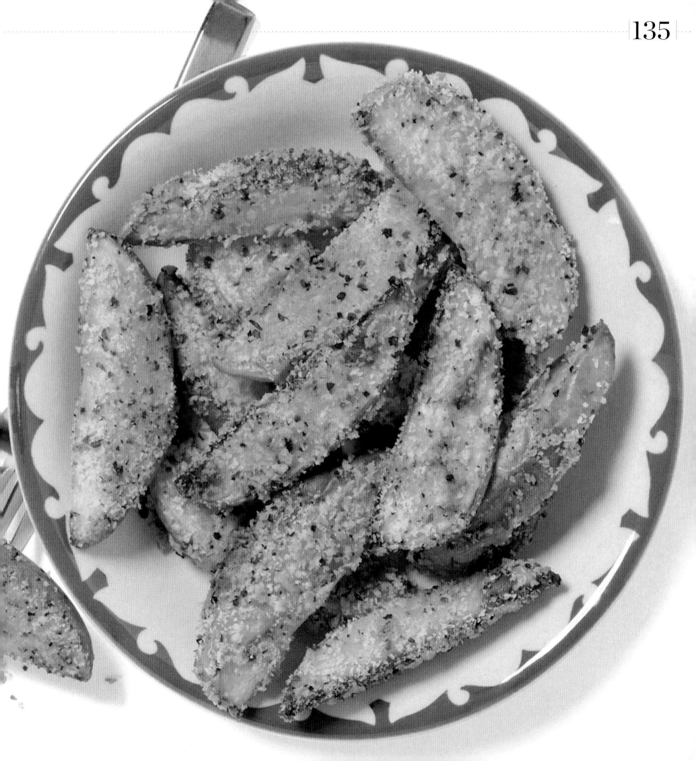

CONFETTI COUSCOUS

PREP TIME: 20 MINUTES + 10 MINUTES COOLING / **COOK TIME:** 10 MINUTES / **MAKES** 4 SERVINGS

This side dish is colorful and festive enough to serve at a holiday meal. Feel free to use different combinations of dried fruit, including jumbo raisins, dried cherries, and dried plums.

MAKE IT A MEAL

3 ounces grilled chicken breast, sprinkled with lemon juice and oregano
140 CALORIES

420
CALORIES
PER MEAL
★ ★

MAKE IT A MEAL

2 ounces grilled flank steak
110 CALORIES

390
CALORIES
PER MEAL
★ ★

2	cups low-sodium chicken or vegetable broth
1	cup whole wheat couscous
2	tablespoons golden raisins
2	teaspoons ground cumin
½	teaspoon salt
¼	cup slivered almonds
¼	cup finely diced red bell pepper
2	tablespoons dried cranberries
¼	cup thinly sliced scallion
¼	cup finely chopped dried apricots
3	tablespoons chopped fresh mint
2	tablespoons olive oil
1	tablespoon fresh lemon juice
1	tablespoon minced fresh ginger
1	clove garlic, minced

1. **BRING** the broth to a gentle boil in a medium saucepan over medium heat. Stir in the couscous, raisins, cumin, and salt. Cover and remove from the heat. Let stand until the couscous is soft, about 5 minutes. Uncover, fluff with a fork, and let cool for 10 minutes.

2. **MEANWHILE,** place the almonds in a skillet and cook over medium heat, shaking the pan often, for 3 to 5 minutes, or until lightly toasted.

3. **GENTLY** stir the toasted almonds, bell pepper, cranberries, scallions, apricots, mint, oil, lemon juice, ginger, and garlic into the couscous.

PER SERVING (1 serving = 1 cup)

Calories	Total Fat	Saturated Fat	Sodium	Carbohydrate	Dietary Fiber	Protein	Calcium
280	11 g	1.5 g	370 mg	39 g	6 g	8 g	6%

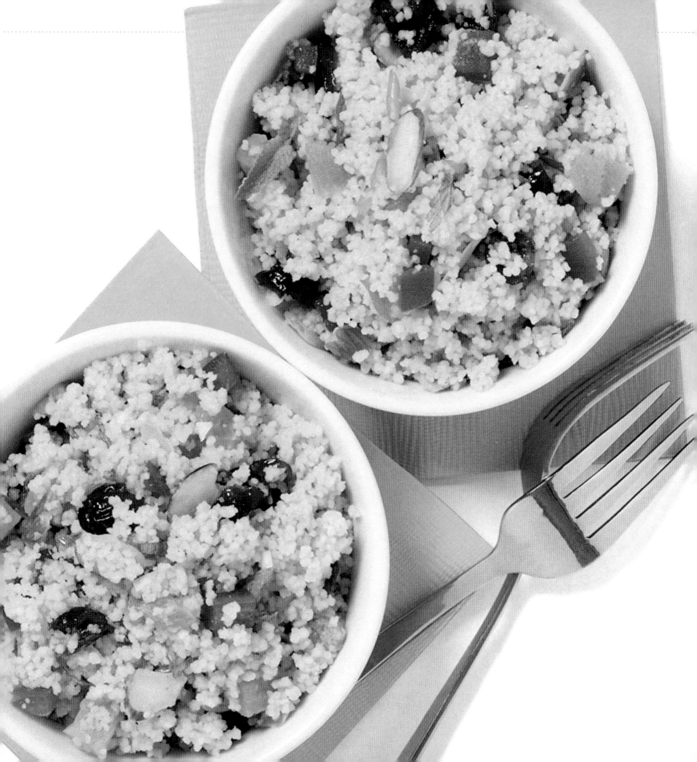

PASTA WITH ZUCCHINI RIBBONS AND SUN-DRIED TOMATO PESTO

PREP TIME: 20 MINUTES / **COOK TIME:** 12 MINUTES / **MAKES** 6 SERVINGS

Zucchini is one of those vegetables with year-round appeal, and swirling it with spaghetti and a chunky sun-dried tomato pesto will guarantee that this dinner will be requested again. Making thin ribbons of zucchini instead of half-moon slices gives zucchini a whole new look.

PESTO

- 1 cup low-sodium vegetable broth
- ½ cup dry-pack sun-dried tomatoes
- 1 tablespoon pine nuts
- 2 teaspoons balsamic vinegar
- 2 teaspoons extra-virgin olive oil
- ¼ cup fresh basil leaves
- ¼ cup fresh flat-leaf parsley leaves
- ⅓ cup crumbled reduced-fat feta cheese

1. TO MAKE THE PESTO: Heat the broth in a microwaveable dish for 1 minute. Place the sun-dried tomatoes in a food processor and process until chopped. Add the warm broth, pine nuts, vinegar, and oil. Pulse on and off 5 or 6 times, then process until evenly blended (do not puree), about 10 seconds. Add the basil and parsley. Process until chopped and blended, about 5 seconds. Add the cheese and pulse to blend. Set the pesto aside.

2. TO MAKE THE PASTA: Bring a large pot of water to a boil over high heat. Add the spaghetti and cook according to package directions. Drain and return to the pot.

3. MEANWHILE, use a vegetable peeler to cut long strips off the zucchini until the seeds begin to show. Discard the seedy centers. You should have about 5 cups of zucchini ribbons.

MAKE IT A MEAL

3 ounces baked fillet of sole
100 CALORIES

1 small (1 ounce) whole wheat roll dipped in ½ teaspoon olive oil
100 CALORIES

420
CALORIES
PER MEAL
★ ★

MAKE IT A MEAL

3 ounces grilled chicken-mushroom sausage
130 CALORIES

1 cup honeydew melon cubes
60 CALORIES

410
CALORIES
PER MEAL
★ ★ ★

PER SERVING (1 serving = 1½ cups)

Calories	Total Fat	Saturated Fat	Sodium	Carbohydrate	Dietary Fiber	Protein	Calcium
220	5 g	1 g	400 mg	38 g	7 g	9 g	8%

PASTA

8	ounces whole wheat spaghetti
3	small zucchini
1	teaspoon olive oil
1	leek (white and light green parts), well washed, halved lengthwise, and thinly sliced crosswise (about 1½ cups)
3	cloves garlic, minced
½	teaspoon coarse salt
½	teaspoon freshly ground black pepper

4. HEAT the oil in a large nonstick skillet over medium heat. Add the leek, garlic, salt, and pepper. Cook, stirring, for 3 minutes, or until the leek softens. Add the zucchini ribbons and stir to coat with the seasonings. Cook for 3 minutes, or until the zucchini softens slightly. Add the pesto to the pan. Cook, stirring, for 1 minute to heat through.

5. ADD the zucchini mixture to the drained spaghetti and toss well. Serve hot or at room temperature.

BROCCOLI RABE WITH GARLIC AND OIL

PREP TIME: 5 MINUTES / **COOK TIME:** 8 MINUTES / **MAKES** 4 SERVINGS

Broccoli rabe has a sharp, slightly bitter flavor that is very different from common broccoli. Blanching the broccoli rabe before sautéeing helps the greens soften and maintain their vibrant color.

1	large bunch broccoli rabe (about 1½ pounds), woody stems discarded
1	tablespoon extra-virgin olive oil
6	cloves garlic, sliced
1	medium onion, sliced
⅛	teaspoon red-pepper flakes
1	tablespoon grated Parmesan cheese
¼	teaspoon salt

1. **BRING** a large pot of lightly salted water to a boil. Add the broccoli rabe, return to a boil, and cook for 2 minutes to blanch and set the color. Drain well.

2. **HEAT** the oil in a large nonstick skillet over medium-high heat. Add the garlic, onion, and pepper flakes, and cook 4 to 5 minutes, or until the onion is softened and the garlic starts to brown.

3. **ADD** the broccoli rabe, Parmesan, and salt, and cook, tossing, for 1 minute to heat through.

PER SERVING (1 serving = 1 cup)

Calories	Total Fat	Saturated Fat	Sodium	Carbohydrate	Dietary Fiber	Protein	Calcium
100	4 g	0.5 g	220 mg	12 g	1 g	7 g	10%

GREEN BEANS AMANDINE

PREP TIME: 10 MINUTES / **COOK TIME:** 10 MINUTES / **MAKES** 4 SERVINGS

Dress up your steamed beans once in a while! Simple and delicious.

1	pound green beans, cut into 2" lengths
1	tablespoon unsalted butter
¼	cup slivered almonds
⅛	teaspoon coarse salt
⅛	teaspoon freshly ground black pepper

1. BRING 1" of water to a boil in a medium saucepan over high heat. Add the beans, cover, and steam for 10 minutes, or until the beans are crisp-tender.

2. MEANWHILE, combine the butter and almonds in a small saucepan. Cook, stirring, over medium-low heat for 5 minutes, or until the almonds and butter are nicely browned. Remove from the heat.

3. DRAIN the beans and transfer to a serving dish. Season with the salt and pepper, then toss with the browned almonds and butter. Serve hot.

MAKE IT A MEAL

3 ounces poached salmon
180 CALORIES

⅔ cup cooked whole wheat couscous
120 CALORIES

400
CALORIES PER MEAL
★ ★ ★

MAKE IT A MEAL

3 ounces grilled London broil
170 CALORIES

1 small (4-ounce) baked potato
110 CALORIES

½ cup raspberries
30 CALORIES

410
CALORIES PER MEAL
★ ★ ★ ★

PER SERVING (1 serving = 1 cup)

Calories	Total Fat	Saturated Fat	Sodium	Carbohydrate	Dietary Fiber	Protein	Calcium
100	6 g	2 g	85 mg	10 g	5 g	4 g	6%

STIR-FRIED ASIAN CHOYS

PREP TIME: 15 MINUTES / **COOK TIME:** 15 MINUTES / **MAKES** 4 SERVINGS

Stir-fried Asian choys (vegetables) make a quick and tasty addition to any meal. Besides the familiar bok choy, look for choy sum (Chinese cabbage), gai lum (Chinese broccoli), and gai choy (Chinese mustard greens). A combination of choys makes for a flavorful and interesting side dish.

- 2 pounds Asian choys (vegetables), one type or a combination
- 2 teaspoons canola oil
- 2 cloves garlic, minced
- 1 teaspoon minced fresh ginger
- 1 tablespoon water
- 1 tablespoon sake (rice wine) or other dry white wine
- 2 teaspoons reduced-sodium soy sauce
- 1 teaspoon toasted sesame oil

1. **TRIM** and wash the choys. If using bok choy, separate the white stems from the green leaves. Cut the stems into ¼"-thick slices and keep separate. Chop the bok choy leaves and other vegetables.

2. **HEAT** the canola oil in a large nonstick skillet or wok over medium-high heat. Add the garlic and ginger, and cook, stirring, for 1 minute or until very fragrant.

3. **IF** using bok choy, add the stem slices and stir-fry for 3 minutes, or until crisp-tender. Add the water, sake, and soy sauce. When sizzling, add the other greens. Cook and stir until just wilted.

4. **DRIZZLE** the toasted sesame oil over the choys and toss until blended. Serve hot.

STIR-FRIED ASIAN CHOYS WITH BLACK BEAN SAUCE *(variation)*

REPLACE the water with 1 tablespoon black bean sauce.

OMIT the toasted sesame oil.

PER SERVING (1 serving = 1 cup) Stir-Fried Asian Choys with Black Bean Sauce (1 serving = 1 cup)

Calories	Total Fat	Saturated Fat	Sodium	Carbohydrate	Dietary Fiber	Protein	Calcium
70	4 g	0 g	350 mg	5 g	2 g	3 g	20%
60	3 g	0 g	380 mg	6 g	2 g	3 g	20%

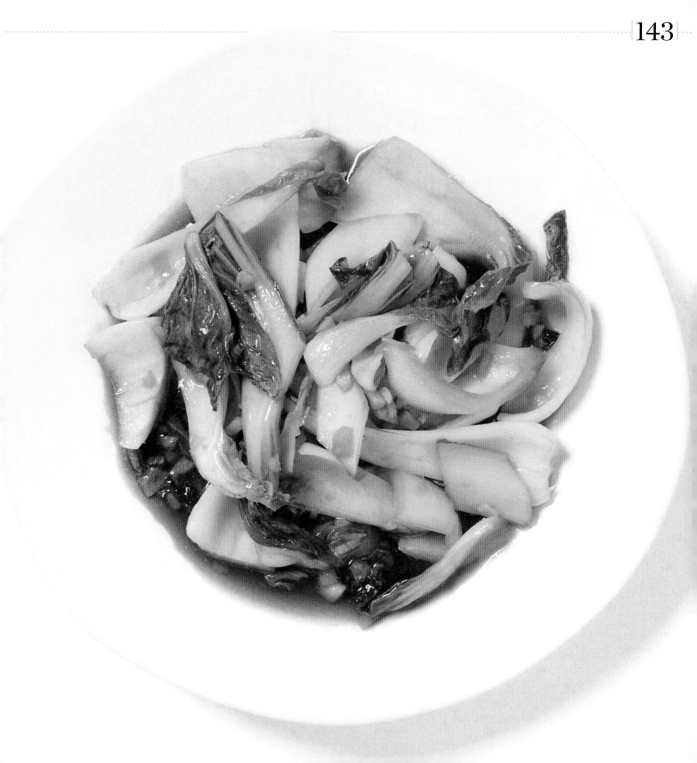

MAKE
IT A
MEAL

3 ounces roasted
lean leg of lamb
160 CALORIES

1 cup steamed
green beans
topped with
1 tablespoon
sliced almonds
70 CALORIES

1 small (4")
whole wheat pita
70 CALORIES

400
CALORIES
PER MEAL
★ ★ ★ ★

MAKE
IT A
MEAL

Salad made with
2 cups mixed baby
greens, ¼ cup
rinsed and drained
kidney beans,
¼ cup rinsed and
drained chickpeas,
1 tablespoon
chopped walnuts,
1 teaspoon olive
oil, 1½ teaspoons
balsamic vinegar
235 CALORIES

1 small (4")
whole wheat pita
70 CALORIES

405
CALORIES
PER MEAL
★ ★ ★

ROASTED TOMATOES STUFFED WITH QUINOA AND HERBS

PREP TIME: 20 MINUTES / **COOK TIME:** 27 MINUTES / **MAKES** 4 SERVINGS

This impressive-looking side dish comes together quickly with just a little chopping. These gorgeous tomatoes can be served hot or made ahead and served at room temperature. And the recipe can easily be doubled for entertaining.

¼ cup quinoa, rinsed

⅔ cup low-sodium vegetable broth

4 tomatoes (about 1⅔ pounds)

⅛ teaspoon freshly ground black pepper

2 tablespoons crumbled reduced-fat feta cheese

2 tablespoons finely chopped fresh basil

2 tablespoons finely chopped fresh parsley

1 tablespoon finely chopped fresh mint

1 teaspoon extra-virgin olive oil

1 teaspoon fresh lemon juice

¼ teaspoon coarse salt

1. **PREHEAT** the oven to 400°F.

2. **COMBINE** the quinoa and broth in a small saucepan. Bring to a boil over medium-high heat and stir well. Reduce to a simmer, cover, and cook for 10 to 15 minutes, or until the quinoa is tender and the broth has been absorbed.

3. **MEANWHILE,** slice the top quarter off the tomatoes and set aside. Use a spoon to scoop out the seeds and pulp from the tomatoes, leaving a sturdy shell. Discard the seeds and pulp. Place the tomatoes in an 8" x 8" baking dish. Season with the pepper.

4. **COMBINE** the cheese, basil, parsley, mint, oil, lemon juice, and salt in a medium bowl. Cut around the stem on the reserved tomato tops and discard. Finely chop the tomato tops and add them to the filling.

5. **WHEN** the quinoa has finished cooking, stir it into the filling. Stuff each tomato shell with a generous ⅓ cup of filling. Bake the tomatoes for 12 minutes, or until warmed through.

PER SERVING (1 serving = 1 stuffed tomato)

Calories	Total Fat	Saturated Fat	Sodium	Carbohydrate	Dietary Fiber	Protein	Calcium
100	3 g	0.5 g	210 mg	15 g	3 g	4 g	4%

ROASTED ROOT VEGETABLES

PREP TIME: 10 MINUTES / **COOK TIME:** 1 HOUR 20 MINUTES / **MAKES** 4 SERVINGS

Braising the vegetables first in a covered baking dish means they can be roasted using very little oil. When shopping for gravy (suggested in the first Make It a Meal option), choose a brand that is lowest in sodium, or make your own and use just a touch of salt to bring out the flavor.

1 medium parsnip, peeled and cut into ½" pieces

1 medium carrot, cut into ½" pieces

1 medium Yukon gold potato, cut into ½" chunks

1 medium sweet potato, peeled and cut into ½" chunks

1 medium yellow onion, cut into 16 wedges

1 medium red onion, cut into 16 wedges

½ medium fennel bulb, cut into ½" slices

8 cloves garlic, peeled

1 tablespoon olive oil

1 teaspoon salt-free herb blend

¾ teaspoon salt

½ teaspoon freshly ground black pepper

½ cup low-sodium vegetable broth

1. PREHEAT the oven to 425°F. Spray a deep 13" x 9" baking dish with cooking spray.

2. COMBINE the parsnip, carrot, potato, sweet potato, yellow onion, red onion, fennel, and garlic in a large bowl. Drizzle with the oil. Sprinkle with the herb blend, salt, and pepper. Mix to distribute the oil and seasonings.

3. TRANSFER the vegetables to the baking dish and pour in the broth. Cover the pan with foil. Bake for 30 minutes. Uncover and stir the vegetables. Bake uncovered for 50 minutes or until the vegetables are soft and lightly browned.

PER SERVING (1 serving = 1½ cups)

Calories	Total Fat	Saturated Fat	Sodium	Carbohydrate	Dietary Fiber	Protein	Calcium
170	4 g	0.5 g	580 mg	32 g	6 g	3 g	8%

MAKE IT A MEAL

3 ounces roast turkey breast with ¼ cup turkey gravy
140 CALORIES

1 small baked apple stuffed with 1 teaspoon chopped walnuts and 1 teaspoon golden raisins
105 CALORIES

415
CALORIES PER MEAL
★ ★ ★

MAKE IT A MEAL

4 ounces packaged seasoned firm tofu (any flavor)
130 CALORIES

1 small baked apple stuffed with 1 teaspoon chopped walnuts and 1 teaspoon golden raisins
105 CALORIES

405
CALORIES PER MEAL
★ ★ ★

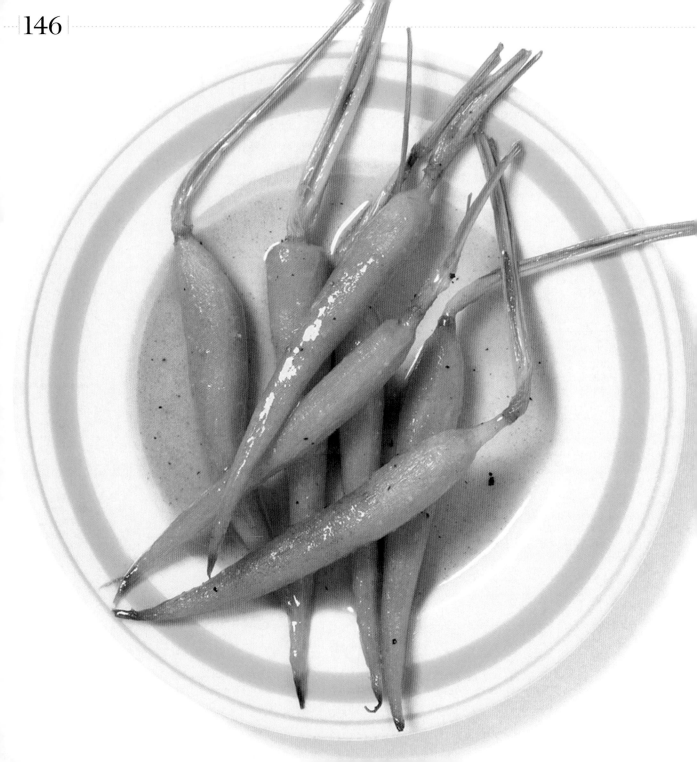

ORANGE AND HONEY–GLAZED CARROTS

PREP TIME: 5 MINUTES / **COOK TIME:** 40 MINUTES / **MAKES** 4 SERVINGS

Baby cut carrots, created from larger carrots, are a rich source of the antioxidant beta-carotene. To substitute full-size carrots, peel and cut into rounds or matchsticks.

1	pound baby carrots
1	cup water
⅔	cup orange juice
3	tablespoons honey
2	tablespoons unsalted butter, cut into bits
½	teaspoon salt
⅛	teaspoon freshly ground black pepper

COMBINE the carrots, water, orange juice, honey, butter, salt, and pepper in a large nonstick skillet. Bring the mixture to a boil over medium-high heat, reduce to a simmer, and cook for 38 to 40 minutes, stirring occasionally, until the carrots are tender and the liquid has reduced to a syrup.

MAKE IT A MEAL

3 ounces cooked turkey cutlet
110 CALORIES

½ cup wild rice/ brown rice pilaf
140 CALORIES

420
CALORIES PER MEAL
★

MAKE IT A MEAL

3 ounces roasted pork loin
120 CALORIES

1 small (4-ounce) baked potato
110 CALORIES

400
CALORIES PER MEAL
★

PER SERVING (1 serving = ½ cup)

Calories	Total Fat	Saturated Fat	Sodium	Carbohydrate	Dietary Fiber	Protein	Calcium
170	6 g	3.5 g	350 mg	29 g	3 g	2 g	4%

7

VEGETARIAN

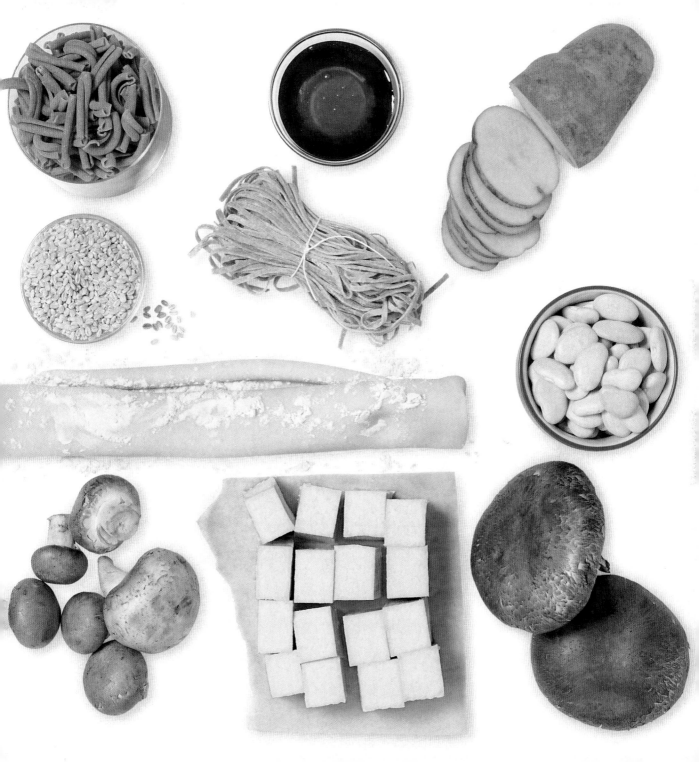

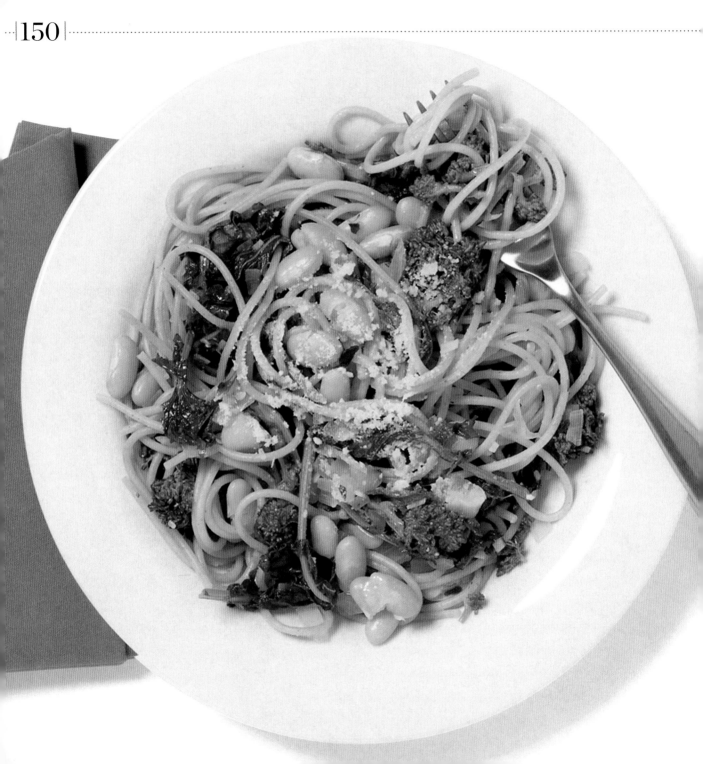

SPAGHETTI WITH BROCCOLI RABE AND WHITE BEANS

PREP TIME: 30 MINUTES / **COOK TIME:** 20 MINUTES / **MAKES** 4 SERVINGS

Broccoli rabe, also called rapini, is a bitter Italian green. If you're not a fan, substitute an equal amount of kale or broccolini. If you're a fan of spicy food, add more red-pepper flakes than the ¼ teaspoon called for here.

8	ounces whole wheat spaghetti
1	tablespoon extra-virgin olive oil
1	onion, chopped
4	cloves garlic, minced
½	teaspoon coarse salt
¼	teaspoon red-pepper flakes
1	bunch (1¼ pounds) broccoli rabe, tough ends trimmed, coarsely chopped
1½	cups low-sodium vegetable broth
1	can (15.5 ounces) cannellini beans, rinsed and drained
2	teaspoons balsamic vinegar
2	tablespoons + ¼ cup grated Romano cheese

1. BRING a large pot of water to a boil over high heat. Add the spaghetti and cook according to package directions. Drain the spaghetti and return to the cooking pot.

2. MEANWHILE, heat the oil in a large nonstick skillet over medium heat. Add the onion, garlic, salt, and pepper flakes. Cook for 2 minutes, stirring, until the onion begins to soften.

3. STIR in the broccoli rabe and broth. Cover and cook, stirring occasionally, for 6 to 10 minutes, or until the broccoli rabe has darkened in color. Stir in the beans and vinegar, and cook to heat through.

4. POUR the broccoli rabe mixture over the cooked spaghetti, and toss to combine. Stir in 2 tablespoons of the cheese and toss well. Garnish each portion with 1 tablespoon of the remaining cheese.

MAKE IT A MEAL

5 tomato slices (about ¼" thick) drizzled with ½ teaspoon olive oil
40 CALORIES

410 CALORIES PER MEAL
★ ★

MAKE IT A MEAL

5 asparagus spears drizzled with ½ teaspoon olive oil and roasted
40 CALORIES

410 CALORIES PER MEAL
★ ★ ★

PER SERVING (1 serving = 1¾ cups)

Calories	Total Fat	Saturated Fat	Sodium	Carbohydrate	Dietary Fiber	Protein	Calcium
370	6 g	2 g	510 mg	64 g	11 g	18 g	20%

PASTA WITH CHEESY PESTO SAUCE

PREP TIME: 30 MINUTES / **COOK TIME:** 30 MINUTES / **MAKES** 4 SERVINGS

A quick meal that takes advantage of summer's bountiful vegetables, penne is tossed with a creamy ricotta pesto sauce and finished with fresh tomatoes and Parmesan.

8   ounces whole wheat penne pasta

2   cups fresh basil leaves

2   tablespoons pine nuts

2   teaspoons minced garlic

4   tablespoons fat-free, reduced-sodium vegetable broth

½   teaspoon coarse salt

¼   teaspoon freshly ground black pepper

½   cup fat-free ricotta cheese

2   teaspoons extra-virgin olive oil

1   leek, white part only, well washed, halved lengthwise, and thinly sliced

2   small zucchini (8 ounces each), halved lengthwise and cut crosswise into ½"-thick slices

1   can (14 ounces) water-packed artichoke heart quarters, drained and rinsed

1   cup grape tomatoes, halved

4   teaspoons grated Parmesan cheese

1. BRING a large pot of water to a boil. Add the penne and cook according to package directions. Drain and return to the pot.

2. MEANWHILE, combine the basil, pine nuts, ½ teaspoon of the garlic, 3 tablespoons of the broth, the salt, and pepper to a blender or food processor. Process until smooth. Add the ricotta and blend or process. Set aside.

3. HEAT the oil in a large nonstick skillet over medium heat. Add the leek and the remaining 1½ teaspoons garlic and cook, stirring, for 1 minute or until fragrant. Add the zucchini and the remaining 1 tablespoon broth and cook, stirring, for 5 minutes, or until the zucchini is crisp-tender.

4. STIR the ricotta mixture and artichoke hearts into the vegetables, and cook for 2 minutes, or until the sauce is simmering. Pour the vegetable and sauce mixture over the pasta and toss well. Garnish each serving with one-fourth of the tomatoes and 1 teaspoon of Parmesan.

PER SERVING (1 serving = 2 cups, ¼ cup tomatoes, 1 teaspoon Parmesan)

Calories	Total Fat	Saturated Fat	Sodium	Carbohydrate	Dietary Fiber	Protein	Calcium
390	8 g	1 g	850 mg	65 g	11 g	17 g	15%

GNOCCHI WITH GARLIC, OIL, AND ROMANO CHEESE

PREP TIME: 5 MINUTES / **COOK TIME:** 10 MINUTES / **MAKES** 4 SERVINGS

You can make your own gnocchi, but it's much easier to buy them ready-made and frozen, refrigerated, or in a shelf-stable pouch. They're delicious with a light garlic-shallot sauce alone, as in the first meal option, or combined with white beans and fresh diced tomatoes as in the second meal.

12	ounces frozen potato gnocchi
2	tablespoons extra-virgin olive oil
½	cup thinly sliced shallots
5	cloves garlic, thinly sliced
¼	cup chopped fresh basil
¼	cup grated Romano cheese
¼	teaspoon salt
¼	teaspoon freshly ground black pepper

1. BRING a large pot of water to a boil. Add the gnocchi and cook according to package directions. Reserve 3 tablespoons of the cooking water and drain.

2. HEAT the oil in a large nonstick skillet over medium-high heat. Add the shallots and garlic, and cook, stirring often, for 2 to 3 minutes, or until starting to brown. Add the gnocchi and cook, tossing, for 1 minute to heat through. Remove from the heat and stir in the basil, cheese, reserved cooking water, salt, and pepper. Serve hot.

MAKE IT A MEAL

Salad made with 2 cups arugula, 1 teaspoon olive oil, 1 teaspoon lemon juice **50 CALORIES**

½ cup Italian ice **60 CALORIES**

390 CALORIES PER MEAL
★ ★

MAKE IT A MEAL

Add ¼ cup chopped tomato and ¼ cup rinsed and drained cannellini beans to the gnocchi **60 CALORIES**

1 cup escarole sautéed in ½ teaspoon olive oil **30 CALORIES**

½ cup raspberries **30 CALORIES**

400 CALORIES PER MEAL
★ ★

PER SERVING (1 serving = ¾ cup)

Calories	Total Fat	Saturated Fat	Sodium	Carbohydrate	Dietary Fiber	Protein	Calcium
280	10 g	3 g	630 mg	40 g	2 g	8 g	10%

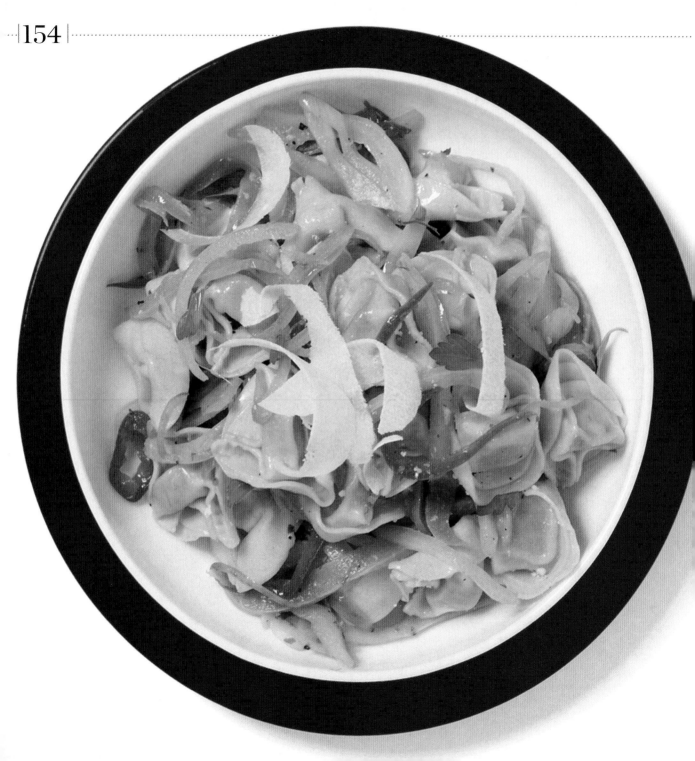

TORTELLINI WITH RED, YELLOW, AND ORANGE BELL PEPPERS

PREP TIME: 15 MINUTES / **COOK TIME:** 18 MINUTES / **MAKES** 4 SERVINGS

This colorful dish can be made with any combination of bell peppers, but be sure to include a red pepper for a healthy shot of beta-carotene. Spinach or tricolor tortellini add even more color.

8	ounces cheese tortellini
2	tablespoons extra-virgin olive oil
1	onion, thinly sliced
6	cloves garlic, sliced
1	teaspoon dried oregano
½	cup thinly sliced fennel
1	red bell pepper, thinly sliced
1	yellow bell pepper, thinly sliced
1	orange bell pepper, thinly sliced
¼	cup chopped fresh parsley
¼	cup grated Parmesan cheese
¼	teaspoon salt
¼	teaspoon freshly ground black pepper

1. BRING a large pot of water to a boil. Add the tortellini and cook according to package directions. Reserve ¼ cup of the cooking water and drain.

2. MEANWHILE, heat the oil in a large nonstick skillet over medium-high heat. Add the onion, garlic, and oregano, and cook, stirring occasionally, for 1 to 2 minutes, or until the onion and garlic start to soften. Stir in the fennel and cook for 1 minute. Add the bell peppers and cook, stirring occasionally, for 8 to 9 minutes, or until the peppers are softened and the onion begins to brown.

3. STIR in the tortellini and the reserved cooking water and cook for 1 minute to heat through. Remove the skillet from the heat and stir in the parsley, cheese, salt, and black pepper.

MAKE IT A MEAL

4 ounces white wine
100 CALORIES

410
CALORIES PER MEAL
★

MAKE IT A MEAL

1 biscotti (⅔ ounce)
90 CALORIES

400
CALORIES PER MEAL
★

PER SERVING (1 serving = 1½ cups)

Calories	Total Fat	Saturated Fat	Sodium	Carbohydrate	Dietary Fiber	Protein	Calcium
310	13 g	4 g	430 mg	38 g	4 g	11 g	20%

SPINACH LASAGNA ROLL-UPS

PREP TIME: 20 MINUTES + 5 MINUTES STANDING / **COOK TIME:** 55 MINUTES / **MAKES** 6 SERVINGS

All the flavors you love in spinach lasagna, but in a fun and easily portion-controlled roll-up.

6	lasagna noodles
1	package (10 ounces) frozen chopped spinach, thawed and squeezed dry
1	container (15 ounces) part-skim ricotta cheese
1	large egg
2	tablespoons grated Parmesan cheese
1	tablespoon Italian seasoning
¼	teaspoon garlic salt
1	tablespoon olive oil
½	medium onion, chopped
2	cloves garlic, minced
1	can (28 ounces) crushed tomatoes with Italian seasonings
½	cup water
¼	teaspoon salt
1	cup shredded part-skim mozzarella cheese

1. **PREHEAT** the oven to 350°F. Coat a 3"-deep 3-quart baking dish with cooking spray.

2. **BRING** a large pot of water to a boil. Add the lasagna noodles and cook according to package directions. Drain well.

3. **MEANWHILE,** combine the spinach, ricotta, egg, Parmesan, Italian seasoning, and garlic salt in a medium bowl and blend well.

4. **HEAT** the oil in a medium saucepan over medium heat. Add the onion and garlic, and cook, stirring occasionally, for 4 to 5 minutes, or until the onion has softened and is starting to brown. Stir in the tomatoes, water, and salt. Bring the mixture to a low boil, reduce to a simmer, and cook for 5 minutes to warm. Keep the tomato sauce warm while you roll up the noodles.

5. **WORKING** with one at a time, place a noodle on a cutting board. Scoop ½ cup of the spinach-ricotta mixture onto the noodle and spread it evenly with a small spatula. Roll up the noodle, patting in any filling that starts to squeeze out. Place the roll on its side (not end up) in the baking dish. Repeat with the remaining noodles and spinach-ricotta filling.

6. **POUR** the tomato sauce over the roll-ups. Cover the baking dish with a lid or foil. Bake for 45 minutes, or until the sauce is bubbling. Remove from the oven, uncover, and sprinkle with the mozzarella. Let stand for 5 minutes before serving.

PER SERVING (1 serving = 1 roll-up)

Calories	Total Fat	Saturated Fat	Sodium	Carbohydrate	Dietary Fiber	Protein	Calcium
380	13 g	6 g	730 mg	41 g	4 g	23 g	50%

MULTIMUSHROOM PIZZA

PREP TIME: 15 MINUTES / **COOK TIME:** 33 MINUTES / **MAKES** 6 SERVINGS

No need to limit yourself to the rather common button and cremini mushrooms in this dish: See what other interesting wild mushrooms your market may have.

1	tablespoon extra-virgin olive oil
8	ounces button mushrooms, sliced
8	ounces cremini (brown) mushrooms, sliced
1	medium onion, chopped
1	teaspoon dried oregano
¼	teaspoon salt
¼	teaspoon freshly ground black pepper
4	cloves garlic, minced
1	thin-crust Boboli pizza shell (10 ounces)
2	plum tomatoes, cut into 12 slices
½	cup shredded part-skim mozzarella cheese
⅓	cup grated Parmesan cheese

1 PREHEAT the oven to 400°F. Coat a baking sheet with cooking spray.

2. HEAT the oil in a large nonstick skillet over medium-high heat. Add the mushrooms, onion, oregano, salt, and pepper, and cook, stirring occasionally, for 9 to 10 minutes, or until starting to brown. Add the garlic and cook for 3 minutes, or until the mushrooms are browned. Remove from the heat.

3. PLACE the pizza shell on the baking sheet. Arrange the tomato slices over the shell in a single layer. Top with the mushroom mixture, mozzarella, and Parmesan. Bake for 17 to 20 minutes, until the crust is crisp and the cheese is melted and lightly browned. Remove from the oven and let cool briefly before cutting into 6 wedges.

PER SERVING (1 serving = 1 wedge)

Calories	Total Fat	Saturated Fat	Sodium	Carbohydrate	Dietary Fiber	Protein	Calcium
230	8 g	2.5 g	470 mg	29 g	5 g	13 g	20%

SPINACH MACARONI AND CHEESE

PREP TIME: 10 MINUTES + 5 MINUTES STANDING / **COOK TIME:** 40 MINUTES / **MAKES** 4 SERVINGS

Frozen butternut squash forms the base of this dish's cheesy sauce, sneaking in fiber, flavor, and extra nutrients.

MAKE IT A MEAL

Waldorf Salad:
½ cup chopped apple, 1 tablespoon diced celery, 2 teaspoons chopped walnuts, 2 tablespoons low-fat plain yogurt
80 CALORIES

410
CALORIES
PER MEAL
★ ★ ★ ★

MAKE IT A MEAL

1 slice (2") angel food cake
70 CALORIES

400
CALORIES
PER MEAL
★ ★

1⅓ cups whole grain elbow macaroni

1 package (12 ounces) frozen winter squash puree, thawed

1 cup reduced-fat (2%) evaporated milk

¼ cup shredded Monterey Jack cheese

⅔ cup shredded reduced-fat sharp Cheddar cheese

2 teaspoons brown mustard

½ teaspoon coarse salt

⅛ teaspoon freshly ground black pepper

¼ cup reduced-fat sour cream

1 package (10 ounces) frozen chopped spinach, thawed and squeezed dry

2 tablespoons panko bread crumbs

1. PREHEAT the oven to 350°F. Coat an 8" x 8" baking pan with cooking spray.

2. BRING a medium pot of water to a boil. Add the macaroni and cook according to the package directions. Drain and return to the cooking pot.

3. MEANWHILE, combine the squash puree and evaporated milk in a medium saucepan. Whisk until smooth and bring the mixture to a simmer over medium heat. Cook, stirring occasionally, for 6 minutes to thicken the mixture. Remove from the heat and stir in the Jack cheese, Cheddar, mustard, salt, and pepper. Mix until the cheeses are melted. Stir in the sour cream and spinach.

4. ADD the spinach-cheese mixture to the macaroni and mix well, breaking up any clumps of spinach. Transfer the macaroni mixture to the baking pan, spreading it evenly. Sprinkle with the panko crumbs. Bake for 15 to 20 minutes, or until crispy on top and bubbling. Let cool for 5 minutes before cutting into 4 squares.

PER SERVING (1 serving = one 4" x 4" square)

Calories	Total Fat	Saturated Fat	Sodium	Carbohydrate	Dietary Fiber	Protein	Calcium
330	10 g	5 g	580 mg	46 g	7 g	20 g	60%

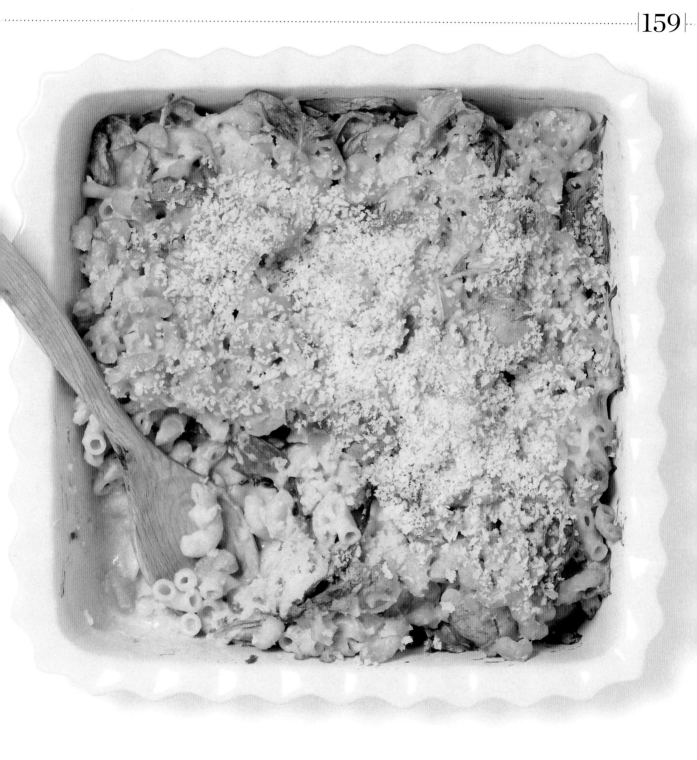

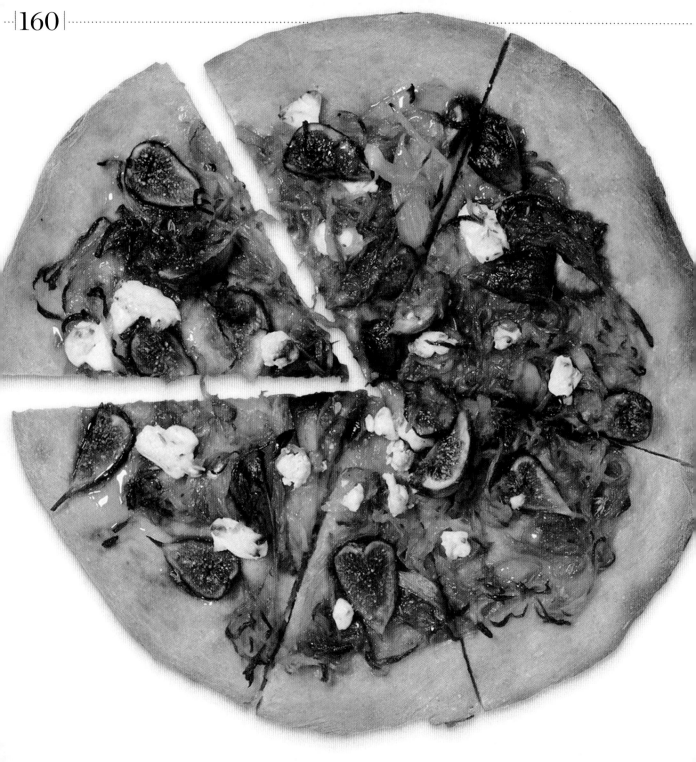

PIZZA WITH GOAT CHEESE, CARAMELIZED FIGS, AND ONIONS

PREP TIME: 15 MINUTES + 1 HOUR RISING / **COOK TIME:** 22 MINUTES / **MAKES** 6 SERVINGS

If you can find it, "00" Italian flour, sold at Italian and specialty stores and Web sites, gives the crust a chewy and authentic texture. The wheat germ makes the dough easier to roll out. To maintain freshness, store wheat germ in the refrigerator.

1	cup bread flour or "00" Italian flour
½	cup white whole wheat flour
¼	cup wheat germ
1½	teaspoons active dry yeast
1	teaspoon salt
¾	cup warm water
2½	teaspoons olive oil
1	large onion, thinly sliced
½	teaspoon sugar
4	fresh black figs, quartered
2	tablespoons balsamic vinegar
3	ounces soft goat cheese, crumbled
1½	tablespoons honey
¼	teaspoon dried thyme

1. COMBINE the flours, wheat germ, yeast, and salt in a bowl. Stir in the warm water and 1½ teaspoons of the oil. Knead for 5 minutes using the dough hook of a mixer until the dough is smooth and elastic, about 8 minutes. Place the dough in a bowl. Cover and allow to rise for 1 hour.

2. MEANWHILE, heat the remaining 1 teaspoon oil in a large nonstick skillet over medium-high heat. Add the onion and sugar, and cook, stirring occasionally, for 5 minutes, or until the onions are lightly browned. Reduce the heat to medium-low and add the figs and vinegar. Simmer for 2 minutes, or until the vinegar has almost evaporated. Set the onion-fig mixture aside.

3. PREHEAT the oven to 450°F. Pat the dough into a 14" circle and place on a large baking sheet. Distribute the onion-fig mixture evenly over the dough. Top with the goat cheese. Bake the crust for 15 minutes or until the cheese melts and the dough is lightly browned.

4. MEANWHILE, combine the honey and thyme in a small microwaveable bowl. Microwave for 15 seconds to make the honey liquid. Set aside, infusing the honey with thyme flavor.

5. REMOVE the pizza from the oven, drizzle with the honey-thyme mixture, and cut the pizza into 6 wedges.

PER SERVING (1 serving = one 7" wedge)

Calories	Total Fat	Saturated Fat	Sodium	Carbohydrate	Dietary Fiber	Protein	Calcium
260	6 g	2.5 g	440 mg	44 g	4 g	9 g	6%

MAKE IT A MEAL

2 cups broccoli rabe sautéed with 1 minced clove garlic and 1 teaspoon olive oil
60 CALORIES

½ cup frozen yogurt
100 CALORIES

420 CALORIES PER MEAL
★

MAKE IT A MEAL

Salad made with 2 cups arugula or lettuce, 1 teaspoon olive oil, 1½ teaspoons balsamic vinegar
55 CALORIES

One 100-calorie ice cream bar
100 CALORIES

415 CALORIES PER MEAL
★ ★

VEGETABLE LO MEIN

PREP TIME: 20 MINUTES / **COOK TIME:** 15 MINUTES / **MAKES** 4 SERVINGS

Shredded tofu and dry tofu are available at many Chinese markets. Although less flavorful and with a softer texture, firm tofu cut into thin strips or Japanese shirataki tofu noodles can be substituted.

1 cup low-sodium vegetable broth

3 tablespoons reduced-sodium soy sauce

2 tablespoons fresh lemon juice

1 tablespoon cornstarch

2 teaspoons honey

3 carrots, halved crosswise and cut lengthwise into thin strips

1 cup halved green beans

2 teaspoons peanut oil

3 cloves garlic, minced

1 piece (1") fresh ginger, minced

2 cups shredded savoy or napa cabbage

1 cup snow peas

3 scallions, cut into 1" pieces

1 package (7 ounces) seasoned shredded tofu or seasoned dry tofu cut into thin strips

1. WHISK together the broth, soy sauce, lemon juice, cornstarch, and honey in a small bowl. Set aside.

2. COOK the carrots and green beans with 2 tablespoons of water in a microwaveable bowl for 2 minutes.

3. COAT a wok or deep skillet with cooking spray, add the peanut oil, and heat over high heat. Add the garlic and ginger, and cook, stirring constantly, for about 30 seconds, or until beginning to soften. Mix in the carrots, green beans, cabbage, snow peas, and scallions, and cook, stirring constantly, for 10 minutes or until they are crisp-tender. Add small amounts of water as necessary to prevent sticking or burning.

4. STIR the broth mixture to recombine and add to a pan with the shredded tofu. Simmer over medium heat for 5 minutes, stirring occasionally, until the sauce is thickened. Remove from the heat.

PER SERVING (1 serving = 2 cups vegetables, ½ cup noodles)

Calories	Total Fat	Saturated Fat	Sodium	Carbohydrate	Dietary Fiber	Protein	Calcium
340	8 g	1 g	680 mg	45 g	7 g	15 g	10%

6 ounces fresh (or 3 ounces dried) Chinese or other spinach lo mein style noodles

1 teaspoon toasted sesame oil

1 teaspoon grated lemon zest

1 teaspoon toasted sesame seeds

5. MEANWHILE, cook the noodles in a medium pan of boiling water according to package directions or until al dente, about 2 minutes. Drain.

6. GENTLY toss the noodles with the vegetable-tofu mixture. Drizzle with the sesame oil and sprinkle with the lemon zest and sesame seeds.

VEGETABLE FRIED BROWN RICE WITH EGG SCRAMBLES AND TOMATO

PREP TIME: 10 MINUTES / **COOK TIME:** 14 MINUTES / **MAKES** 4 SERVINGS

What a great way to use leftover rice, and in a dish that is far healthier and tastier than what you're likely to get with Chinese takeout. Any type of frozen mixed vegetables—including traditional (peas, carrots, and corn), Asian blend, broccoli and cauliflower combo, and others—can be used.

4	teaspoons canola oil
2	large eggs, lightly beaten
1	medium onion, chopped
1	tablespoon grated fresh ginger
2	cloves garlic, minced
1	cup frozen mixed vegetables
1	medium tomato, chopped
4	cups cold cooked brown rice, preferable day-old
3	tablespoons reduced-sodium soy sauce
1	tablespoon hoisin sauce

1. HEAT 1 teaspoon of the oil in a large nonstick skillet over medium-high heat. Add the eggs and cook, without stirring, turning once, for 2 to 3 minutes, or until firm. Break into smaller pieces with a wooden spoon and transfer to a bowl.

2. RETURN the skillet to the heat and add the remaining 3 teaspoons oil. Stir in the onion, ginger, and garlic, and cook, stirring, for 2 minutes or until the onion is starting to soften. Add the mixed vegetables and cook for 1½ minutes to begin to soften. Stir in the tomato and cook for 2 to 3 minutes, or until beginning to collapse. Add the rice and cook, stirring, for 2 to 3 minutes to heat through. Mix in the cooked eggs, soy sauce, and hoisin sauce, and cook, stirring, for 1 minute to heat through. Serve hot.

MAKE IT A MEAL

½ cup steamed edamame in the shell
50 CALORIES

½ cup steamed bok choy
10 CALORIES

410 CALORIES PER MEAL
★ ★ ★

MAKE IT A MEAL

2 ounces extra-firm tofu tossed with ½ cup steamed bok choy
60 CALORIES

410 CALORIES PER MEAL
★ ★ ★

PER SERVING (1 serving = 1½ cups)

Calories	Total Fat	Saturated Fat	Sodium	Carbohydrate	Dietary Fiber	Protein	Calcium
350	9 g	1.5 g	590 mg	56 g	6 g	11 g	6%

BUDDHA'S DELIGHT

PREP TIME: 30 MINUTES / **COOK TIME:** 20 MINUTES / **MAKES** 4 SERVINGS

This Chinese restaurant classic can be made with almost any combination of vegetables. For even cooking, cut all the vegetables to about the same size.

¾	cup low-sodium vegetable broth
¼	cup hoisin sauce
1	tablespoon reduced-sodium soy sauce
2	teaspoons cornstarch
1	tablespoon canola oil
1	package (14 ounces) light firm tofu, drained and cut into ½" cubes
1	tablespoon toasted sesame oil
1	onion, chopped
1	tablespoon grated fresh ginger
8	ounces mushrooms, sliced
¾	pound asparagus, cut into 1" pieces
2	carrots, sliced
1	red bell pepper, cut into thin strips
½	pound snow peas
4	scallions, chopped

1. **COMBINE** the broth, hoisin sauce, soy sauce, and cornstarch in a medium bowl.

2. **HEAT** the canola oil in a large nonstick skillet over medium-high heat. Add the tofu and cook, stirring occasionally, for 6 to 7 minutes, or until lightly golden. Transfer to a plate.

3. **HEAT** the sesame oil in the same skillet over medium-high heat. Add the onion and ginger, and cook, stirring often, for 1 minute. Add the mushrooms and cook for 4 minutes, or until starting to soften and brown slightly.

4. **STIR** in the asparagus, carrots, and bell pepper, and cook for 4 minutes, or until crisp-tender. Add the snow peas and cook for 1 minute, or until bright green. Return the tofu to the pan and cook for 1 minute. Stir the broth mixture to recombine, add to the skillet, and bring to a boil. Cook for 2 minutes, or until the sauce thickens. Remove from the heat and stir in the scallions.

MAKE
IT A
MEAL

1 almond cookie
(½ ounce)
90 CALORIES

1 medium orange
70 CALORIES

400
CALORIES
PER MEAL
★ ★ ★

MAKE
IT A
MEAL

½ cup green tea
ice cream
140 CALORIES

380
CALORIES
PER MEAL
★ ★ ★

PER SERVING (1 serving = 2 cups)

Calories	Total Fat	Saturated Fat	Sodium	Carbohydrate	Dietary Fiber	Protein	Calcium
240	10 g	1 g	500 mg	27 g	6 g	14 g	25%

VEGETARIAN MA PO TEMPEH

PREP TIME: 20 MINUTES / **COOK TIME:** 22 MINUTES / **MAKES** 4 SERVINGS

Tempeh is a fermented soybean cake that originated in Indonesia. Look for it in the vegetarian section of the refrigerated food case at your market or at a health or natural foods store.

MAKE
IT A
MEAL

½ cup cooked
brown rice
110 CALORIES

½ cup fresh
fruit salad
50 CALORIES

410
CALORIES
PER MEAL
★ ★

MAKE
the variation
A MEAL

½ cup cooked
brown rice
110 CALORIES

½ cup fresh
fruit salad
50 CALORIES

410
CALORIES
PER MEAL
★ ★

1 tablespoon peanut oil

3 cloves garlic, finely chopped

2 tablespoons finely chopped ginger

1 medium onion, finely chopped

1 medium red bell pepper, cut into ½"-wide strips

1 package (10 ounces) sliced cremini (brown) mushrooms

1 can (8 ounces) sliced water chestnuts, drained

1 can (8 ounces) bamboo shoots, drained

8 ounces tempeh, cut into ½" cubes

1 cup low-sodium vegetable broth

1 tablespoon Thai chili-garlic sauce (sriracha)

1 tablespoon reduced-sodium soy sauce

1 tablespoon sugar

½ teaspoon finely ground Sichuan peppercorns

2 teaspoons cornstarch blended with 2 tablespoons water

4 scallions, finely chopped

1. HEAT the oil in a wok or large skillet over medium heat. Add the garlic and ginger, and stir-fry for 1 minute. Add the onion, bell pepper, mushrooms, water chestnuts, bamboo shoots, and tempeh. Cook for 1 minute.

2. WHISK together the broth, chili-garlic sauce, soy sauce, sugar, and peppercorns in a small bowl. Add to the wok. Cover and cook the tempeh-vegetable mixture for 18 minutes, stirring occasionally, until the vegetables are tender and the tempeh has absorbed some of the liquid.

3. STIR the cornstarch mixture to recombine, then add to the wok and cook for 2 minutes to thicken the sauce. Serve sprinkled with the scallions.

MA PO TOFU *(variation)*
SUBSTITUTE 1 pound extra-firm tofu, cut into 1" cubes, for the tempeh

PER SERVING (1 serving = 1¼ cups) Ma Po Tofu (1 serving = 1¼ cups)

Calories	Total Fat	Saturated Fat	Sodium	Carbohydrate	Dietary Fiber	Protein	Calcium
250	10 g	2 g	280 mg	29 g	5 g	16 g	10%
250	11 g	1.5 g	280 mg	26 g	5 g	16 g	25%

CUBAN RICE AND BEANS

PREP TIME: 10 MINUTES / **COOK TIME:** 39 MINUTES / **MAKES** 4 SERVINGS

Beans, here black and pinto, wear two hats in the world of nutrition. They are considered vegetables, with plenty of vitamins and fiber, and also are thought of as protein foods.

4	teaspoons extra-virgin olive oil
1	medium onion, thinly sliced
1	large red bell pepper, sliced
3	cloves garlic, minced
1	teaspoon dried basil
1	teaspoon ground cumin
½	teaspoon ground coriander
16	grape tomatoes
5	teaspoons white wine vinegar
1	can (15 ounces) no-salt-added black beans, rinsed and drained
1	can (15 ounces) no-salt-added pinto beans, rinsed and drained
¾	teaspoon salt
¼	teaspoon freshly ground black pepper
½	cup rice

1. HEAT the oil in a large saucepan over medium-high heat. Add the onion, bell pepper, garlic, basil, cumin, and coriander. Cook, stirring occasionally, for 5 minutes, or until beginning to soften.

2. ADD the tomatoes and cook for 3 minutes, or until beginning to collapse. Add the vinegar and cook for 30 seconds to evaporate. Mix in the black and pinto beans, bring to a boil, reduce to a simmer, cover, and cook for 30 minutes, stirring occasionally, until the vegetables are very tender and the mixture is fairly thick. Season with the salt and pepper.

3. MEANWHILE, cook the rice according to package directions.

4. SERVE the bean mixture over the rice.

MAKE IT A MEAL

Sangria spritzer made with ¾ cup sangria and ¾ cup seltzer
120 CALORIES

420 CALORIES PER MEAL
★ ★

MAKE IT A MEAL

5 steamed asparagus spears
20 CALORIES

1 small slice (1 ounce) Italian bread
80 CALORIES

400 CALORIES PER MEAL
★ ★

PER SERVING (1 serving = 1 cup beans, ½ cup rice)

Calories	Total Fat	Saturated Fat	Sodium	Carbohydrate	Dietary Fiber	Protein	Calcium
300	5 g	0.5 g	460 mg	51 g	11 g	12 g	10%

VEGETABLE DUMPLINGS WITH DIPPING SAUCE

PREP TIME: 45 MINUTES / **COOK TIME:** 20 MINUTES / **MAKES** 4 SERVINGS

Look for dumpling wrappers in the refrigerated or freezer section of a market that carries Asian ingredients. They're like wonton wrappers, but they're round. Modify the vegetable ingredients to suit your taste.

4	ounces extra-firm tofu
½	cup torn napa or savoy cabbage
½	cup torn bok choy leaves
2	tablespoons bean sprouts
2	fresh shiitake mushrooms, stems discarded, caps halved
1	scallion, cut into 3 pieces
1	small carrot, cut into chunks
1	piece (1") fresh ginger, finely chopped
1	clove garlic, minced
1	large egg, lightly beaten
2	teaspoons hoisin-garlic sauce (such as Soy Vay Asian Glaze) or regular hoisin sauce
1	teaspoon dry sherry
1	teaspoon toasted sesame oil
¼	teaspoon freshly ground black pepper
32	round dumpling wrappers

1. **SHRED** the tofu using the coarse holes of a grater. Arrange on several layers of paper towels to drain.

2. **COMBINE** the cabbage, bok choy, bean sprouts, mushrooms, scallion, and carrot in a food processor. Pulse on and off to coarsely chop. Place the mixture in a bowl and stir in the ginger and garlic.

3. **ADD** the drained tofu, egg, hoisin-garlic sauce, sherry, sesame oil, and pepper to the vegetables and mix well.

4. **PLACE** 1 scant tablespoon of the vegetable mixture in the center of a dumpling wrapper. Dip your finger in some water and dampen the edges of the wrapper. Fold in half and pinch with your fingers to seal the edges. (Or pleat the dumpling into a purse shape if desired.)

PER SERVING (1 serving = 8 dumplings, 2 tablespoons sauce)

Calories	Total Fat	Saturated Fat	Sodium	Carbohydrate	Dietary Fiber	Protein	Calcium
340	11 g	2 g	540 mg	46 g	3 g	14 g	10%

2 tablespoons peanut butter (creamy or chunky)

1 tablespoon tahini (sesame paste)

¼ cup water

½ tablespoon rice vinegar

1 teaspoon reduced-sodium soy sauce

½ teaspoon sugar

5. COAT a steamer basket or insert with cooking spray and place in a large pot over 3" of water. Bring the water to a boil over high heat. Working in batches, place a single layer of dumplings in the basket, cover, and steam for 10 minutes, or until cooked through. Keep the cooked dumplings warm until all the dumplings are steamed.

6. MEANWHILE, mix together the peanut butter and tahini. Stir in the water, vinegar, soy sauce, and sugar. Serve the sauce with the warm dumplings.

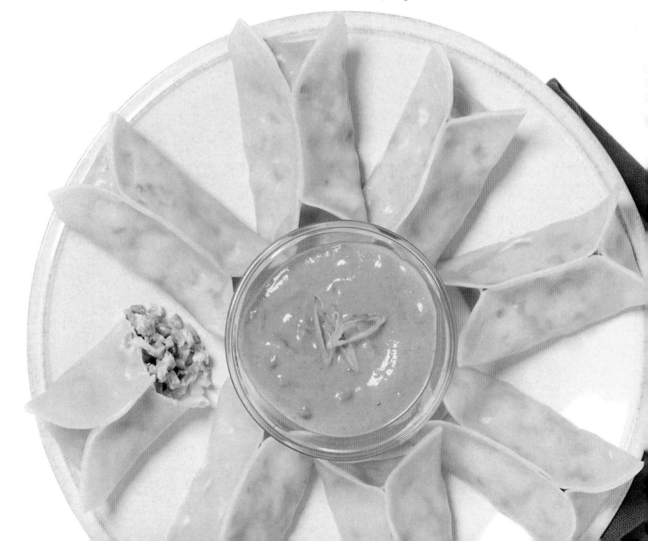

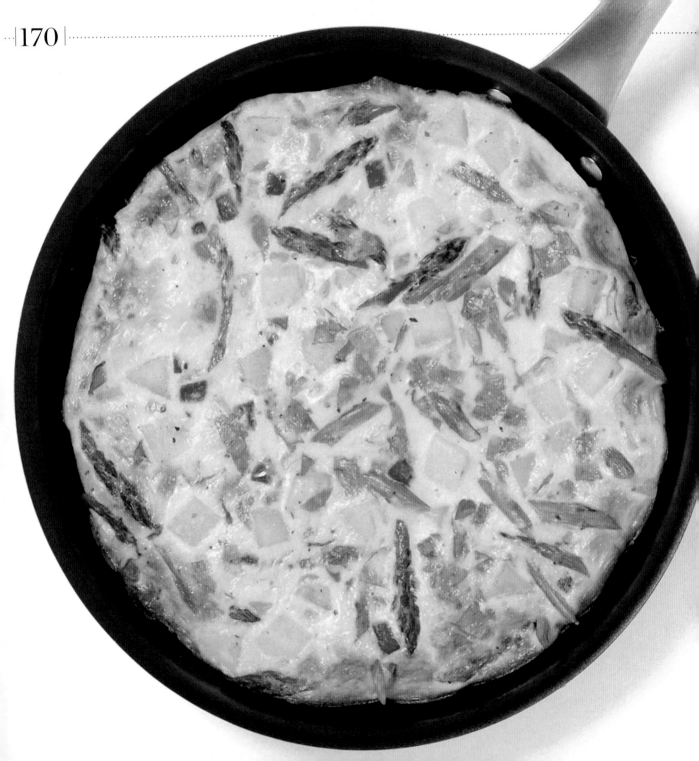

FRITTATA WITH ASPARAGUS, BASIL, AND ROMANO CHEESE

PREP TIME: 15 MINUTES / **COOK TIME:** 28 MINUTES / **MAKES** 4 SERVINGS

The extra egg whites in this recipe serve to increase portion size without adding a lot of calories. In eggs, most of the calories are in the yolk. Vary the frittata with different types of vegetables and/or cheese.

1	large russet (baking) potato (12 ounces), peeled and cut into ½" cubes
4	large eggs
4	large egg whites
½	cup fat-free milk
¼	cup grated Romano cheese
¼	cup chopped fresh basil
¼	teaspoon salt
¼	teaspoon freshly ground black pepper
1	tablespoon extra-virgin olive oil
1	onion, chopped
1	red bell pepper, chopped
2	cloves garlic, minced
½	pound asparagus, cut into 1" pieces

1. PREHEAT the broiler.

2. PLACE the potato in a saucepan with enough cold water to cover by 2". Bring the water to a boil and cook for 10 minutes, or until the potato cubes are tender but still hold their shape. Drain and set aside.

3. MEANWHILE, beat together the whole eggs, egg whites, milk, cheese, basil, salt, and pepper in a medium bowl.

4. HEAT the oil in a 10" broilerproof nonstick skillet over medium-high heat. Add the onion, bell pepper, and garlic, and cook for 2 to 3 minutes, stirring occasionally, until the vegetables start to soften. Add the asparagus and cook until crisp-tender, 3 to 4 minutes. Stir in the potatoes and cook for 1 minute.

5. REDUCE the heat to medium, pour in the egg mixture, and stir gently to combine. Cook for 7 to 8 minutes, or until the eggs are set. Transfer the skillet to the broiler and cook 5" from the heat for 1 to 2 minutes to brown the top. Let the frittata stand for 5 minutes before cutting into 4 wedges.

MAKE IT A MEAL

Medium piece (2 ounces) foccacia
150 CALORIES

420
CALORIES PER MEAL
★ ★

MAKE IT A MEAL

Salad made with 2 cups mixed baby greens, 10 cherry tomatoes, 1 tablespoon light Italian dressing, 2 tablespoons plain croutons
95 CALORIES

1 cup light cranberry juice
40 CALORIES

405
CALORIES PER MEAL
★ ★ ★

PER SERVING (1 serving = 1 wedge)

Calories	Total Fat	Saturated Fat	Sodium	Carbohydrate	Dietary Fiber	Protein	Calcium
270	11 g	3.5 g	430 mg	27 g	4 g	18 g	20%

ITALIAN PEPPERS, ONIONS, AND EGGS

PREP TIME: 10 MINUTES / **COOK TIME:** 16 MINUTES / **MAKES** 4 SERVINGS

Use any combination of peppers in this colorful dish, including red, orange, yellow, or a mix of baby peppers. Avoid overcooking the eggs in order to keep them moist.

6	large eggs
2	large egg whites
½	cup fat-free milk
¾	teaspoon salt
¼	teaspoon freshly ground black pepper
2	teaspoons olive oil
1	medium onion, sliced
1	medium red bell pepper, thinly sliced
1	medium green bell pepper, thinly sliced
½	teaspoon dried basil
4	cloves garlic, minced
2	teaspoons balsamic vinegar

1. WHISK together the whole eggs, egg whites, milk, ½ teaspoon of the salt, and ⅛ teaspoon of the pepper in a medium bowl.

2. HEAT 1 teaspoon of the oil in a large nonstick skillet over medium-high heat. Add the onion, bell peppers, and basil, and cook for 7 to 8 minutes, stirring occasionally, until softened. Stir in the garlic and the remaining salt and pepper and cook for 3 minutes, or until softened. Add the vinegar and cook, stirring, for 30 seconds to evaporate. Transfer the mixture to a bowl.

3. RETURN the skillet to medium-high heat and add the remaining 1 teaspoon oil. Pour in the egg mixture and cook for 1½ to 2 minutes, using a silicone spatula to gently push the egg mixture toward the center as it sets on the bottom but stays very wet on top. Fold in the onion and pepper mixture, cooking another 1 to 2 minutes, or until the eggs are completely set. Serve hot.

PER SERVING (1 serving = 1¼ cups)

Calories	Total Fat	Saturated Fat	Sodium	Carbohydrate	Dietary Fiber	Protein	Calcium
180	10 g	2.5 g	590 mg	10 g	2 g	13 g	10%

SAVORY BLACK BEAN PATTIES

PREP TIME: 15 MINUTES + UP TO 1 HOUR CHILLING / **COOK TIME:** 9 MINUTES / **MAKES** 4 SERVINGS

Dried beans, including black beans, soybeans, and others, are extremely high in fiber, as well as rich in protein and other nutrients. If you choose to use canned beans for this recipe, you'll need two 15-ounce cans. Pinto beans or white beans also can be used here. Make slider-size burgers by forming 8 small patties and serving them on slider buns.

1½   teaspoons olive oil

1   medium onion, finely chopped

2   cloves garlic, finely chopped

2   tablespoons dried porcini mushroom slices

3   cups cooked or rinsed and drained canned black beans

⅓   cup panko bread crumbs

1   large egg

3   tablespoons finely chopped fresh cilantro

1   teaspoon Thai chili-garlic sauce (sriracha)

1½   teaspoons ground cumin

¾   teaspoon salt

½   teaspoon freshly ground black pepper

1. HEAT the oil in a large skillet over medium heat. Add the onion and garlic, and cook for 3 minutes, or until the onion is softened. Remove from the heat.

2. PROCESS the dried mushrooms in a food processor until finely chopped. Add the beans and process just until finely chopped; do not puree. Transfer to a large mixing bowl. Add the sautéed onion mixture, panko, egg, cilantro, chili-garlic sauce, cumin, salt, and pepper. Mix well. Refrigerate for at least 15 minutes and up to 1 hour.

3. FORM the bean mixture into 4 patties. Coat a large skillet with cooking spray. Place over medium heat, add the patties, and cook for 3 minutes, or until lightly browned and crisp on the bottom. Turn over, gently press down with a spatula to flatten slightly, and cook for 3 minutes, or until lightly browned and crisp on the second side. You may need to cook the patties in two batches.

SAVORY EDAMAME PATTIES *(variation)*

SUBSTITUTE shelled edamame for the black beans. Cook the edamame according to package directions before processing.

MAKE
IT A
MEAL

Serve each patty on a whole wheat hamburger bun with 2 slices tomato, 2 lettuce leaves, 1 tablespoon ketchup
145 CALORIES

415
CALORIES
PER MEAL
★ ★ ★

MAKE
the variation
A MEAL

½ cup rice pilaf
140 CALORIES

390
CALORIES
PER MEAL
★ ★ ★

PER SERVING (1 serving = 1 patty) Savory Edamame Patties (1 serving = 1 patty)

Calories	Total Fat	Saturated Fat	Sodium	Carbohydrate	Dietary Fiber	Protein	Calcium
270	4.5 g	1 g	510 mg	43 g	13 g	16 g	6%
250	8 g	0.5 g	560 mg	26 g	8 g	17 g	10%

PORTOBELLO BURGER WITH GRILLED TOMATO

PREP TIME: 15 MINUTES / **COOK TIME:** 15 MINUTES / 4 SERVINGS

Try these festive burgers when you have a vegetarian on your guest list. They're tasty and hearty enough to please the palates of meat lovers also.

8	thin slices cucumber (from ½ small)
3	tablespoons red wine vinegar
5	teaspoons extra-virgin olive oil
2	teaspoons sugar
2	cloves garlic, minced
1	tablespoon Dijon mustard
1	teaspoon Worcestershire sauce
4	portobello mushrooms (4 ounces each), stems removed
½	teaspoon salt
⅛	teaspoon freshly ground black pepper
½	cup shredded part-skim mozzarella cheese
1	medium tomato, cut into 4 thick slices
4	whole wheat hamburger buns
4	thin slices red onion (from ½ small)

1. PREHEAT a grill to medium-high.

2. COMBINE the cucumber, 1 tablespoon of the vinegar, 1 teaspoon of the oil, and the sugar in a bowl. Set aside to marinate while you prepare the burgers.

3. COMBINE the garlic, mustard, Worcestershire sauce, 3 teaspoons (or 1 tablespoon) of the oil, and the remaining 2 tablespoons vinegar in a small bowl. Brush the portobellos with this vinegar mixture and sprinkle with the salt and pepper. Set the mushrooms gill-side down on a grill rack that has been coated with cooking spray. Grill for 6 minutes, until starting to soften. Turn over and top with the mozzarella. Grill for 6 to 7 minutes, or until tender. Meanwhile, brush the tomato slices with the remaining 1 teaspoon oil and grill for 1 minute per side.

4. SET a bun bottom on each of 4 plates. Top each with 1 tomato slice, 1 onion slice, 1 portobello, 2 cucumber slices, and the bun tops.

MAKE IT A MEAL

Salad made with 2 cups mixed baby greens and 10 sprays salad dressing spray
30 CALORIES

½ cup frozen yogurt
100 CALORIES

410
CALORIES PER MEAL
★ ★

MAKE IT A MEAL

1 medium red bell pepper, halved, brushed with ½ teaspoon olive oil, grilled, and sliced
60 CALORIES

½ cup Italian ice
60 CALORIES

400
CALORIES PER MEAL
★ ★

PER SERVING (1 serving = 1 burger)

Calories	Total Fat	Saturated Fat	Sodium	Carbohydrate	Dietary Fiber	Protein	Calcium
280	12 g	3 g	690 mg	34 g	6 g	13 g	15%

GRILLED TOFU STEAKS OVER ARUGULA AND TOMATO SALAD

PREP TIME: 10 MINUTES + 30 MINUTES MARINATING / **COOK TIME:** 16 MINUTES / **MAKES** 4 SERVINGS

Use firm or extra-firm tofu. Silken tofu is too soft for grilling. To give this dish an Asian flavor, use rice vinegar in place of balsamic and substitute sesame oil for some of the olive oil.

1	package (14 ounces) light firm tofu
2	tablespoons balsamic vinegar
2	cloves garlic, minced
3	tablespoons fresh lemon juice
3	ounces baguette, cut into ½" cubes
8	cups baby arugula
4	plum tomatoes, cut into 8 wedges each
3	tablespoons chopped shallots
5	teaspoons extra-virgin olive oil
1	teaspoon Dijon mustard
1	teaspoon honey
½	teaspoon salt
¼	teaspoon freshly ground black pepper

1. **PLACE** the tofu on a stack of several paper towels and gently press out excess moisture for about 1 minute. Cut into 4 slices.

2. **COMBINE** the vinegar, garlic, and 1 tablespoon of the lemon juice in a shallow glass or ceramic dish (that will hold the tofu snugly in one layer). Add the tofu slices, turning to coat. Let marinate for 30 minutes.

3. **MEANWHILE,** preheat the oven to 350°F. Spread the bread cubes on a large baking sheet and bake for 8 to 10 minutes, or until lightly browned and crisp. Set aside to cool.

4. **COMBINE** the arugula, tomatoes, and bread cubes in a large bowl. Mix the shallots, oil, mustard, honey, salt, pepper, and remaining 2 tablespoons lemon juice in a small bowl. Pour the shallot mixture over the arugula mixture and toss well. Divide among 4 plates.

5. **COAT** a nonstick grill pan with cooking spray and heat over medium-high heat. Remove the tofu from the marinade and add to the grill pan. Grill the tofu for 3 minutes per side or until well marked and hot. Serve the grilled tofu over the salad.

MAKE IT A MEAL

½ cup cooked whole wheat penne
90 CALORIES

3 gingersnaps
90 CALORIES

420 CALORIES PER MEAL
★ ★

MAKE IT A MEAL

½ cup wild rice/ brown basmati rice pilaf
140 CALORIES

1 clementine
30 CALORIES

410 CALORIES PER MEAL
★ ★

PER SERVING (1 serving = 1 tofu steak, 2½ cups salad)

Calories	Total Fat	Saturated Fat	Sodium	Carbohydrate	Dietary Fiber	Protein	Calcium
240	9 g	1 g	530 mg	27 g	3 g	14 g	45%

MIDDLE EASTERN PITZA

PREP TIME: 10 MINUTES / **COOK TIME:** 17 MINUTES / **MAKES** 4 SERVINGS

Toasting the pitas before adding the toppings helps keep them crisp when they bake. For a drier topping, allow the tomatoes to drain for several minutes before combining with the other ingredients.

¼ cup tomato paste

3 tablespoons water

¾ teaspoon ground cumin

⅛ teaspoon ground cinnamon

⅛ teaspoon cayenne pepper

4 large (6½") whole wheat pitas, toasted

2 plum tomatoes, chopped

1 medium green bell pepper, chopped

2 scallions, chopped

¾ cup crumbled reduced-fat feta cheese

1 tablespoon fresh lemon juice

1 tablespoon extra-virgin olive oil

¼ cup chopped fresh parsley

1. PREHEAT the oven to 400°F.

2. MIX the tomato paste, water, cumin, cinnamon, and cayenne in a small bowl, stirring until smooth. Spread the mixture over one side of each pita and set on a baking sheet.

3. COMBINE the tomatoes, bell pepper, scallions, cheese, lemon juice, and oil in a bowl. Spoon the mixture over the pitas. Bake for 15 to 17 minutes, or until the tomatoes and bell pepper soften. Serve sprinkled with the parsley.

PER SERVING (1 serving = 1 pitza)

Calories	Total Fat	Saturated Fat	Sodium	Carbohydrate	Dietary Fiber	Protein	Calcium
240	8 g	3 g	730 mg	33 g	6 g	11 g	10%

SUMMER SQUASH GRATIN ON A BARLEY BED

PREP TIME: 20 MINUTES / **COOK TIME:** 1 HOUR 10 MINUTES / **MAKES** 4 SERVINGS

Be sure to squeeze as much moisture as possible out of the squash so the dish doesn't get too watery. For a different flavor, use basil or oregano in place of the herbes de Provence.

⅔	cup pearled barley
1⅓	cups water
1	teaspoon unsalted butter
1	teaspoon olive oil
1	large yellow onion, finely chopped
1½	pounds summer squash (zucchini, yellow squash, pattypan, and others), grated and squeezed dry
2	wedges Laughing Cow Light cheese, cut into small pieces
2	tablespoons all-purpose flour
½	teaspoon herbes de Provence or dried thyme
½	teaspoon salt
½	teaspoon freshly ground black pepper
½	cup low-fat or fat-free milk
2	large eggs
½	cup shredded reduced-fat Cheddar cheese

1. **PLACE** the barley and water in a medium saucepan. Bring to a boil over medium-high heat. Reduce to a simmer, cover, and cook for 30 minutes, or until the barley is cooked to al dente.

2. **PREHEAT** the oven to 350°F. Coat a 2½-quart round baking dish with cooking spray.

3. **MEANWHILE,** coat a large skillet with cooking spray and heat over medium heat. Add the butter and oil. Add the onion and cook for 5 minutes, or until softened. Mix in the squash and cook for 5 minutes, or until crisp-tender. Remove from the heat and stir in the Laughing Cow cheese. Stir in the flour, herbes de Provence, salt, and pepper.

4. **PLACE** the cooked barley in the baking dish. Top with the squash mixture.

5. **WHISK** the milk and eggs together in a small bowl. Pour over the squash mixture. Stir gently to combine, without disturbing the barley layer. Sprinkle with the Cheddar.

6. **BAKE** for 40 minutes, or until the cheese is lightly browned and the edges of the gratin begin to brown.

MAKE IT A MEAL

2 mini brownie bites (such as Hostess)
110 CALORIES

390
CALORIES
PER MEAL
★ ★

MAKE IT A MEAL

½ cup frozen yogurt
100 CALORIES

380
CALORIES
PER MEAL
★ ★

PER SERVING (1 serving = 1½ cups)

Calories	Total Fat	Saturated Fat	Sodium	Carbohydrate	Dietary Fiber	Protein	Calcium
280	8 g	3 g	580 mg	41 g	8 g	15 g	20%

TOMATO AND PEPPER TART

PREP TIME: 20 MINUTES / **COOK TIME:** 50 MINUTES / **MAKES** 6 SERVINGS

Using prepared pie dough makes this recipe easy enough for a weeknight. Caramelized sweet onions, brightly colored peppers, and tomatoes dance in a crispy crust with creamy goat cheese and a sprinkling of fresh herbs.

MAKE IT A MEAL

Salad made with 2 cups romaine lettuce, 1 medium tomato cut into wedges, ¼ cup grated carrot, 2 tablespoons seasoned croutons, and 2 tablespoons light Caesar dressing
145 CALORIES

395
CALORIES PER MEAL
★

MAKE IT A MEAL

1 cup steamed green beans with 1 tablespoon chopped walnuts and 1 teaspoon walnut oil
130 CALORIES

380
CALORIES PER MEAL
★ ★

- 1 sweet onion, thinly sliced
- ¼ teaspoon coarse salt
- ⅛ teaspoon freshly ground black pepper
- ⅓ cup low-sodium vegetable broth
- 1 refrigerated pie crust (7.5 ounces)
- 1 large egg, beaten
- 3 ounces soft goat cheese
- 1 yellow bell pepper, diced
- 2 plum tomatoes, cut crosswise into ¼"-thick slices
- 1 tablespoon fresh rosemary or 1½ teaspoons dried
- ½ teaspoon fresh thyme or ¼ teaspoon dried

1. PREHEAT the oven to 450°F.

2. COAT a large nonstick skillet with cooking spray and heat over medium heat. Add the onion, salt, and black pepper. Cook for 5 minutes, stirring occasionally, until the onion just begins to brown. Add 2 tablespoons of the broth to prevent the onion from burning. Cook and stir for another 5 minutes. Repeat, adding another 2 tablespoons of the broth and stirring for 5 minutes. Add the remaining broth, cook, and stir for 2 to 3 minutes, until the onion is golden and soft. Set the mixture aside.

3. PLACE an 11" tart pan with a removable bottom on a baking sheet and fit the pie crust into the pan. Brush the crust with 1 tablespoon of the beaten egg. Prick the bottom of the crust several times with a fork. Bake for 8 minutes to set the crust. Remove the crust and reduce the oven temperature to 400°F.

4. COMBINE the remaining egg and goat cheese in a small bowl. Beat with an electric mixer to blend. Spread the goat cheese mixture into the tart shell. Add a layer of onions. Top the onions with a single layer of bell pepper, then a layer of tomato slices arranged so that the peppers can still be seen. Sprinkle the top with the rosemary and thyme. Spray the top of the tart with cooking spray.

5. BAKE for 20 to 25 minutes, until the vegetables are tender and the crust is golden. Let rest for 10 minutes before slicing into 6 wedges. Serve the tart warm or at room temperature.

PER SERVING (1 serving = one 5" wedge)

Calories	Total Fat	Saturated Fat	Sodium	Carbohydrate	Dietary Fiber	Protein	Calcium
250	14 g	7 g	310 mg	24 g	1 g	6 g	6%

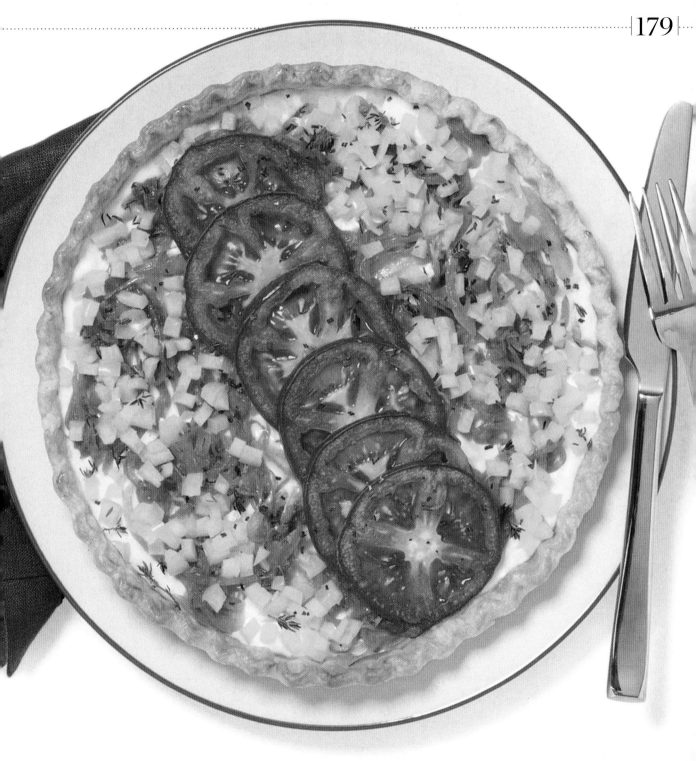

RATATOUILLE NAPOLEON

PREP TIME: 20 MINUTES + 15 MINUTES STANDING / **COOK TIME:** 40 MINUTES / **MAKES** 4 SERVINGS

Inspired by the flavors of Provence, layers of summer vegetables come together nicely in this vegetarian meal. Very versatile, it can be served warm or made in advance and served at room temperature.

1	large eggplant (about 1 pound), peeled and cut lengthwise into ½"-thick slices
3	small zucchini, cut lengthwise into ¼"-thick slices
4	plum tomatoes
1	can (15.5 ounces) cannellini beans, rinsed and drained
1	teaspoon fresh rosemary or ½ teaspoon dried
1	teaspoon olive oil
1	leek (white and pale green parts), well washed, halved lengthwise, and thinly sliced crosswise
4	cloves garlic, minced
¾	teaspoon coarse salt

1. PREHEAT the oven to 450°F. Line 2 baking sheets with foil and coat the foil with cooking spray.

2. PLACE the eggplant slices on one baking sheet (they can overlap). Place the zucchini slices on the second baking sheet. Coat the tops of the eggplant and zucchini with cooking spray. Bake for 18 to 20 minutes, or until lightly golden and tender. Remove the vegetables from the oven and reduce the oven temperature to 350°F.

3. MEANWHILE, cut the tomatoes crosswise into ½"-thick slices and place on paper towels to drain. Combine the beans and rosemary in a food processor and process until smooth (the mixture will be thick).

4. COAT a large nonstick skillet with cooking spray and heat over medium heat. Add the oil, leek, garlic, ½ teaspoon of the salt, and ¼ teaspoon of the pepper. Cook for 7 minutes, stirring often, until the leek is soft. Remove from the heat and stir in the basil.

5. ASSEMBLE the napoleon: Coat an 8" x 8" baking dish with cooking spray. Layer the eggplant slices in the bottom of the baking dish. (Overlap large slices if they don't fit in one layer.) Season the eggplant with ⅛ teaspoon of the salt and ⅛ teaspoon of the pepper. Drop the bean mixture by spoonfuls onto the eggplant and spread it into a single layer. Sprinkle the olives evenly over the bean layer, then top with half of the leek mixture.

PER SERVING (1 serving = one 4" x 4" square)

Calories	Total Fat	Saturated Fat	Sodium	Carbohydrate	Dietary Fiber	Protein	Calcium
230	6 g	1 g	720 mg	38 g	9 g	8 g	10%

½ teaspoon freshly ground black pepper

½ cup thinly sliced fresh basil

¼ cup pitted kalamata olives (about 12), quartered lengthwise

4 standard-size sheets frozen phyllo dough, thawed

6. **ADD** the zucchini slices, gently pressing them into a flat layer. Season the zucchini with the remaining ⅛ teaspoon each salt and pepper. Make a layer of tomato slices. Top with the remaining leek mixture.

7. **PLACE** the phyllo on a work surface. Spray 1 sheet with cooking spray and gently form the phyllo into a ball, just as you would crumple up a piece of paper. Place the phyllo ball in one corner of the baking dish so that it will nicely garnish a portion once baked. Repeat with the remaining phyllo, making 4 phyllo garnishes on top of the dish. Bake for 20 minutes, or until the phyllo is golden and the tomatoes are tender. Let rest for 15 minutes.

8. **SLICE** through the vegetables with a very sharp knife to cut the napoleon into 4 squares. Use a spatula to lift out the squares. If making the dish ahead of time, do not slice until serving time.

8

SEAFOOD

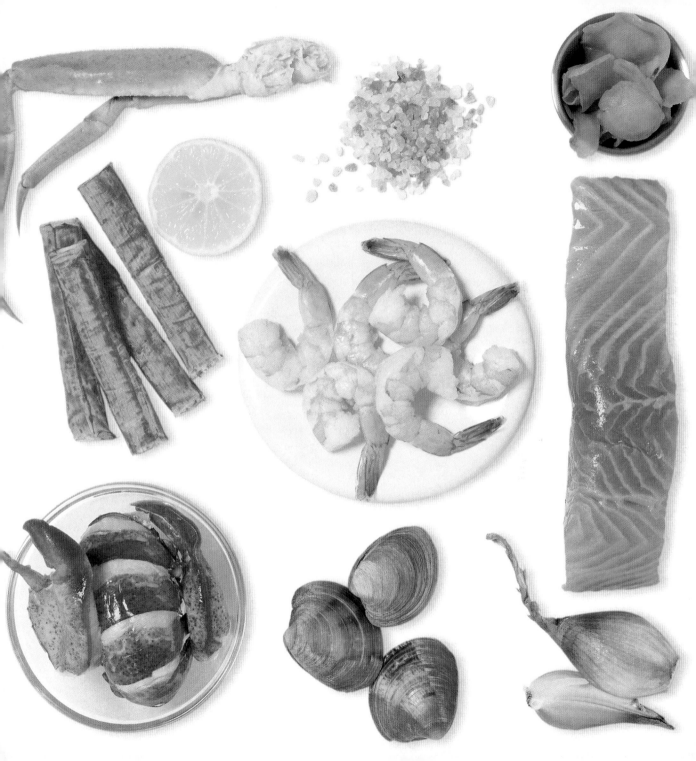

GRILLED TUNA AND PORTOBELLOS WITH WASABI DRESSING

PREP TIME: 15 MINUTES / **COOK TIME:** 15 MINUTES / **MAKES** 4 SERVINGS

Meaty tuna and earthy portobellos are grilled to perfection and served over a bed of peppery watercress. The Japanese-inspired sauce is made with spicy wasabi powder and a touch of sesame. It does double duty as the marinade and the dressing.

½ cup light mayonnaise

2 tablespoons reduced-sodium soy sauce

2 tablespoons wasabi powder

2 tablespoons rice vinegar

1 tablespoon fresh lemon juice

2 tablespoons water

2 tablespoons sugar

2 teaspoons toasted sesame oil

4 tuna steaks (4 ounces each), about 1" thick

3 portobello mushroom caps (about 9 ounces total)

1. **PREHEAT** the grill to high. Combine the mayonnaise, soy sauce, wasabi powder, vinegar, lemon juice, water, sugar, and sesame oil in a small bowl.

2. **PAT** the tuna dry with paper towels and place in a shallow bowl. Coat with ¼ cup of the wasabi sauce. Let sit for 10 minutes while the grill heats. Meanwhile, brush ¼ cup of the wasabi sauce over both sides of the portobellos. Set the remaining sauce aside to use as a dressing.

3. **PLACE** the mushrooms gill-side up on a grill rack that's been coated with cooking spray. Grill for 6 minutes. Turn the mushrooms over and at the same time add the tuna to the grill. Grill the mushrooms for 5 minutes longer, until tender. Grill the tuna for 3 minutes, flip, and cook for 1 minute for rare and 2 minutes for medium-rare. Transfer the mushrooms and tuna to a cutting board.

4. **WHEN** cool enough to handle, cut the mushrooms into ½"-wide strips. Cut the tuna into ¼"-wide strips.

PER SERVING (1 serving = 2 cups salad [including mushrooms], 3 ounces cooked fish, 2 tablespoons sauce)
Grilled Wild Salmon and Wasabi Sauce over Watercress (1 serving = 2 cups salad + 3 ounces cooked fish + 2 tablespoons sauce)

Calories	Total Fat	Saturated Fat	Sodium	Carbohydrate	Dietary Fiber	Protein	Calcium
330	14 g	2.5 g	610 mg	19 g	3 g	30 g	8%
360	20 g	3 g	620 mg	17 g	2 g	25 g	8%

4   cups watercress or pea shoots

1   cup precut carrot matchsticks

3   scallions, thinly sliced, or ¼ cup thinly sliced red onion

1   tablespoon sesame seeds, toasted

5. TO ASSEMBLE THE SALADS: Place 1 cup of watercress or pea shoots on each of 4 plates. Top each with ¼ cup carrots. Evenly divide the tuna and mushroom slices among the salad plates, fanning the slices over the watercress. Drizzle about 2 tablespoons of the reserved wasabi sauce over each salad. Garnish with the scallions and sesame seeds.

GRILLED WILD SALMON AND WASABI SAUCE OVER WATERCRESS
(variation)

SUBSTITUTE 1 pound wild salmon fillet for the tuna (same cooking time).

OMIT the mushrooms.

ADD 1 cup snow peas, halved on the diagonal, to the salad (sprinkle over the carrots in Step 5).

CURRIED TUNA SALAD ROLLS WITH FIG CHUTNEY

PREP TIME: 20 MINUTES / MAKES 4 SERVINGS

Light mayonnaise is creamier than low-fat mayo and helps blend the flavors in this luncheon dish. Look for fig marmalade in the international aisle of the market or in a specialty or Middle Eastern food store.

MAKE IT A MEAL

1 medium (1½ ounces) French roll
110 CALORIES

400 CALORIES PER MEAL
★ ★ ★

MAKE IT A MEAL

2 mini brownie bites (such as Hostess)
110 CALORIES

400 CALORIES PER MEAL
★ ★ ★

3	cans (5 ounces each) water-packed white tuna, drained
½	cup chopped apple, any variety
¼	cup dried currants
¼	cup chopped walnuts
⅓	cup light mayonnaise
2	tablespoons low-fat or fat-free plain yogurt
2	tablespoons chopped red onion
1	tablespoon curry powder
4	large leaves soft lettuce, such as Bibb, green leaf, or Boston
2	tablespoons fig marmalade or apricot jam
1	tablespoon cider vinegar

1. **COMBINE** the tuna, apple, currants, walnuts, mayonnaise, yogurt, onion, and curry powder in a large bowl.

2. **DIVIDE** the tuna mixture among the lettuce leaves (about ½ cup each). Roll up, tucking in the sides if desired.

3. **MIX** the fig marmalade or apricot jam and cider vinegar in a small bowl. Dollop 2 teaspoons of the fig chutney on top of each lettuce roll.

PER SERVING (1 serving = 1 tuna roll, 2 teaspoons chutney)

Calories	Total Fat	Saturated Fat	Sodium	Carbohydrate	Dietary Fiber	Protein	Calcium
290	14 g	2 g	460 mg	20 g	2 g	23 g	6%

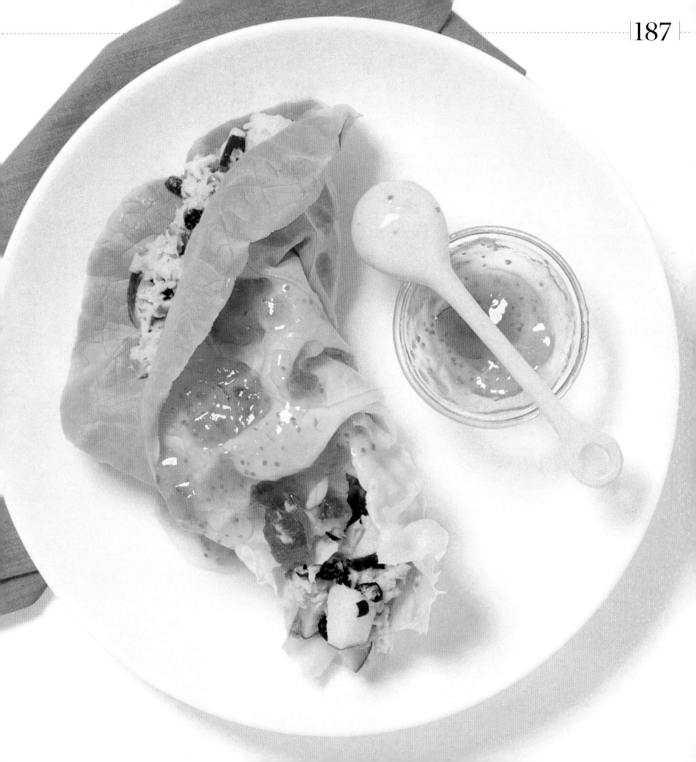

CAPER-SHALLOT TUNA CAKES

PREP TIME: 15 MINUTES / **COOK TIME:** 11 MINUTES / **MAKES** 4 SERVINGS

Yellowfin tuna is more abundant and less expensive than bluefin tuna, a favorite in sushi and sashimi. This recipe will work with other types of fresh and even canned fish. Smaller cakes are perfect party fare.

MAKE IT A MEAL

½ whole wheat English muffin
70 CALORIES

Salad made with 2 cups romaine lettuce, 4 cherry tomatoes, and 1 teaspoon olive oil
70 CALORIES

420
CALORIES PER MEAL
★ ★ ★

MAKE IT A MEAL

1 small (4-ounce) baked potato with 1 teaspoon unsalted whipped butter
135 CALORIES

415
CALORIES PER MEAL
★ ★ ★

6 tablespoons low-fat mayonnaise

2 tablespoons sweet pickle relish

2 teaspoons Dijon mustard

2 slices (1 ounce each) whole wheat bread, torn into big pieces

1 pound yellowfin tuna, finely chopped

1 large egg

¼ cup chopped fresh basil

¼ cup finely chopped shallots

1 tablespoon nonpareil capers, drained

½ teaspoon salt

¼ teaspoon freshly ground black pepper

5 teaspoons olive oil

1. COMBINE the mayonnaise, pickle relish, and mustard in a small bowl.

2. PLACE the bread in a food processor and pulse to form fine crumbs. Transfer to a medium bowl. Stir in the tuna, egg, basil, shallots, capers, salt, and pepper, and mix well. Form the mixture into 8 cakes ½" to ¾" thick.

3. HEAT the oil in a large nonstick skillet over medium heat. Add the tuna cakes and cook for 6 minutes without turning, until golden on the bottom. Turn the cakes and cook for 4 to 5 minutes, or until golden on the second side and cooked through. Serve the cakes with the sauce alongside.

PER SERVING (1 serving = 2 tuna cakes, 2 tablespoons sauce)

Calories	Total Fat	Saturated Fat	Sodium	Carbohydrate	Dietary Fiber	Protein	Calcium
280	11 g	2.5 g	770 mg	14 g	1 g	30 g	4%

LATTICE-TOP TUNA POT PIE

PREP TIME: 15 MINUTES / **COOK TIME:** 47 MINUTES / **MAKES** 4 SERVINGS

By putting crust just on the top of the pie, you save more than 100 calories per serving. Try this recipe with chicken or crabmeat in place of the tuna and any combo of frozen vegetables.

1	tablespoon unsalted butter
1	medium onion, finely chopped
2	tablespoons all-purpose flour
½	teaspoon salt
½	teaspoon freshly ground black pepper
1	cup low-fat milk
½	teaspoon salt-free garlic-herb seasoning
2	cans (5 to 7 ounces) water-packed light tuna, drained and flaked
2	cups frozen mixed vegetables
2	tablespoons chopped fresh parsley
½	tube (8 ounces) crescent roll dough

1. **PREHEAT** the oven to 350°F. Coat a 2-quart round baking dish with cooking spray.

2. **MELT** the butter in a medium saucepan over medium heat. Add the onion and cook for 5 minutes, stirring often, until softened. Sprinkle the flour, salt, and pepper over the onion and mix well. Add the milk and garlic-herb seasoning. Bring to a boil, reduce to a simmer, and cook for 2 minutes to thicken the sauce. Remove from the heat and stir in the tuna, mixed vegetables, and parsley. Spoon the tuna mixture into the baking dish.

3. **ROLL** out the crescent dough on a lightly floured board into a 10" x 6" rectangle. Cut the rectangle crosswise into 8 strips (about 1¼" wide). Weave 6 of the strips to form a lattice pattern on top of the pot pie. Place the remaining two strips around the inside edge of the dish to form a border.

4. **BAKE** for 40 minutes, or until the crust is browned and crisp and the filling is bubbling.

MAKE
IT A
MEAL

Mini (0.6 ounce)
dark chocolate
candy bar
90 CALORIES

420
CALORIES
PER MEAL
★ ★

MAKE
IT A
MEAL

1 cup strawberries
50 CALORIES

380
CALORIES
PER MEAL
★ ★ ★

PER SERVING (1 serving = 1¼ cups)

Calories	Total Fat	Saturated Fat	Sodium	Carbohydrate	Dietary Fiber	Protein	Calcium
330	12 g	4.5 g	670 mg	30 g	2 g	24 g	15%

GRILLED SALMON WITH RED PEPPER AND KALAMATA TAPENADE

PREP TIME: 10 MINUTES / **COOK TIME:** 10 MINUTES / **MAKES** 4 SERVINGS

Grilling salmon is a quick way to a satisfying and company-worthy meal. Our version is cooked very simply, then dressed up with a colorful homemade tapenade. Choose salmon fillets of uniform thickness so that they all cook in the same amount of time.

KALAMATA TAPENADE

- ½ cup chopped red bell pepper (about ½ medium)
- ¼ cup pitted kalamata olives (about 11)
- 2 tablespoons chopped fresh flat-leaf parsley
- 2 teaspoons olive oil
- 1 teaspoon fresh lemon juice
- 1 teaspoon capers, drained
- 1 clove garlic, halved
- ⅛ teaspoon freshly ground black pepper

SALMON

- 4 pieces (4 ounces each) salmon fillet
- 1 teaspoon olive oil
- ¼ teaspoon dried oregano
- ½ lemon

1. PREHEAT the grill to high.

2. TO MAKE THE KALAMATA TAPENADE: Combine the bell pepper, olives, parsley, oil, lemon juice, capers, garlic, and black pepper in a food processor. Process until smooth. Transfer to a small serving bowl and set aside.

3. TO MAKE THE SALMON: Place the salmon pieces, skin-side down, on a grill rack that has been coated with cooking spray. Brush the top sides with the oil and sprinkle with the oregano. Grill, uncovered, for 5 minutes. Carefully flip the fish over using two spatulas. Grill for 4 to 5 minutes, or until the fish just begins to flake in the center (test by flipping one piece back over and using a fork to flake it). Transfer to a serving platter and squeeze the lemon juice over the top of each piece.

4. SERVE family style, passing the tapenade alongside.

PER SERVING (1 serving = 1 salmon fillet, 2 tablespoons tapenade)

Calories	Total Fat	Saturated Fat	Sodium	Carbohydrate	Dietary Fiber	Protein	Calcium
260	17 g	3 g	270 mg	3 g	1 g	23 g	2%

SALMON PASTA PRIMAVERA

PREP TIME: 20 MINUTES / **COOK TIME:** 25 MINUTES / **MAKES** 6 SERVINGS

This dish works equally well with a short cut pasta like penne or fusilli. For a creamier sauce, stir the Parmesan cheese into the dish before serving.

1   pound skinless salmon fillet

8   ounces spaghetti

1   cup baby carrots, quartered lengthwise

1   cup 1" pieces asparagus

1   cup fresh or frozen haricots verts or baby string beans

1   tablespoon olive oil

2   cloves garlic

1   cup fresh or frozen peas

1   can (15 ounces) no-salt-added diced tomatoes

½   cup low-sodium vegetable broth

2   teaspoons salt-free Italian seasoning

½   teaspoon salt

¼   teaspoon freshly ground black pepper

½   cup grated Parmesan cheese

1. **COAT** a nonstick skillet with cooking spray and heat over medium-high heat. Add the salmon and cook for 9 to 10 minutes, turning once, until browned and the fish flakes easily with a fork. Transfer to plate and keep warm.

2. **BRING** a large pot of water to a boil. Cook the pasta according to package directions. Drain and place in a large serving bowl.

3. **MEANWHILE,** fill a large bowl with ice and cold water. Place the carrots and ¼ cup of water in a small micro-waveable bowl and microwave for 2 minutes. Drain the carrots and place in the ice water to stop the cooking. Microwave the asparagus with ¼ cup of water for 90 seconds, drain, and add to the ice water. Microwave the haricots verts with ¼ cup of water for 1 minute, drain, and place in the ice water.

4. **HEAT** the oil in a large skillet over medium heat. Add the garlic and cook for 1 minute. Drain the vegetables from the bowl of ice water. Add to the skillet along with the peas. Cook for 3 minutes to warm through. Add the tomatoes, broth, Italian seasoning, salt, and pepper. Cook for 5 minutes to heat through.

5. **ADD** the vegetable mixture to the drained pasta. Gently flake the salmon into 1" chunks, add to the pasta and vegetables, and gently toss. Top each serving with 1 rounded tablespoon Parmesan.

MAKE IT A MEAL

½ cup honeydew melon cubes
30 CALORIES

400 CALORIES PER MEAL
★ ★ ★

MAKE IT A MEAL

2 small (4½") sesame breadsticks
40 CALORIES

410 CALORIES PER MEAL
★ ★ ★

PER SERVING (1 serving = 2½ cups)

Calories	Total Fat	Saturated Fat	Sodium	Carbohydrate	Dietary Fiber	Protein	Calcium
370	12 g	3 g	390 mg	40 g	5 g	26 g	15%

SALMON FISH TACOS WITH HAWAIIAN CABBAGE SLAW

PREP TIME: 10 MINUTES / **COOK TIME:** 10 MINUTES / **MAKES** 4 SERVINGS

While the origin of fish tacos is hotly debated, with Mexico, Hawaii, and Southern California all laying claim, their popularity is beyond question. We give a nod to Hawaii by topping salmon with a tangy Hawaiian cabbage slaw. Our recipe variation leans toward its Mexican roots with a guacamole garnish on tilapia. (Be sure to wear plastic gloves when handling fresh jalapeños.)

MAKE IT A MEAL

½ cup juice-packed canned pineapple chunks
50 CALORIES

410
CALORIES
PER MEAL
★ ★ ★

MAKE the variation A MEAL

½ cup juice-packed canned pineapple chunks
50 CALORIES

380
CALORIES
PER MEAL
★ ★ ★

2	cups shredded or chopped green cabbage
½	small red onion, shredded or chopped
1	teaspoon minced jalapeño chile pepper
	Juice of ½ lime
2	teaspoons vegetable oil
1	teaspoon sugar
½	teaspoon salt
1	tablespoon chili powder
½	teaspoon ground cumin
½	teaspoon garlic powder
¾	pound salmon fillet
4	flour tortillas (7"–8")
½	cup fat-free (0%) plain Greek yogurt
4	tablespoons chopped fresh cilantro

1. COMBINE the cabbage, onion, jalapeño, lime juice, 1 teaspoon of the oil, the sugar, and ¼ teaspoon of the salt in a medium bowl. Refrigerate the slaw until ready to serve.

2. PREHEAT the broiler.

3. STIR together the chili powder, cumin, garlic powder, remaining ¼ teaspoon salt, and remaining 1 teaspoon oil to form a paste. Rub onto both sides of the salmon fillet. Broil the salmon about 8" from the heat for 4 minutes per side or until cooked through but still moist. When cool enough to handle, flake the salmon with a fork (discard the skin).

4. WARM the tortillas for 2 minutes in the oven or 10 seconds in a skillet over medium heat.

5. STIR ¼ cup of the yogurt into the cabbage slaw. Top each tortilla with ⅓ cup flaked salmon, ½ cup cabbage slaw, 1 tablespoon yogurt, and 1 tablespoon cilantro.

TILAPIA FISH TACOS WITH GUACAMOLE *(variation)*

SUBSTITUTE ½ cup guacamole for the cabbage slaw, using 2 tablespoons per taco.

SUBSTITUTE 1 pound of tilapia fillets for the salmon.

PER SERVING (1 serving = 1 taco) Tilapia Fish Tacos with Guacamole (1 serving = 1 taco)

Calories	Total Fat	Saturated Fat	Sodium	Carbohydrate	Dietary Fiber	Protein	Calcium
360	16 g	3 g	670 mg	31 g	3 g	24 g	10%
330	10 g	2.5 g	700 mg	29 g	3 g	29 g	10%

PAN-SEARED COD WITH GLAZED TOMATOES

PREP TIME: 5 MINUTES / **COOK TIME:** 22 MINUTES / **MAKES** 4 SERVINGS

Once popular fried and in fish sticks, scrod (young cod) and cod can be difficult to find. Mahi mahi, snapper, and other fish with a firm white flesh make suitable substitutes. The sweet-sour flavor of the glazed tomatoes plays off the clean taste of the fish.

3 teaspoons olive oil

2 cloves garlic, minced

1 pint grape or cherry tomatoes

¼ cup water

½ teaspoon salt

¼ teaspoon freshly ground black pepper

¼ cup balsamic vinegar

1 tablespoon sugar

4 scrod or cod fillets (4 ounces each)

1. **PREHEAT** the oven to 350°F.

2. **HEAT** 1 teaspoon of the oil in a large skillet over medium heat. Add the garlic and cook, stirring, for 1 minute. Add the tomatoes, water, salt, and pepper. Cook over medium heat for 10 minutes, stirring occasionally, until the tomatoes are soft and collapsed. Add the balsamic vinegar and sugar, and cook for 4 minutes, or until the vinegar has almost completely evaporated.

3. **RUB** all sides of the fillets with the remaining 2 teaspoons oil. Coat a large ovenproof skillet with cooking spray and place over medium heat. Place the fish in the skillet and sear on each side for 2 minutes. Place the skillet in the oven and bake for 3 minutes, or until the fish is cooked through and flakes easily with a fork.

4. **SERVE** the fish topped with the glazed tomatoes.

MAKE IT A MEAL

1 small (4 ounces) baked potato with 1 teaspoon unsalted whipped butter **135 CALORIES**

½ cup light vanilla ice cream **100 CALORIES**

405 CALORIES PER MEAL ★ ★

MAKE IT A MEAL

⅔ cup cooked brown rice **150 CALORIES**

Salad made with 1½ cups baby spinach, 1 diced medium tomato, 1 teaspoon olive oil, 1½ teaspoons balsamic vinegar **85 CALORIES**

405 CALORIES PER MEAL ★ ★

PER SERVING (1 serving = 1 fish fillet, ¼ cup tomatoes)

Calories	Total Fat	Saturated Fat	Sodium	Carbohydrate	Dietary Fiber	Protein	Calcium
170	4.5 g	0.5 g	360 mg	9 g	1 g	21 g	4%

HALIBUT PACKETS WITH ORANGE AND ASPARAGUS

PREP TIME: 20 MINUTES + 1 MINUTE STANDING / **COOK TIME:** 12 MINUTES / **MAKES** 4 SERVINGS

Cooking in a packet (en papillote in French) steams the contents while infusing them with the flavor of the seasoning. Try this cooking method with delicate fish, such as sole, as well as firmer fish, such as salmon.

MAKE IT A MEAL

1 small (4") whole wheat pita
70 CALORIES

½ cup honeydew cubes
30 CALORIES

380 CALORIES PER MEAL
★ ★

MAKE the variation A MEAL

⅔ cup cooked couscous
120 CALORIES

390 CALORIES PER MEAL
★ ★

¼ cup orange juice

¼ cup finely chopped shallots

2 teaspoons balsamic vinegar

2 teaspoons Dijon mustard

2 teaspoons grated orange zest

½ teaspoon salt

¼ teaspoon freshly ground black pepper

4 teaspoons extra-virgin olive oil

4 skinless halibut fillets (6 ounces each)

1 pound asparagus

½ cup diced tomato

1. **PREHEAT** the oven to 450°F. Cut 4 sheets of parchment (12" x 20" each) in half, short side to short side. Open back up and coat the sheet with cooking spray.

2. **COMBINE** the orange juice, shallots, vinegar, mustard, orange zest, salt, and pepper in a small bowl. Slowly whisk in 3 teaspoons of the oil.

3. **PLACE** a halibut fillet on half of each sheet of parchment. Toss the asparagus spears with the remaining 1 teaspoon oil and divide them among the pieces of parchment, placing them next to the halibut. Spoon the orange juice mixture over the fillets and asparagus, dividing it evenly among the packets. Sprinkle each with 2 tablespoons of tomato. Fold the parchment loosely over the filling and fold the edges in to seal the packet.

4. **PLACE** the packets on a large baking sheet. Bake for 10 to 12 minutes, or until the packets are puffed. Remove from the oven and carefully vent the top of each with the tip of a sharp knife. Let rest for 1 minute, place a packet on each of 4 serving plates, and carefully fold back the parchment.

PER SERVING (1 serving = 1 packet)
Halibut Packets with Lemon and Zucchini (1 serving = 1 fillet +1 cup zucchini)

Calories	Total Fat	Saturated Fat	Sodium	Carbohydrate	Dietary Fiber	Protein	Calcium
280	9 g	1.5 g	450 mg	10 g	3 g	38 g	10%
270	9 g	1.5 g	460 mg	8 g	2 g	37 g	10%

HALIBUT PACKETS WITH LEMON AND ZUCCHINI *(variation)*

SUBSTITUTE 2 tablespoons lemon juice for the orange juice.

SUBSTITUTE lemon zest for the orange zest.

SUBSTITUTE 4 cups diced zucchini (about 1 pound) for the asparagus.

ADD 1 teaspoon dried oregano.

CRISP CATFISH WITH LEMON TARTAR SAUCE

PREP TIME: 15 MINUTES / **COOK TIME:** 13 MINUTES / **MAKES** 4 SERVINGS

Cooking spray has just enough fat to help crisp the coating of these fish fillets without adding measurable fat or calories. Try this recipe with other flat fillets like sole.

3	tablespoons light mayonnaise
2	tablespoons sweet pickle relish
2	tablespoons fat-free plain yogurt
1	teaspoon grated lemon zest
2	tablespoons all-purpose flour
1	teaspoon paprika
2	large egg whites, lightly beaten
½	cup yellow cornmeal
4	catfish fillets (4 ounces each)
½	teaspoon salt
¼	teaspoon freshly ground black pepper

1. **PREHEAT** the oven to 450°F. Coat a large baking sheet with cooking spray.

2. **TO MAKE THE TARTAR SAUCE:** Combine the mayonnaise, pickle relish, yogurt, and lemon zest in a small bowl.

3. **COMBINE** the flour and paprika in a shallow bowl or pie plate. Place the egg whites in a second shallow bowl and the cornmeal in a third. Sprinkle the catfish with the salt and pepper. Working with one at a time, dredge both sides of the fillets in the flour, shaking off any excess. Dip in the egg whites and then in the cornmeal. Set on the baking sheet.

4. **LIGHTLY** coat the catfish fillets with cooking spray and bake for 7 minutes. Turn the catfish over, coat with cooking spray, and bake for 5 to 6 minutes, or until the fish is cooked through and crisp. Serve topped with the tartar sauce.

PER SERVING (1 serving = 1 fillet, 1¾ tablespoons tartar sauce)

Calories	Total Fat	Saturated Fat	Sodium	Carbohydrate	Dietary Fiber	Protein	Calcium
270	13 g	3 g	530 mg	18 g	2 g	21 g	2%

SWORDFISH SATAY WITH WARM PEANUT SAUCE

PREP TIME: 15 MINUTES + 30 MINUTES SOAKING / **COOK TIME:** 7 MINUTES / **MAKES** 4 SERVINGS

Swordfish satay follows the lead of classic chicken satay served in Thai restaurants everywhere. The peanut sauce can be made ahead of time and refrigerated until needed, then simply reheated in the microwave.

PEANUT SAUCE

¼	cup creamy peanut butter
3	tablespoons hot water
1	tablespoon light coconut milk
1	tablespoon fresh lime juice
1	teaspoon Thai fish sauce
1	teaspoon reduced-sodium soy sauce
1	teaspoon light brown sugar
1	clove garlic, minced
1	teaspoon grated fresh ginger

SATAY

2	cloves garlic, minced
1	tablespoon grated fresh ginger
1	teaspoon turmeric
½	teaspoon light brown sugar
1	tablespoon reduced-sodium soy sauce
1	tablespoon light coconut milk
1	tablespoon fresh lime juice
1½	pounds swordfish steak, skin discarded, cut into ¾" chunks

1. **SOAK** eight 10" wooden skewers in water for at least 30 minutes.

2. **TO MAKE THE PEANUT SAUCE:** Combine the peanut butter, hot water, coconut milk, lime juice, fish sauce, soy sauce, brown sugar, garlic, and ginger in a microwaveable bowl and whisk until smooth. Microwave for 30 seconds. Whisk and repeat. Set aside.

3. **PREHEAT** the grill to high.

4. **TO MAKE THE SATAY:** Whisk together the garlic, ginger, turmeric, brown sugar, soy sauce, coconut milk, and lime juice in a medium nonmetal bowl. Add the swordfish to the marinade and toss well to coat. Let marinate for 10 minutes while the grill heats.

5. **DIVIDE** the swordfish chunks evenly among the 8 skewers (discard the marinade). Place the skewers on a grill rack that has been coated with cooking spray. Grill for 2 to 3 minutes, flip and grill for 2 to 3 minutes longer, or until the fish is well marked and cooked through. Serve hot with the peanut sauce for dipping.

MAKE IT A MEAL

1 small zucchini brushed with ½ teaspoon sesame oil and grilled **40 CALORIES**

½ cup juice-packed canned pineapple chunks **50 CALORIES**

420
CALORIES PER MEAL
★ ★ ★

MAKE IT A MEAL

10 cherry tomatoes **30 CALORIES**

¼ cup mango sorbet **60 CALORIES**

420
CALORIES PER MEAL
★ ★ ★

PER SERVING (1 serving = 2 skewers, about 2 tablespoons sauce)

Calories	Total Fat	Saturated Fat	Sodium	Carbohydrate	Dietary Fiber	Protein	Calcium
330	15 g	4 g	500 mg	8 g	1 g	38 g	2%

QUICK CIOPPINO

PREP TIME: 15 MINUTES / **COOK TIME:** 32 MINUTES / **MAKES** 4 SERVINGS

Cioppino is a fisherman's stew made from the catch of the day. You can vary the ingredients based on your taste and which fish and shellfish are fresh at the market.

MAKE
IT A
MEAL

1 small
(1 ounce) slice
Italian bread
80 CALORIES

410
CALORIES
PER MEAL
★ ★

MAKE
IT A
MEAL

½ cup sorbet
80 CALORIES

410
CALORIES
PER MEAL
★ ★

1	tablespoon extra-virgin olive oil
1	onion, chopped
½	bulb fennel, chopped
3	cloves garlic, minced
1	teaspoon chopped fresh thyme
⅛	teaspoon lightly crushed saffron threads
½	pound red potatoes, cut into ½" cubes
1	can (14.5 ounces) diced tomatoes
1	bottle (8 ounces) clam juice
1	pound small mussels, scrubbed and debearded
½	pound peeled and deveined large shrimp
½	pound tilapia fillet, cut into 1" pieces

1. **HEAT** the oil in a large soup pot over medium-high heat. Add the onion, fennel, garlic, thyme, and saffron, and cook for 4 to 5 minutes, stirring occasionally, until starting to soften.

2. **ADD** the potatoes and cook for 2 minutes. Stir in the tomatoes and clam juice. Bring to a boil, reduce to a simmer, cover, and cook for 20 minutes, or until the potatoes are fork-tender.

3. **INCREASE** the heat to medium and bring back to a boil. Stir in the mussels, shrimp, and tilapia. Re-cover, return to a boil, and cook for 5 minutes, or until the mussels open and the seafood is cooked through. (Discard any mussels that do not open.)

PER SERVING (1 serving = 2 cups)

Calories	Total Fat	Saturated Fat	Sodium	Carbohydrate	Dietary Fiber	Protein	Calcium
330	8 g	1.5 g	820 mg	23 g	3 g	39 g	10%

SASHIMI-MELON CUBES WITH CARAMELIZED SOY SAUCE

PREP TIME: 20 MINUTES / **COOK TIME:** 7 MINUTES / **MAKES** 4 SERVINGS

This colorful appetizer is the perfect starter for a warm-weather dinner. Red watermelon can be used if yellow is not available, but the color contrast will not be as striking. Or, if you do use red watermelon, opt for white-flesh sushi-grade fish instead of tuna for visual appeal.

2	tablespoons reduced-sodium soy sauce
2	tablespoons sugar
½	pound sushi-grade tuna, cut into 20 blocks (1" x ½")
¾	pound yellow watermelon, trimmed and cut into 20 (1") cubes
20	chives, cut into 8" lengths

1. **COMBINE** the soy sauce and sugar in a small saucepan or skillet. Simmer over low heat for 7 minutes, or until the sauce is thick enough to coat the back of a spoon.

2. **PLACE** a tuna block on top of a watermelon cube. Gently tie a chive around the watermelon and tuna. Place on a serving tray. Just before serving, drizzle with the caramelized soy.

PER SERVING (1 serving = 5 cubes)

Calories	Total Fat	Saturated Fat	Sodium	Carbohydrate	Dietary Fiber	Protein	Calcium
110	0.5 g	0 g	310 mg	11 g	0 g	14 g	2%

MAKE IT A MEAL

3 ounces grilled flank steak
170 CALORIES

½ cup cooked Japanese or medium-grain white rice
120 CALORIES

2 cups raw spinach, steamed
20 CALORIES

420
CALORIES PER MEAL
★ ★

MAKE IT A MEAL

1 cup steamed edamame in the shell
100 CALORIES

¼ cup wasabi peas
140 CALORIES

10 unsalted brown rice crackers
70 CALORIES

420
CALORIES PER MEAL
★ ★ ★ ★

SUSHI TRIO

PREP TIME: 1 HOUR + 20 MINUTES COOLING / **COOK TIME:** 40 MINUTES / **MAKES** 4 SERVINGS

Once you get the hang of it, making your own sushi is easy and less expensive than buying it. If you don't have a bamboo mat, a small silicone baking mat works well and is easier to clean. Look for wasabi mayonnaise in the condiment or international section of your market or in an Asian grocery store.

MAKE
IT A
MEAL

1 cup miso soup
40 CALORIES

390
CALORIES
PER MEAL
★ ★

MAKE
IT A
MEAL

¼ cup shelled
edamame
50 CALORIES

400
CALORIES
PER MEAL
★ ★ ★

SUSHI RICE
- 1 cup short-grain brown rice
- 2 tablespoons rice vinegar
- 1 tablespoon sugar
- ½ teaspoon salt

SMOKED SALMON HAND ROLLS
- 2 sheets nori, halved crosswise
- ½ cup sushi rice
- 2 teaspoons wasabi mayonnaise
- 4 ounces smoked salmon, cut into 12 thin strips
- 2 scallions, finely chopped
- 1 hard-cooked egg, finely chopped
- 2 teaspoons salmon roe

1. TO MAKE THE SUSHI RICE: Cook the rice according to package directions. Remove from the heat.

2. MEANWHILE, combine the rice vinegar, sugar, and salt, and sprinkle over the cooked rice. Gently fold the rice to combine with the vinegar mixture, using a wooden spoon or rice paddle. Transfer the rice to a large plate and let cool to room temperature, about 20 minutes.

3. TO MAKE THE SMOKED SALMON HAND ROLLS: Place half a nori sheet diagonally on a cutting board with the point of one corner facing you. Place 2 tablespoons of the sushi rice in the middle of the nori sheet. Dip your fingers in water and use them to spread the rice so that it is 1" from each of the long sides and ½" from each of the short sides of the sheet. Spread ½ teaspoon of the wasabi mayonnaise over the rice. Lay 3 strips of smoked salmon on the rice vertically from the point facing you. Sprinkle 1 teaspoon of the chopped scallions alongside the salmon strips. Sprinkle 1 rounded teaspoon of the chopped egg alongside the scallions. Sprinkle ½ teaspoon of the salmon roe alongside the chopped egg. Fold up the corner of the nori sheet that's closest to you and place it over most of the fillings. Roll the nori starting from the right or left corner. The sushi will resemble a flat-bottom cone. Repeat with the remaining nori sheets and fillings.

PER SERVING (1 serving = 1 hand roll, 6 pieces California roll, 6 pieces tuna roll)

Calories	Total Fat	Saturated Fat	Sodium	Carbohydrate	Dietary Fiber	Protein	Calcium
350	8 g	1.5 g	810 mg	49 g	5 g	21 g	8%

CALIFORNIA ROLLS

- 2 sheets nori, halved crosswise
- 1 cup + 2 tablespoons sushi rice
- 2 tablespoons + 2 teaspoons mashed avocado or guacamole
- 3 ounces imitation crab or kamaboko fish cake, cut into thin strips
- ½ small cucumber, peeled, seeded, and cut into thin strips

TUNA ROLLS

- 2 sheets nori, halved crosswise
- 1 cup + 2 tablespoons sushi rice
- 4 ounces bluefin or other sushi-grade tuna, cut into ¼" strips

  Wasabi paste

  Pickled ginger

  Reduced-sodium soy sauce

4. TO MAKE THE CALIFORNIA ROLLS: Place half a nori sheet crosswise on a bamboo sushi mat or piece of foil with the long side facing you. Place a generous ¼ cup of sushi rice on the nori. Dip your fingers in water and use them to spread the rice to the edge of the nori on one long side and both short sides and about ¼" in from the second long side. Spread 2 teaspoons of avocado or guacamole over the rice. Place 2 rows of crab or kamaboko strips lengthwise down the center of the rice. If a single strip is too short, place 2 strips end to end so that the crab extends from one edge of the nori to the other. Place 2 rows of cucumber strips next to the crab, piecing them together as needed to extend from one edge to the other. Wet your fingertips or a brush to moisten the ¼" border along the long side of the nori. Starting on the long side nearest you, use the sushi mat to roll up the nori, pressing the moistened edge to hold the roll together. Cut crosswise into 6 pieces. Repeat with the remaining nori and fillings.

5. TO MAKE THE TUNA ROLLS: Place half a nori sheet crosswise on a bamboo sushi mat or piece of foil with the long side facing you. Place a generous ¼ cup of sushi rice on the nori. Dip your fingers in water and use them to spread the rice to the edge of the nori on one long side and both short sides and about ¼" in from the second long side. Place 2 rows of tuna strips lengthwise down the center of the rice. If a single strip is too short, place 2 strips end to end so that the tuna extends from one edge of the nori to the other. Starting on the long side nearest you, use the sushi mat to roll up the nori, pressing the moistened edge to hold the roll together. Cut crosswise into 6 pieces. Repeat with the remaining nori and fillings.

6. SERVE the rolls with wasabi paste, pickled ginger, and reduced-sodium soy sauce to taste.

STEAMED MUSSELS WITH WHITE WINE AND GARLIC

PREP TIME: 15 MINUTES / **COOK TIME:** 12 MINUTES / **MAKES** 4 SERVINGS

All types of shellfish are naturally lower in calories because they have so little fat. Crusty bread and spaghetti—both whole wheat for extra fiber—are perfect side dishes for soaking up the sauce.

1	tablespoon extra-virgin olive oil
1	onion, chopped
1	rib celery, chopped
6	cloves garlic, minced
1	cup white wine
¼	cup water
2	pounds mussels (40 medium, about 3" long), scrubbed and debearded
¼	cup chopped fresh basil

1. **HEAT** the oil in a large pot over medium-high heat. Add the onion, celery, and garlic, and cook, stirring often, for 3 to 4 minutes, or until the onion starts to soften and the garlic just starts to brown.

2. **ADD** the wine and water. Bring the mixture to a boil and cook for 3 minutes. Add the mussels, cover tightly, and cook for 4 to 5 minutes, until the mussels open (discard any that do not open). Stir in the basil and serve the mussels with the broth spooned over them.

PER SERVING (1 serving = 10 mussels)

Calories	Total Fat	Saturated Fat	Sodium	Carbohydrate	Dietary Fiber	Protein	Calcium
170	5 g	1 g	260 mg	9 g	1 g	11 g	6%

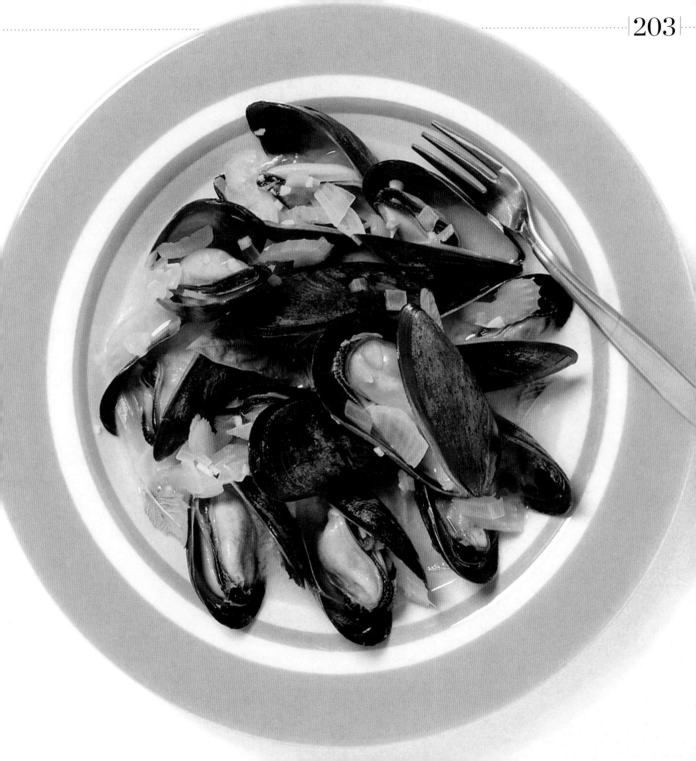

SHRIMP SCAMPI WITH ARTISANAL PASTA

PREP TIME: 10 MINUTES / **COOK TIME:** 14 MINUTES / **MAKES** 4 SERVINGS

A restaurant favorite, lemony shrimp scampi is easy to make at home. Offered alongside pasta (handmade for an indulgent touch, or regular curly fusilli) plus a simple salad, this dinner is sure to be a hit.

MAKE IT A MEAL

Salad made with 2 cups baby arugula and 1 tablespoon balsamic vinegar
20 CALORIES

410 CALORIES PER MEAL
★ ★

MAKE IT A MEAL

1 medium tomato, sliced and sprinkled with sea salt
20 CALORIES

410 CALORIES PER MEAL
★ ★

- ½ pound imported handmade pasta
- 2 teaspoons butter
- 2 teaspoons olive oil
- 5 cloves garlic, minced
- 1 shallot, minced
- ½ teaspoon coarse salt
- ¼ teaspoon freshly ground black pepper
  Pinch of red-pepper flakes
- 3 tablespoons fresh lemon juice
- ⅓ cup bottled clam juice or reduced-sodium chicken broth
- 1 teaspoon grated lemon zest
- 1 pound peeled and deveined large shrimp, tails removed
- ¼ cup finely chopped fresh flat-leaf parsley

1. **BRING** a large pot of water to a boil. Add the pasta and cook according to package directions. Reserve ½ cup of pasta cooking water, drain the pasta, and return it to the pot.

2. **MEANWHILE,** melt the butter with the oil in a large nonstick skillet over medium heat. Add the garlic, shallot, salt, black pepper, and pepper flakes. Cook for 3 minutes, stirring, until the shallot is softened. Add the lemon juice and clam juice. Increase the heat and bring to a simmer. Cook for 2 minutes to reduce slightly.

3. **ADD** the lemon zest and shrimp. Cook for 4 minutes, stirring once or twice, until the shrimp are pink and cooked through. Pour the shrimp mixture over the pasta and toss well. Add small amounts of the reserved pasta water as needed to thin the sauce. Serve garnished with the parsley.

PER SERVING (1 serving = 1¼ cups)

Calories	Total Fat	Saturated Fat	Sodium	Carbohydrate	Dietary Fiber	Protein	Calcium
390	7 g	2 g	470 mg	48 g	2 g	31 g	10%

SHRIMP ARRABBIATA

PREP TIME: 10 MINUTES / **COOK TIME:** 9 MINUTES / **MAKES** 4 SERVINGS

Arrabbiata is a spicy Italian sauce that usually pairs tomatoes and hot pepper, along with olive oil, herbs, and garlic. Try this dish with whole grain spaghetti to bump up the fiber.

- 8 ounces linguine
- 2 tablespoons extra-virgin olive oil
- ¾ pound peeled and deveined large shrimp
- ½ teaspoon salt
- 4 cloves garlic, minced
- 1 teaspoon dried oregano
- ¼ teaspoon red-pepper flakes
- 1 can (14.5 ounces) petite-cut diced tomatoes
- 1 tablespoon tomato paste
- 3 tablespoons chopped fresh basil

1. **BRING** a large pot of water to a boil. Add the linguine and cook according to package directions. Drain.

2. **MEANWHILE,** heat 1 tablespoon of the oil in a large nonstick skillet over medium-high heat. Sprinkle the shrimp with ¼ teaspoon of the salt and add to the skillet. Cook, turning once, for 1½ to 2 minutes per side, or until pink and cooked through. Transfer to a plate.

3. **ADD** the remaining 1 tablespoon oil to the skillet and heat over medium-high heat. Add the garlic, oregano, and pepper flakes, and cook for 45 seconds, or until the garlic is fragrant and just beginning to brown. Add the tomatoes and tomato paste, and cook for 3 minutes, stirring occasionally, until slightly thickened. Add the shrimp and remaining ¼ teaspoon salt and cook for 1 minute to heat the shrimp through. Remove from the heat and stir in the basil.

4. **SERVE** the linguine topped with the shrimp mixture.

MAKE
IT A
MEAL

½ cup marinated artichoke hearts
60 CALORIES

380
CALORIES
PER MEAL
★

MAKE
IT A
MEAL

4 ounces
white wine
100 CALORIES

420
CALORIES
PER MEAL

PER SERVING (1 serving = 1 cup pasta, ¾ cup shrimp mixture)

Calories	Total Fat	Saturated Fat	Sodium	Carbohydrate	Dietary Fiber	Protein	Calcium
320	8 g	1.5 g	600 mg	48 g	3 g	13 g	4%

DEVILED CRAB CAKES

PREP TIME: 20 MINUTES / **COOK TIME:** 20 MINUTES / **MAKES** 4 SERVINGS

This restaurant favorite is a snap to prepare at home. Be sure to use the best-quality crabmeat you can find.

¼ cup finely chopped fresh parsley

1 shallot, finely chopped (about ¼ cup)

2 large eggs, lightly beaten

2 tablespoons light mayonnaise

2 teaspoons Dijon mustard

2 teaspoons fresh lemon juice

¾ teaspoon seasoning salt

¼ teaspoon hot sauce

1 pound lump crabmeat

½ cup panko bread crumbs

1 lemon, cut into 8 wedges

1. **COMBINE** the parsley, shallot, eggs, mayonnaise, mustard, lemon juice, seasoning salt, and hot sauce in a large bowl and mix well. Stir in the crabmeat. Add the panko and gently mix until just combined.

2. **DIVIDE** the crab cake mixture into 12 even portions (¼ cup each) and form into balls.

3. **COAT** a large nonstick skillet with cooking spray and heat over medium heat. Add 6 balls of crab mixture to the pan. Coat the top of each portion with cooking spray, then gently press down on each with a spatula to flatten to about ½" thick. Cook for 3 to 5 minutes, until the crab cakes are golden on the bottom.

4. **FLIP** the crab cakes and cook for 3 to 5 minutes, or until cooked through. Transfer the crab cakes to a plate and cover with foil to keep warm. Repeat with the remaining balls of crab mixture to make 6 more cakes.

5. **SERVE** the crab cakes with the lemon wedges.

PER SERVING (1 serving = 3 crab cakes)

Calories	Total Fat	Saturated Fat	Sodium	Carbohydrate	Dietary Fiber	Protein	Calcium
190	4 g	0 g	840 mg	8 g	0 g	28 g	15%

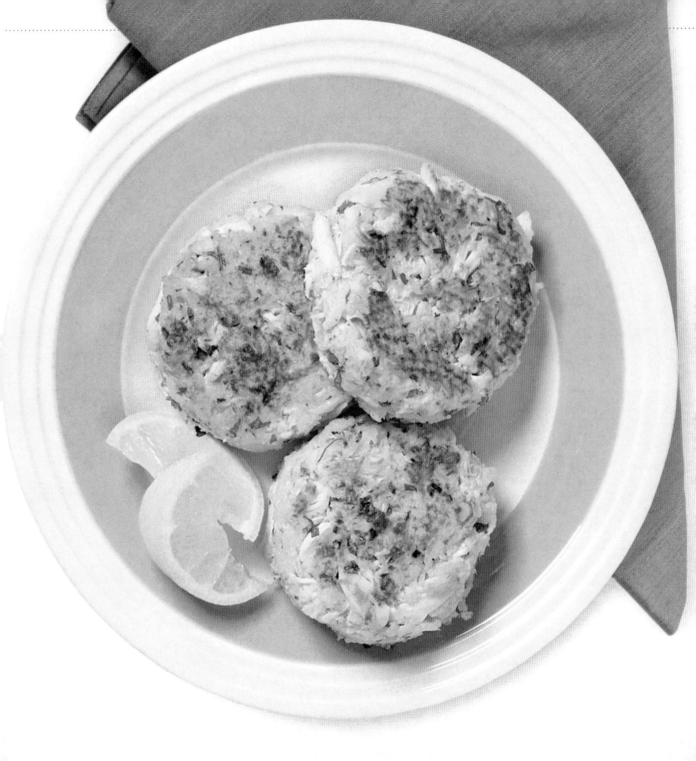

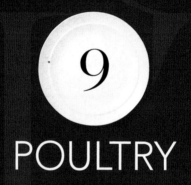

9

POULTRY

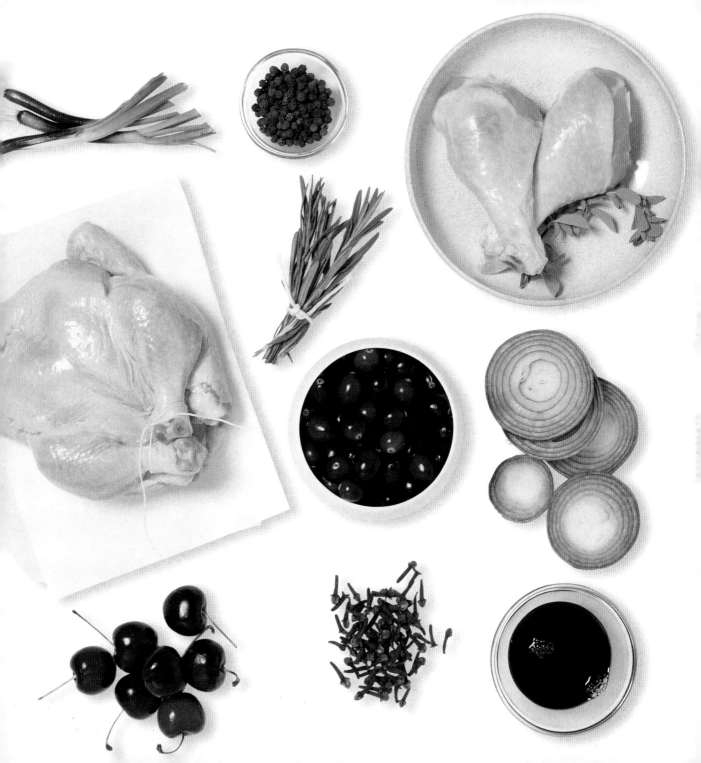

PAN-ROASTED CHICKEN BREAST WITH BALSAMIC REDUCTION

PREP TIME: 10 MINUTES / **COOK TIME:** 14 MINUTES / **MAKES** 4 SERVINGS

Keep individually wrapped chicken breasts in the freezer for a quick and elegant dish like this one. For a different flavor, use oregano in place of the thyme and honey instead of currant jelly.

MAKE IT A MEAL

½ cup cooked orzo
100 CALORIES

½ cup baked acorn squash
60 CALORIES

400
CALORIES PER MEAL
★

MAKE IT A MEAL

½ cup cooked white rice
100 CALORIES

½ cup steamed green peas
70 CALORIES

410
CALORIES PER MEAL
★

3   teaspoons extra-virgin olive oil
4   boneless, skinless chicken breast halves (4 ounces each)
⅜   teaspoon salt
¼   teaspoon freshly ground black pepper
⅓   cup chopped shallots
½   teaspoon chopped fresh thyme
½   cup fat-free, reduced-sodium chicken broth
½   cup balsamic vinegar
1   tablespoon sugar
3   tablespoons currant jelly
2   tablespoons chopped fresh basil

1. PREHEAT the oven to 350°F. Coat a baking sheet with cooking spray.

2. HEAT 2 teaspoons of the oil in a large nonstick skillet over medium-high heat. Sprinkle the chicken with ¼ teaspoon of the salt and ⅛ teaspoon of the pepper. Add the chicken to the skillet and cook for 2 minutes per side, or until browned. Transfer the chicken to the baking sheet and place in the oven. Bake for 8 to 10 minutes, or until a thermometer inserted into the thickest portion of the breast registers 170°F.

3. MEANWHILE, return the skillet to the heat and add the remaining 1 teaspoon oil. Stir in the shallots and thyme, and cook, stirring often, for 1 minute. Add the broth, vinegar, and sugar. Bring to a boil and cook, stirring occasionally, for 4 minutes, or until slightly thickened and reduced by about half. Stir in the jelly until dissolved. Remove from the heat and stir in the basil and the remaining ⅛ teaspoon salt and ⅛ teaspoon pepper. Serve the chicken with the balsamic reduction spooned on top.

PER SERVING (1 serving = 1 chicken breast, 2 tablespoons sauce)

Calories	Total Fat	Saturated Fat	Sodium	Carbohydrate	Dietary Fiber	Protein	Calcium
240	6 g	1 g	340 mg	21 g	0 g	24 g	2%

GREEK CHICKEN SKILLET DINNER

PREP TIME: 10 MINUTES / **COOK TIME:** 22 MINUTES / **MAKES** 4 SERVINGS

This easy skillet meal will satisfy your craving for Greek flavors with seasoned chicken and savory orzo with spinach, tomatoes, mint, and feta cheese.

1	tablespoon olive oil
¾	pound boneless, skinless chicken breasts, cut into bite-size chunks
2	cloves garlic, minced
½	teaspoon dried oregano
1	pint grape tomatoes
2½	cups fat-free, reduced-sodium chicken broth
2	tablespoons fresh lemon juice
1	cup orzo
1	package (6 ounces) baby spinach
3	scallions, finely chopped
2	tablespoons finely chopped fresh mint
¼	cup crumbled reduced-fat feta cheese

1. HEAT the oil in a large, deep nonstick skillet over medium heat. Add the chicken, garlic, and oregano. Cook, stirring, for 5 minutes. Add the tomatoes and cook for 5 minutes, stirring occasionally, until the chicken is almost fully cooked. Transfer the mixture to a bowl and set aside.

2. COMBINE 2 cups of the broth, the lemon juice, and the orzo in the same skillet. Bring to a boil over high heat. Reduce to a simmer, cover, and cook for 8 minutes, or until the orzo has absorbed the broth and is nearly tender.

3. RETURN the chicken and tomatoes to the skillet. Top with the spinach (don't worry, it will cook down a lot), pour the remaining ½ cup broth on top, and re-cover the skillet. Cook for 2 minutes to wilt the spinach. Stir in the scallions, mint, and cheese. Serve hot.

MAKE IT A MEAL

⅓ cup lemon sorbet
70 CALORIES

410
CALORIES
PER MEAL
★ ★

MAKE IT A MEAL

Salad made with ½ cup sliced cucumber, 1 teaspoon olive oil, 1 teaspoon lemon juice, ¼ teaspoon oregano
50 CALORIES

390
CALORIES
PER MEAL
★ ★

PER SERVING (1 serving = 1¼ cups)

Calories	Total Fat	Saturated Fat	Sodium	Carbohydrate	Dietary Fiber	Protein	Calcium
340	6 g	1.5 g	530 mg	42 g	5 g	30 g	10%

CHICKEN PROVENÇAL

PREP TIME: 5 MINUTES / **COOK TIME:** 51 MINUTES / **MAKES** 4 SERVINGS

This stew from the south of France makes a warming dinner on a cold winter night and is equally suited to pairing with a light salad for a spring supper. Black olives are more traditional in this dish, but we like the flavor imparted by green olives.

1	pound boneless, skinless chicken thighs
½	teaspoon olive oil
2	cloves garlic, minced
1	cup no-salt-added canned diced tomatoes
1	cup no-salt-added canned tomato sauce
½	cup fat-free, reduced-sodium chicken broth
½	cup dry white wine
1½	teaspoons herbes de Provence
1	teaspoon anchovy paste
½	teaspoon salt
¼	teaspoon freshly ground black pepper
¼	cup chopped fresh parsley
¼	cup sliced pitted green olives

1. CUT the chicken into 1½" pieces, trimming away and discarding excess fat. Set aside.

2. HEAT the oil in a medium saucepan on medium heat. Add the garlic and cook for 1 minute. Add the chicken, tomatoes, tomato sauce, broth, wine, herbes de Provence, anchovy paste, salt, and pepper. Stir to combine. Bring to a boil over medium-high heat. Reduce to a simmer and cook for 50 minutes to thicken the sauce, stirring occasionally and adjusting the heat as needed to maintain a gentle simmer.

3. STIR in the parsley and olives.

PER SERVING (1 serving = 1 cup)

Calories	Total Fat	Saturated Fat	Sodium	Carbohydrate	Dietary Fiber	Protein	Calcium
230	7 g	1 g	790 mg	10 g	2 g	24 g	4%

CHICKEN FRANÇAISE

PREP TIME: 10 MINUTES / **COOK TIME:** 20 MINUTES / **MAKES** 4 SERVINGS

Quick-cooking chicken cutlets are topped with a buttery, lemony sauce in this restaurant-fancy dish.

CHICKEN

2	tablespoons olive oil
2	tablespoons all-purpose flour
1	large egg
1	tablespoon water
4	thin-sliced chicken breast cutlets (about 14 ounces total)
	Pinch of freshly ground black pepper

SAUCE

3	tablespoons unsalted butter, cut into slices
1	teaspoon all-purpose flour
½	cup fat-free, reduced-sodium chicken broth
¼	cup white wine
2	tablespoons fresh lemon juice
¼	teaspoon coarse salt
⅛	teaspoon freshly ground black pepper
¼	cup chopped fresh flat-leaf parsley

1. TO COOK THE CHICKEN: Heat the oil in a large cast-iron or nonstick skillet over medium-high heat.

2. PLACE the flour on a small plate or piece of waxed paper. On a second small plate, whisk the egg with the water until well combined and thinned. Dredge each chicken cutlet in the flour (shaking off the excess), then quickly dip each side in the egg and place in the hot skillet. Sprinkle the top side of the chicken with the pepper and cook for 3 to 4 minutes, or until the bottom is crispy and nicely browned. Turn the cutlets over and cook for 3 to 4 minutes on the second side, until the chicken is cooked through at the thickest point (check by cutting into one piece). Transfer the chicken pieces to a plate lined with paper towels and cover with foil to keep warm.

3. TO MAKE THE SAUCE: Add the butter and flour to the same skillet and whisk over medium-high heat until melted. Add the broth, wine, lemon juice, salt, and pepper. Bring to a boil over high heat and cook for 5 to 8 minutes, stirring occasionally, until the sauce is reduced to about ⅓ cup.

4. WHEN the sauce has reduced and thickened, return the chicken cutlets to the skillet. Flip them to coat with the sauce and cook for 1 to 2 minutes to rewarm. Transfer the chicken to a platter, pour the sauce over all, and sprinkle with the parsley.

MAKE IT A MEAL

1 small (1 ounce) whole wheat roll
80 CALORIES

½ cup steamed broccoli
25 CALORIES

405
CALORIES PER MEAL
★

MAKE IT A MEAL

1 cup steamed carrots
50 CALORIES

1 cup strawberries
50 CALORIES

400
CALORIES PER MEAL
★ ★ ★

PER SERVING (1 serving = 1 chicken cutlet, 1½ tablespoons sauce)

Calories	Total Fat	Saturated Fat	Sodium	Carbohydrate	Dietary Fiber	Protein	Calcium
300	18 g	7 g	260 mg	5 g	0 g	25 g	2%

CHICKEN CURRY WITH VEGETABLES

PREP TIME: 35 MINUTES / **COOK TIME:** 20 MINUTES / **MAKES** 4 SERVINGS

This aromatic dish is flavored with garam masala, an Indian spice blend containing cinnamon and cardamom. For a different and equally delicious flavor, use a tablespoon of curry powder— sweet or hot, the choice is yours—in place of the garam masala, turmeric, coriander, and cumin. This curry freezes and reheats well, making it perfect for the brown bag gourmet.

MAKE IT A MEAL

½ cup cooked brown basmati rice
110 CALORIES

390
CALORIES PER MEAL
★ ★ ★

MAKE IT A MEAL

½ piece (1½ ounces) naan
100 CALORIES

½ cup fresh pineapple chunks
40 CALORIES

420
CALORIES PER MEAL
★ ★ ★

1   teaspoon canola oil
1   pound boneless, skinless chicken breasts, cut into ¾" pieces
½   onion, finely chopped
4   cloves garlic, minced
1   tablespoon grated fresh ginger
1   jalapeño chile pepper, seeded and finely chopped (wear plastic gloves when handling)
1½ teaspoons garam masala
¾   teaspoon turmeric
½   teaspoon ground coriander
½   teaspoon ground cumin
½   teaspoon coarse salt
¾   cup fat-free, reduced-sodium chicken broth
1   large head cauliflower, cut into bite-size florets (about 8½ cups)

1. COAT a large saucepan with cooking spray and place over medium-high heat. Add the oil and chicken, and cook, stirring, for 4 minutes, until almost cooked through. Transfer to a plate.

2. REDUCE the heat to medium and add the onion, garlic, ginger, jalapeño, garam masala, turmeric, coriander, cumin, and salt. Stir well to combine. Add the broth and cook for 3 minutes, or until the onion begins to soften.

3. STIR in the cauliflower and green beans. Cover and cook for 8 minutes, stirring once, until the vegetables are crisp-tender.

PER SERVING (1 serving = 2 cups curry, 1 tablespoon yogurt)

Calories	Total Fat	Saturated Fat	Sodium	Carbohydrate	Dietary Fiber	Protein	Calcium
280	7 g	3.5 g	490 mg	21 g	8 g	34 g	10%

½   pound green beans,
    cut into 1" pieces
1   cup light coconut milk
1   teaspoon grated lime zest
3   tablespoons finely
    chopped fresh cilantro
⅓   cup fat-free (0%) plain
    Greek yogurt

4. ADD the coconut milk and lime zest. Return the chicken (and any accumulated juices from the plate) to the pan and stir well. Bring to a simmer and cook for 5 minutes, or until the chicken is cooked through and the sauce has reduced slightly.

5. STIR in the cilantro. Garnish each serving with a generous tablespoon of yogurt.

SLOW-COOKER CHICKEN AND APPLE STEW

PREP TIME: 20 MINUTES / **COOK TIME:** 3–6 HOURS / **MAKES** 4 SERVINGS

Although they are a bit higher in fat and calories, chicken thighs are preferable to chicken breasts in slow-cooker dishes. They are particularly moist and tender when cooked on the low setting.

MAKE
IT A
MEAL

½ cup cooked
egg noodles
110 CALORIES

410
CALORIES
PER MEAL
★ ★ ★

MAKE
IT A
MEAL

½ cooked acorn
squash used as
an edible bowl
90 CALORIES

390
CALORIES
PER MEAL
★ ★ ★

1	pound boneless, skinless chicken thighs, halved crosswise, visible fat removed
1	pound baby carrots
2	cups shredded green cabbage
2	Granny Smith or other firm, tart apples, sliced into eighths
1	onion, chopped
1	can (14.5 ounces) fat-free, reduced-sodium chicken broth
½	cup apple cider (farmstand-style)
1	tablespoon finely chopped fresh sage
½	teaspoon salt
½	teaspoon freshly ground black pepper
¼	teaspoon garlic powder
1	tablespoon vegetable oil
1	tablespoon all-purpose flour

1. PLACE the chicken, carrots, cabbage, apples, and onion in a slow cooker. For a firmer texture, add the apples halfway through the cooking period. Combine the broth, cider, sage, salt, pepper, and garlic powder in a medium bowl and add to the slow cooker. Cook the chicken on high for 3 hours or low for 6 hours. Turn off the slow cooker.

2. JUST before serving, heat the oil in a small saucepan over medium-low heat. Stir in the flour and cook for 1 to 2 minutes, or until the flour just begins to darken. Add 1 cup of liquid from the slow cooker and stir to blend. Cook over medium-low heat, stirring, for about 2 minutes, or until the liquid begins to thicken. Gently stir the thickened gravy into the stew in the slow cooker.

PER SERVING (1 serving = 2 cups)

Calories	Total Fat	Saturated Fat	Sodium	Carbohydrate	Dietary Fiber	Protein	Calcium
300	8 g	1.5 g	710 mg	32 g	7 g	25 g	8%

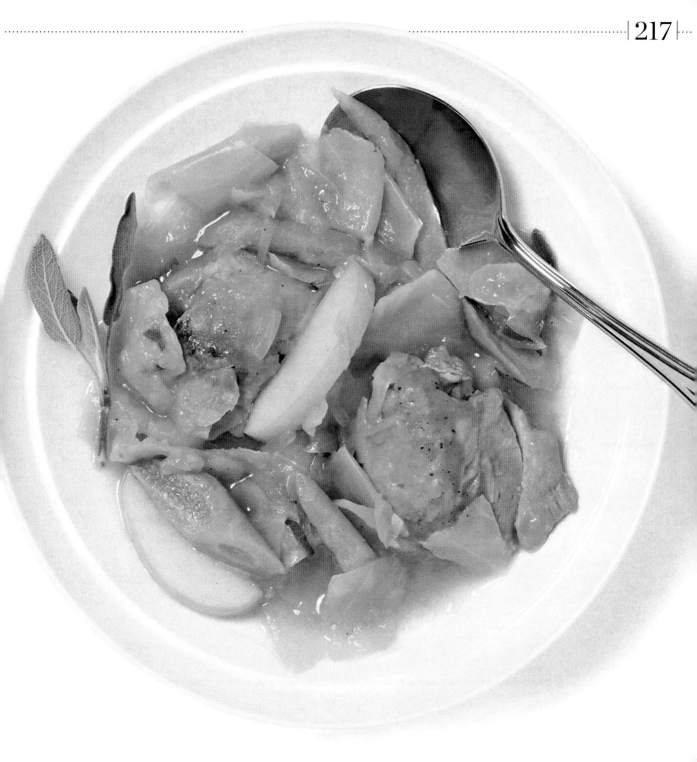

HOMESTYLE CHICKEN AND CAULIFLOWER CASSEROLE

PREP TIME: 10 MINUTES + 5 MINUTES STANDING / **COOK TIME:** 1 HOUR / **MAKES** 6 SERVINGS

Homemade white sauce is combined with sautéed leeks, seasoned chicken, brown rice, and cauliflower to yield a satisfying family-style entrée. Feel free to substitute broccoli for the cauliflower if you prefer.

3	cups cauliflower florets (from about ½ head)
1	can (12 ounces) fat-free evaporated milk
¼	cup all-purpose flour
⅛	teaspoon ground nutmeg
⅛	teaspoon coarse salt
3	cups cooked brown rice (leftover rice is ideal)
2	teaspoons olive oil
¾	pound thin-sliced chicken breast cutlets, cut into 1" pieces
2	leeks, white part only, well washed and cut into thin slices
2	cloves garlic, minced
1	teaspoon garlic salt
½	teaspoon poultry seasoning
¼	teaspoon freshly ground black pepper
1	egg white
½	cup shredded reduced-fat sharp Cheddar cheese

1. PREHEAT the oven to 350°F. Coat a 3-quart baking dish with cooking spray.

2. BRING ½" of water to a boil in a medium saucepan over high heat. Add the cauliflower, cover, and steam for 5 to 8 minutes, or until just crisp-tender. Drain and transfer to a large bowl.

3. COMBINE the evaporated milk, flour, nutmeg, and salt in the same saucepan. Cook over medium heat, whisking constantly, for 5 minutes, or until the sauce thickens. Pour the sauce over the cauliflower. Add the cooked brown rice to the cauliflower and set the bowl aside.

4. HEAT the oil in a large nonstick skillet over medium heat. Add the chicken, leeks, garlic, garlic salt, poultry seasoning, and pepper. Cook, stirring occasionally, for 6 to 8 minutes, or until the chicken is cooked through.

5. TRANSFER the chicken mixture to the bowl with the rice and cauliflower. Add the egg white. Stir well to combine all the ingredients, then transfer to the baking dish. Cover and bake for 15 minutes. Uncover and bake for 20 minutes, or until bubbling around the edges and heated through. Remove from the oven, sprinkle with the cheese, and let sit for 5 minutes before serving.

PER SERVING (1 serving = 1½ cups)

Calories	Total Fat	Saturated Fat	Sodium	Carbohydrate	Dietary Fiber	Protein	Calcium
310	5 g	2 g	410 mg	40 g	4 g	25 g	35%

CHICKEN KATSUDON WITH SNOW PEA SALAD

PREP TIME: 15 MINUTES / **COOK TIME:** 35 MINUTES / **MAKES** 4 SERVINGS

Katsudon (typically made with pork) is one of several donburi (Japanese meals-in-a-bowl). It's Japanese comfort food at its best—and a great way to use leftover rice!

¾   pound thin-sliced chicken breast cutlets

1   tablespoon Smart Balance spread, melted

⅓   cup panko bread crumbs

¼   teaspoon garlic salt

1½   cups fat-free, reduced-sodium chicken broth

¼   cup mirin (sweet rice wine)

2   tablespoons reduced-sodium soy sauce

1   onion, halved and very thinly sliced

2   large eggs, lightly beaten

8   ounces snow peas, lightly steamed

1   cup shredded carrot

1   teaspoon sesame seeds, toasted

3   tablespoons bottled light Asian-style salad dressing

2   cups leftover cooked brown rice, reheated

1   scallion, chopped

1. PREHEAT the oven to 425°F.

2. WORKING with one chicken cutlet at a time, brush one side with some of the melted spread, pat on some of the panko crumbs, and carefully transfer to a nonstick baking sheet. Spray the cutlets with a little cooking spray and sprinkle with the garlic salt. Bake for 20 to 25 minutes, or until golden. Transfer to a cutting board to cool slightly.

3. MEANWHILE, stir together the broth, mirin, and soy sauce in a small saucepan. Bring to a boil over high heat, reduce to a simmer, and add the onion. Simmer for 10 minutes, or until the broth is reduced by about half. Pour the beaten eggs over the broth and onion mixture, but do not stir it. Simmer gently for 1 minute.

4. HALVE the snow peas on the diagonal and toss them with the carrot in a medium bowl. Add the sesame seeds and dressing, and toss well. Set aside.

5. SLICE the cutlets crosswise into 1"-wide strips. Scoop ½ cup of hot rice into each of 4 bowls. Divide the chicken strips among the bowls, laying them on top of the rice. Ladle the egg and onion out of the broth and place it over the chicken (it should not cover all the chicken, so that some chicken remains crispy). Ladle additional broth around the sides of the bowl. Garnish each serving with a little chopped scallion and serve hot with the snow pea salad alongside.

MAKE IT A MEAL

½ cup honeydew melon cubes
30 CALORIES

400
CALORIES PER MEAL
★ ★

MAKE IT A MEAL

½ cup strawberries
30 CALORIES

400
CALORIES PER MEAL
★ ★ ★

PER SERVING (1 serving = ½ cup rice, 2 ounces cooked chicken, ½ cup onion/egg mixture, 1 cup salad)

Calories	Total Fat	Saturated Fat	Sodium	Carbohydrate	Dietary Fiber	Protein	Calcium
370	7 g	2 g	930 mg	43 g	5 g	28 g	8%

SLOW-COOKER COQ AU VIN

PREP TIME: 30 MINUTES / **COOK TIME:** 15 MINUTES + 4–8 HOURS / **MAKES** 6 SERVINGS

There is some prep involved with this slow-cooker recipe, but the results are worth it! With tender chicken, earthy mushrooms, and sweet carrots in a rich red-wine sauce, it has all of the elements of the classic dish. Boneless, skinless chicken thighs are available at most markets and are particularly well-suited to slow cooking. For a lighter flavor, switch to white wine or chicken broth.

MAKE IT A MEAL

½ cup cooked white rice
100 CALORIES

390 CALORIES PER MEAL
★ ★

MAKE IT A MEAL

1 medium slice (1½ ounces) baguette
120 CALORIES

410 CALORIES PER MEAL
★ ★

- 1 teaspoon olive oil
- 2 packages (12 ounces each) mushrooms, quartered
- 1½ teaspoons quick-cooking tapioca
- 1 pound carrots, cut crosswise into ½" slices
- 1 medium onion, finely chopped
- 1 tablespoon minced garlic
- 2 tablespoons real bacon bits or 1 slice cooked and crumbled bacon
- 2 packets (4 grams each) fat-free, salt-free chicken bouillon
- 1 teaspoon dried oregano
- 1 bay leaf
- ½ teaspoon coarse salt
- ½ teaspoon dried thyme
- ¼ teaspoon freshly ground black pepper

1. COAT a large nonstick skillet with cooking spray and place over medium heat. Add the oil and mushrooms, and cook for 5 minutes, stirring often, until the mushrooms start to give off some liquid. Increase the heat to medium-high and cook for 10 minutes, stirring occasionally, until the mushrooms are lightly browned and all of the liquid has evaporated.

2. MEANWHILE, begin layering ingredients into a slow cooker. Sprinkle the tapioca on the bottom of the cooker. Top with the carrots, onion, and garlic. Sprinkle the bacon, bouillon, oregano, bay leaf, salt, thyme, and pepper. Do not mix the ingredients together. Place the chicken thighs on top of the vegetables and seasonings.

PER SERVING (1 serving = 1 chicken thigh, 1 cup sauce/vegetables)

Calories	Total Fat	Saturated Fat	Sodium	Carbohydrate	Dietary Fiber	Protein	Calcium
290	8 g	2 g	440 mg	16 g	3 g	33 g	6%

6 boneless, skinless chicken thighs (2 pounds total, about 5 ounces each), trimmed of visible fat
¾ cup dry red wine
1 tablespoon tomato paste
1 tablespoon Dijon mustard

3. COMBINE the wine, tomato paste, and mustard in a small bowl. When the mushrooms are done cooking, pour the wine mixture into the hot skillet with the mushrooms. Let the liquid come to a simmer, then remove from the heat and pour the mixture over the chicken.

4. COVER and cook on high for 4 hours or low for 8 hours. To serve, push the mushrooms aside and use tongs to lift out the chicken thighs. Stir the vegetables and sauce together. Spoon 1 cup vegetables and sauce over each chicken thigh.

CHICKEN TERIYAKI

PREP TIME: 5 MINUTES + 4 HOURS MARINATING / **COOK TIME:** 14 MINUTES / **MAKES** 4 SERVINGS

Reduced-sodium soy sauce is significantly lower in sodium than regular soy sauce or teriyaki sauce, but it still has plenty, so use it judiciously to enhance flavor.

3	tablespoons reduced-sodium soy sauce
2	tablespoons honey
2	tablespoons natural rice vinegar
¼	teaspoon red-pepper flakes
4	boneless, skinless chicken thighs (4 ounces each), trimmed of visible fat

1. COMBINE the soy sauce, honey, vinegar, and pepper flakes in a bowl. Add the chicken and toss well to coat. Refrigerate for 2 to 4 hours, turning occasionally.

2. PREHEAT the broiler.

3. REMOVE the chicken from the marinade and set on a broiler pan coated with cooking spray. Pour the marinade into a small saucepan and bring to a boil over medium-high heat. Cook for 2 minutes. Remove from the heat and set aside.

4. BROIL the chicken 8" from the heat for 5 to 6 minutes, or until starting to brown. Turn over and broil for 4 minutes. Brush with the reserved marinade and broil for 2 minutes or until a thermometer inserted into the thickest portion registers 170°F.

MAKE
IT A
MEAL

½ cup steamed white rice
100 CALORIES

Salad made with ½ cup seaweed and ½ teaspoon sesame oil
40 CALORIES

1 medium orange
70 CALORIES

410
CALORIES
PER MEAL
★ ★

MAKE
IT A
MEAL

4 pieces (1 ounce each) California roll
170 CALORIES

½ cup steamed broccoli
30 CALORIES

400
CALORIES
PER MEAL
★ ★

PER SERVING (1 serving = 1 thigh)

Calories	Total Fat	Saturated Fat	Sodium	Carbohydrate	Dietary Fiber	Protein	Calcium
200	9 g	2.5 g	520 mg	9 g	0 g	21 g	2%

PAN-GRILLED CHICKEN TACOS WITH CORN AND BLACK BEAN SALSA

PREP TIME: 10 MINUTES / **COOK TIME:** 15 MINUTES / **MAKES** 4 SERVINGS

Chicken thighs are moister than chicken breast—they're a bit higher in fat—and take a couple minutes longer to cook. Trim off extra fat before cooking. If you're watching your sodium, make your own salsa with a combo of fresh corn, rinsed canned black beans, lime juice, tomato, and jalapeño pepper.

¾	small red onion, thinly sliced
½	jalapeño chile pepper, finely chopped (wear plastic gloves when handling)
1	tablespoon fresh lime juice
½	teaspoon ground cumin
½	teaspoon chili powder
½	teaspoon salt
⅛	teaspoon chipotle pepper powder
3	boneless, skinless chicken thighs (4 ounces each), well trimmed
8	corn tortillas (6")
1	cup shredded romaine lettuce
½	cup fat-free corn and black bean salsa

1. **COMBINE** the onion, jalapeño, and lime juice in a small bowl.

2. **MIX** the cumin, chili powder, salt, and chipotle powder in a separate small bowl. Rub the mixture over the chicken. Coat a nonstick grill pan with cooking spray and heat over medium-high heat. Add the chicken and cook for 6 to 7 minutes per side or until a thermometer inserted into the thickest portion registers 170°F. Transfer to a cutting board. When cool enough to handle, cut into strips.

3. **HEAT** the tortillas according to package directions. Top each with 2 tablespoons lettuce, 3 tablespoons chicken strips, 1 tablespoon of the onion mixture, and 1 tablespoon salsa and fold in half. Serve while the tortillas are still warm.

PER SERVING (1 serving = 2 tacos)

Calories	Total Fat	Saturated Fat	Sodium	Carbohydrate	Dietary Fiber	Protein	Calcium
250	8 g	2 g	490 mg	28 g	5 g	19 g	8%

MAKE IT A MEAL

½ cup fat-free refried beans
90 CALORIES

½ cup fresh fruit salad
50 CALORIES

390
CALORIES PER MEAL
★ ★ ★

MAKE IT A MEAL

Salad made with 2 cups romaine lettuce, 1 medium diced tomato, 2 tablespoons sliced black olives, 1 teaspoon olive oil, 1 teaspoon red wine vinegar
100 CALORIES

½ cup fresh fruit salad
50 CALORIES

400
CALORIES PER MEAL
★ ★ ★ ★

CHICKEN QUESADILLAS

PREP TIME: 15 MINUTES + 2 MINUTES STANDING / **COOK TIME:** 20 MINUTES / **MAKES** 4 SERVINGS

It's hard to tell the difference between regular and reduced-fat Cheddar in a cooked dish such as this one. You can add heat by using reduced-fat pepper Jack cheese instead.

2	teaspoons canola oil
1	onion, thinly sliced
3	cloves garlic, minced
⅛	teaspoon salt
2	flour tortillas (10")
8	ounces cooked chicken breast, shredded
¾	cup shredded reduced-fat sharp Cheddar cheese
2	tablespoons chopped fresh cilantro

1. HEAT the oil in a large nonstick skillet over medium-high heat. Add the onion, garlic, and salt. Cook, stirring occasionally, for 9 to 10 minutes, or until the onion is golden.

2. ARRANGE the tortillas on a work surface. Top the half closest to you with the onion mixture. Dividing evenly, top each with the chicken, cheese, and cilantro. Fold the top half of each tortilla over the filling to form a semicircle.

3. WIPE out the skillet and return it to medium heat. Add the quesadillas and cook, turning once, for 9 to 10 minutes, or until the cheese is melted and the outsides are lightly browned. Transfer to a cutting board and let cool for 2 minutes before cutting each quesadilla in half.

PER SERVING (1 serving = ½ quesadilla)

Calories	Total Fat	Saturated Fat	Sodium	Carbohydrate	Dietary Fiber	Protein	Calcium
300	12 g	4 g	510 mg	22 g	2 g	26 g	35%

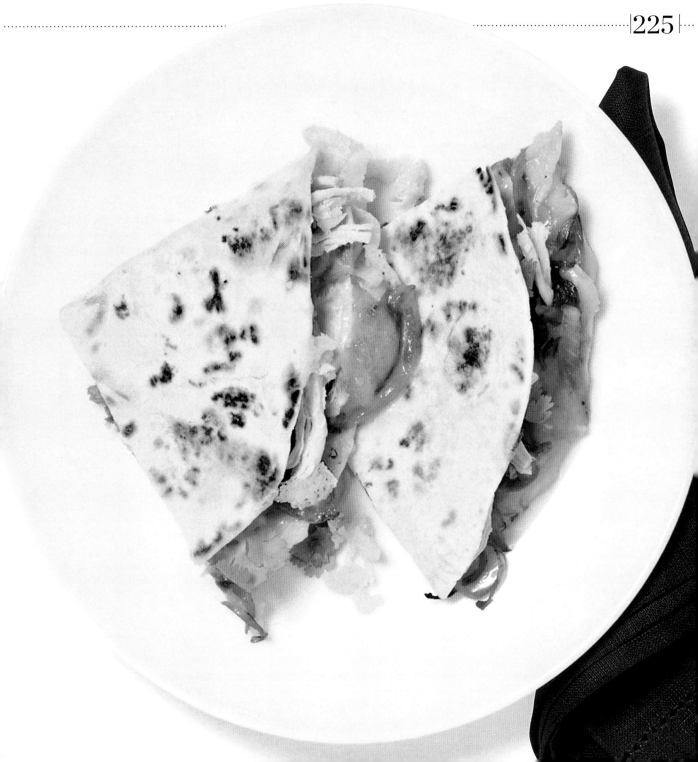

MARGARITA CHICKEN

PREP TIME: 5 MINUTES + 4 HOURS MARINATING / **COOK TIME:** 50 MINUTES / **MAKES** 4 SERVINGS

In this dish, the chicken is cooked with the skin on to help keep it moist. Decrease the cooking time if you choose to make the recipe with boneless, skinless chicken breast or thighs. The tequila can be replaced with additional orange juice, but that will change the flavor of the dish.

1   whole chicken (3 pounds)
½   cup orange juice
¼   cup tequila
    Grated zest and juice of 2 limes
1   tablespoon finely chopped jalapeño chile pepper (wear plastic gloves when handling)
1   tablespoon honey
1   clove garlic, finely chopped
½   teaspoon salt
¼   cup finely chopped fresh cilantro
1   teaspoon cornstarch mixed with 2 tablespoons cold water

1. CUT the chicken into 8 serving pieces: 2 thighs, 2 drumsticks, and 2 breasts cut in half. Reserve the wings and backs for another use. Place the chicken in a resealable plastic bag. Whisk together the orange juice, tequila, lime zest, lime juice, jalapeño, honey, garlic, salt, and 2 tablespoons of the cilantro in a small bowl. Pour over the chicken, seal the bag, and marinate for 2 to 4 hours, turning at least once to distribute the marinade.

2. PREHEAT the oven to 350°F. Place the chicken and marinade in a 13" x 9" baking dish or other baking dish large enough to hold the chicken pieces in one layer. Bake for 45 to 50 minutes, or until a thermometer inserted into the thickest portion of the thigh registers 170°F. Remove and discard the skin from the chicken pieces. Place the chicken on a platter, cover, and keep warm.

3. CAREFULLY pour the pan juices into a small gravy separator and let the fat rise to the top. Pour the juices (but not the fat) into a small microwaveable bowl (if you don't have a gravy separator, pour the juices into a glass measuring cup and use a turkey baster to remove as much of the juice mixture as possible without disturbing the fat layer). Stir the cornstarch mixture into the defatted juices. Microwave for 1 minute and then stir. Serve the chicken sprinkled with the remaining 2 tablespoons cilantro. Serve the sauce on the side.

PER SERVING (1 serving = 2 pieces chicken, 2 tablespoons sauce)

Calories	Total Fat	Saturated Fat	Sodium	Carbohydrate	Dietary Fiber	Protein	Calcium
270	4.5 g	1 g	420 mg	11 g	1 g	38 g	4%

MOROCCAN-SPICED GRILLED CHICKEN WITH ISRAELI COUSCOUS

PREP TIME: 10 MINUTES / **COOK TIME:** 15 MINUTES / **MAKES** 6 SERVINGS

A heady, sweet spice mixture adds exotic flavor to this quick-and-easy grilled chicken. Israeli couscous (sometimes called Moroccan couscous) is larger than the regular variety.

CHICKEN

- ½ teaspoon ground cinnamon
- ½ teaspoon ground cumin
- ½ teaspoon coarse salt
- ¼ teaspoon ground allspice
- ¼ teaspoon cayenne pepper
- ¼ teaspoon ground cloves
- 6 boneless, skinless chicken thighs (about 1¼ pounds total), trimmed of visible fat

COUSCOUS

- 1 tablespoon extra-virgin olive oil
- ½ medium onion, chopped
- 1 medium carrot, chopped
- 2 cloves garlic, minced
- ½ teaspoon ground ginger
- ¼ teaspoon coarse salt
- 1 cup Israeli couscous
- 1½ cups fat-free, reduced-sodium chicken broth
- ¼ cup slivered almonds
- 2 tablespoons raisins

1. TO MAKE THE CHICKEN: Combine the cinnamon, cumin, salt, allspice, cayenne, and cloves in a gallon-size resealable plastic bag. Add the chicken, close the bag, and shake to coat. Set aside.

2. TO MAKE THE COUSCOUS: Heat the oil in a medium nonstick skillet over medium heat. Add the onion, carrot, garlic, ginger, and salt. Cook, stirring, for 2 minutes, or until the onions have softened a bit. Add the couscous and stir to combine with the vegetables. Pour in the broth and stir. Bring to a simmer, reduce the heat to low, cover, and cook for 8 minutes, or until the couscous is tender and the liquid is absorbed. Add the almonds and raisins, and stir thoroughly

3. MEANWHILE, preheat the grill to high. Grill the chicken for 4 minutes per side, or until cooked through.

4. DIVIDE the couscous among 6 plates and top with a chicken thigh.

MAKE IT A MEAL

Salad made with ½ cup sliced cucumber, ½ cup sliced radishes, 1 teaspoon olive oil, ½ teaspoon za'atar (Middle Eastern seasoning) **60 CALORIES**

390 CALORIES PER MEAL ★ ★ ★

MAKE IT A MEAL

1 medium orange **70 CALORIES**

400 CALORIES PER MEAL ★ ★ ★

PER SERVING (1 serving = 1 chicken thigh, ⅔ cup couscous)

Calories	Total Fat	Saturated Fat	Sodium	Carbohydrate	Dietary Fiber	Protein	Calcium
330	14 g	3 g	440 mg	24 g	2 g	26 g	4%

GOLDEN ROAST CHICKEN WITH LEMON, GARLIC, AND ROSEMARY

PREP TIME: 15 MINUTES + 10 MINUTES STANDING / **COOK TIME:** 1 HOUR 25 MINUTES / **MAKES** 6 SERVINGS

Cooking chicken with the skin on helps keep the meat moist. The meat is protected by a thin membrane that prevents fat from soaking in.

MAKE IT A MEAL

½ cup cornbread stuffing
180 CALORIES

1 cup cooked broccoli
50 CALORIES

380
CALORIES PER MEAL
★ ★ ★

MAKE IT A MEAL

1 medium (6½ ounces) sweet potato, baked
100 CALORIES

1 cup cooked broccoli
50 CALORIES

2 small (½ ounce each) chocolate chip cookies
110 CALORIES

410
CALORIES PER MEAL
★ ★ ★

1	tablespoon chopped fresh rosemary
3	cloves garlic, minced
2	teaspoons extra-virgin olive oil
2	teaspoons fresh lemon juice
2	teaspoons grated orange zest
1	teaspoon grated lemon zest
½	teaspoon salt
¼	teaspoon freshly ground black pepper
1	roasting chicken (about 3 pounds)

1. PREHEAT the oven to 400°F. Coat a roasting rack and a 13" x 9" roasting pan with cooking spray.

2. COMBINE the rosemary, garlic, oil, lemon juice, orange and lemon zests, salt, and pepper in a small bowl.

3. REMOVE and discard the giblets and neck from the chicken and trim any excess fat. Loosen the skin over the breast and legs by inserting your fingers between the skin and meat and gently pushing. Rub the rosemary mixture under the loosened skin and over the breast and legs. Tie the legs with kitchen twine and tuck the wing tips under the chicken. Set the chicken on the rack in the roasting pan, breast-side down.

4. ROAST the chicken for 35 minutes. Carefully turn the chicken breast-side up and roast for 48 to 50 minutes longer, or until an instant-read thermometer inserted into the breast registers 180°F and the juices run clear. Transfer the chicken to a cutting board and let rest for 10 minutes before cutting into 6 serving pieces: 2 breast halves, 2 drumsticks, and 2 thighs. Remove the skin before eating.

PER SERVING (1 serving = 1 piece)

Calories	Total Fat	Saturated Fat	Sodium	Carbohydrate	Dietary Fiber	Protein	Calcium
150	4.5 g	1 g	280 mg	1 g	0 g	24 g	2%

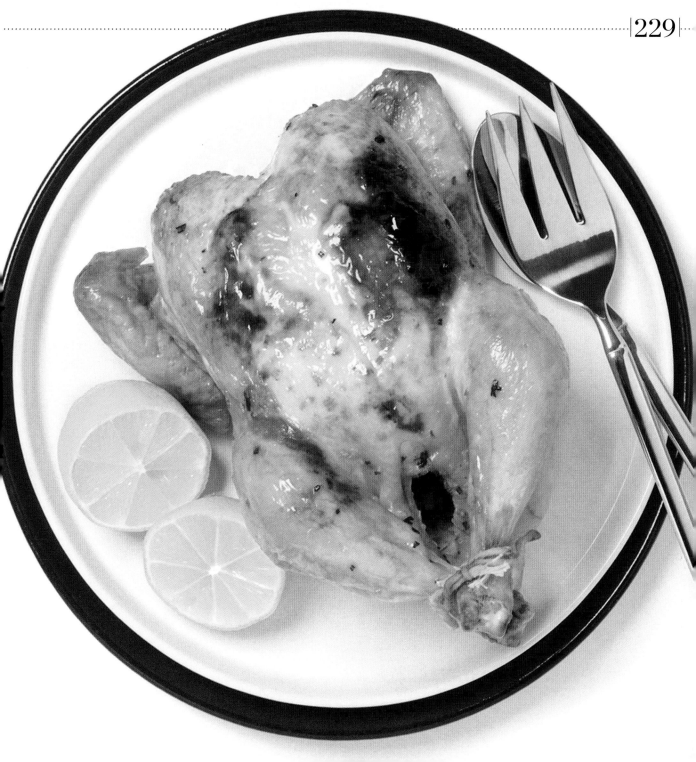

GRILLED SPICE-RUBBED CHICKEN THIGHS

PREP TIME: 5 MINUTES / **COOK TIME:** 24 MINUTES / **MAKES** 4 SERVINGS

This spice rub gives the thighs a traditional Southwestern flavor. The seasoning chart on page 26 can help you choose other classic seasoning combos, or buy a premixed seasoning blend to your liking.

2 teaspoons sugar
1 teaspoon chili powder
1 teaspoon ground coriander
¾ teaspoon ground cumin
½ teaspoon dried oregano
½ teaspoon salt
¼ teaspoon freshly ground black pepper
4 bone-in, skinless chicken thighs (6 ounces each), trimmed of visible fat

1. PREHEAT the grill to medium-high.

2. COMBINE the sugar, chili powder, coriander, cumin, oregano, salt, and pepper in a small bowl. Rub the mixture over both sides of the thighs. Set the chicken on a grill rack that has been coated with cooking spray. Grill for 12 minutes per side or until a thermometer inserted into the thickest portion registers 170°F.

PER SERVING (1 serving = 1 thigh)

Calories	Total Fat	Saturated Fat	Sodium	Carbohydrate	Dietary Fiber	Protein	Calcium
200	10 g	2.5 g	370 mg	2 g	0 g	24 g	2%

STUFFED TURKEY CUTLETS

PREP TIME: 20 MINUTES / **COOK TIME:** 40 MINUTES / **MAKES** 4 SERVINGS

*This recipe is suitable for a weeknight or the holidays, but without the fuss of a big turkey.
If gravy is not your style, remove the foil 10 minutes before the end of cooking time, brush the
tops of the turkey rolls with a little melted butter or margarine, and let them brown slightly.*

1	tablespoon Smart Balance spread
1	rib celery, finely chopped
¼	medium onion, finely chopped
4	slices (1 ounce each) whole wheat bread, cubed or torn into pieces
¼	teaspoon poultry seasoning
¼	teaspoon coarse salt
1	egg white
⅓	cup fat-free, reduced-sodium chicken broth
4	thin turkey breast cutlets (about 4 ounces each)
1	cup jarred turkey gravy

1. PREHEAT the oven to 350°F. Coat a 9" x 9" baking dish with cooking spray.

2. MELT the spread in a small skillet over medium heat. Add the celery and onion, and cook, stirring, for 5 minutes, or until the vegetables are softened. Transfer to a medium bowl. Add the bread cubes, poultry seasoning, and salt, and toss to combine. Stir in the egg white and broth.

3. POUND each piece of turkey between pieces of waxed paper to a ⅛" thickness. Spread ⅓ cup of the stuffing mixture onto each turkey piece toward the wide end. Roll up the turkey and place the rolls seam-side down in the baking dish.

4. COVER with foil and bake for 30 minutes. Remove from the oven, remove the foil, and top each turkey roll with ¼ cup gravy. Return the turkey to the oven for 5 to 10 minutes, or until the gravy is hot and the turkey is cooked through.

MAKE
IT A
MEAL

1 cup baked butternut squash cubes
80 CALORIES

½ medium pear
50 CALORIES

390
CALORIES
PER MEAL
★ ★ ★

MAKE
IT A
MEAL

1 cup roasted Brussels sprouts
60 CALORIES

Fat-free chocolate pudding snack cup
90 CALORIES

410
CALORIES
PER MEAL
★ ★

PER SERVING (1 serving = 1 turkey roll, ¼ cup gravy)

Calories	Total Fat	Saturated Fat	Sodium	Carbohydrate	Dietary Fiber	Protein	Calcium
260	5 g	1.5 g	730 mg	16 g	2 g	34 g	6%

TURKEY IN MOLE SAUCE

PREP TIME: 45 MINUTES / **COOK TIME:** 1 HOUR / **MAKES** 6 SERVINGS

This traditional recipe looks more daunting than it actually is, especially since the blender or food processor makes quick work of the grinding and pureeing. Many brands of unsweetened chocolate are extra rich in heart-healthy phytochemicals.

MAKE
IT A
MEAL

2 warmed corn
tortillas (6")
120 CALORIES

410
CALORIES
PER MEAL
★ ★ ★ ★

MAKE
IT A
MEAL

½ cup cooked
white rice
100 CALORIES

390
CALORIES
PER MEAL
★ ★ ★ ★

8	ancho (dried poblano) peppers
2	dried pasilla peppers
1	dried chipotle pepper or 1 canned chipotle pepper in adobo sauce
2	tablespoons sliced almonds
2	tablespoons unsalted peanuts
2	tablespoons hulled pumpkin seeds
2	tablespoons sesame seeds
1½	teaspoons vegetable oil
1	medium onion, chopped
3	cloves garlic, finely chopped
1	can (14.5 ounces) diced tomatoes
1	fresh tomatillo, husked and diced
¼	cup raisins
1	corn tortilla (6"), crumbled
½	teaspoon anise seeds
½	teaspoon ground cinnamon
½	teaspoon coarse salt
¼	teaspoon ground allspice

1. HEAT a large skillet over medium-high heat. Add the ancho, pasilla, and dried chipotle peppers (if using a canned chipotle, do not add it here) to the skillet, 3 or 4 at a time, and toast for 30 seconds on each side. Place the toasted peppers in a large heatproof bowl and cover with boiling water. Allow to sit for 45 minutes, or until soft.

2. MEANWHILE, place the skillet back over medium heat and add the almonds, peanuts, pumpkin seeds, and sesame seeds. Heat for about 1 minute, until they begin to brown and smell fragrant. Remove from the skillet and set aside.

3. COAT the skillet with cooking spray. Add the oil and heat over medium heat. Add the onion and garlic, and cook for 1 minute. Add the canned chipotle (if using), tomatoes, tomatillo, and raisins. Bring to a simmer over medium heat. Add the tortilla. Simmer for 1 minute. Remove from the heat and transfer to a food processor or blender. Add the toasted nuts, pumpkin seeds, and sesame seeds.

4. COMBINE the anise seeds, cinnamon, salt, allspice, coriander seeds, and black pepper in a spice grinder. Finely grind and add to the processor or blender.

PER SERVING (1 serving = 2 meatballs, ¾ cup sauce)

Calories	Total Fat	Saturated Fat	Sodium	Carbohydrate	Dietary Fiber	Protein	Calcium
290	15 g	4 g	320 mg	23 g	7 g	22 g	6%

¼ teaspoon coriander seeds

¼ teaspoon freshly ground black pepper

1½ ounces unsweetened chocolate, chopped

¼ cup chopped fresh cilantro

1 teaspoon light brown sugar

¾ cup fat-free, reduced-sodium chicken broth

1½ pounds 93% lean ground turkey

5. ADD the chocolate, cilantro, brown sugar, and broth to the processor or blender.

6. DRAIN the peppers. Wearing gloves, remove the stem, seeds, and membranes from the peppers and add the peppers to the processor or blender. Process to a smooth puree (makes 4 cups of mole sauce).

7. PREHEAT the oven to 350°F. Coat a large (at least 3-quart) round baking dish with cooking spray.

8. FORM the ground turkey into 12 meatballs (about ¼ cup each). Spread 1 cup of the mole sauce in the bottom of the baking dish. Gently place the meatballs over the sauce (in more than one layer if necessary). Top the meatballs with the remaining mole sauce. Bake for 1 hour, or until the sauce is bubbling and a thermometer inserted into a meatball registers 160°F.

HOLIDAY CHERRY TURKEY MEAT LOAF

PREP TIME: 25 MINUTES / **COOK TIME:** 1 HOUR / **MAKES** 4 SERVINGS

Great for a holiday weekend, this recipe incorporates the traditional flavors of turkey, sweet potatoes, and pumpkin pie. Sweet potato disks cook at the same time as the meat loaf.

410
CALORIES
PER MEAL
★ ★ ★

(variation)

410
CALORIES
PER MEAL
★ ★

4	sweet potatoes (6½ ounces each)
1	tablespoon olive oil
½	teaspoon pumpkin pie spice
¾	teaspoon salt
1	pound 93% lean ground turkey
1	large egg
½	cup whole wheat bread crumbs (from 1 slice bread)
¼	cup chopped dried tart cherries
¼	cup canned crushed tomatoes
¼	teaspoon freshly ground black pepper
1	cup frozen unsweetened pitted sweet cherries
¼	cup water

1. PREHEAT the oven to 375°F. Peel the sweet potatoes and cut them crosswise into ¼"-thick slices. Brush both sides with the oil and place the slices on a nonstick baking sheet. Sprinkle them with the pumpkin pie spice and ¼ teaspoon of the salt. Bake for 45 to 60 minutes or until lightly browned.

2. MEANWHILE, combine the turkey, egg, bread crumbs, dried cherries, tomatoes, ¼ teaspoon of the salt, and the pepper in a large bowl. Blend thoroughly but gently. Spray a 9" x 5" loaf pan with cooking spray and place the turkey mixture into the pan. Place in the oven along with the sweet potatoes and bake for 45 minutes, or until an instant-read thermometer inserted into the center registers 165°F and the meat is no longer pink.

3. WHILE the meat loaf and sweet potatoes are baking, make the cherry ketchup: Combine the frozen cherries, water, vinegar, ketchup, brown sugar, and the remaining ¼ teaspoon salt in a small saucepan. Tie the cinnamon, allspice, cardamom, and cloves (if using) in a small square of cheesecloth, or place the spices in a tea ball. Add the spice sachet to the saucepan. Cover and simmer the mixture over medium-low heat for 20 minutes to infuse the mixture with the spices. Let cool for 10 minutes and discard the spice sachet. Transfer the mixture to a blender (or use a hand-held blender right in the pan) and process

PER SERVING (1 serving = 1 slice meat loaf, 2 tablespoons cherry ketchup, 12 to 16 sweet potato disks)
Thanksgiving Cranberry Turkey Meat Loaf (1 serving = 1 slice meat loaf, 2 tablespoons cranberry ketchup, 12 to 16 sweet potato disks)

Calories	Total Fat	Saturated Fat	Sodium	Carbohydrate	Dietary Fiber	Protein	Calcium
410	12 g	3 g	680 mg	49 g	7 g	27 g	6%
410	12 g	3 g	680 mg	50 g	6 g	27 g	6%

- 2 tablespoons balsamic vinegar
- 1 tablespoon ketchup
- 1 tablespoon light brown sugar
- 1 small cinnamon stick, broken into small pieces
- 3 allspice berries
- 3 cardamom pods
- 3 cloves (optional)

to a smooth puree. Return the puree to the saucepan and simmer over medium-low heat for 10 minutes, or until the ketchup thickens.

4. CUT the meat loaf into 4 slices, and top with 2 tablespoons of cherry ketchup. Divide the sweet potatoes into 4 portions.

THANKSGIVING CRANBERRY TURKEY MEAT LOAF *(variation)*

SUBSTITUTE sweetened, dried cranberries for the dried cherries and fresh cranberries for the frozen cherries. Increase the brown sugar in the ketchup to 2 tablespoons.

TURKEY PICCATA

PREP TIME: 10 MINUTES / **COOK TIME:** 8 MINUTES / **MAKES** 4 SERVINGS

Invest in a high-quality nonstick skillet so that you can cook turkey and chicken cutlets without having to add a lot of extra fat.

1½ tablespoons all-purpose flour

1 teaspoon dried basil

½ teaspoon ground coriander

⅜ teaspoon salt

¼ teaspoon freshly ground black pepper

4 turkey breast cutlets (4 ounces each)

1 tablespoon extra-virgin olive oil

½ cup fat-free, reduced-sodium chicken broth

3 tablespoons fresh lemon juice

4 teaspoons capers, rinsed and drained

4 teaspoons unsalted butter

1. COMBINE the flour, basil, coriander, ¼ teaspoon of the salt, and ⅛ teaspoon of the pepper in a large bowl. Working with one at a time, dip both sides of the turkey cutlets into the flour mixture, shaking off the excess. Place on a large plate.

2. HEAT the oil in a large nonstick skillet over medium-high heat. Add the turkey and cook for 3 to 4 minutes, turning once, until lightly browned and cooked through. Transfer to a plate.

3. POUR the broth and lemon juice into the skillet and bring to a boil. Cook for 1 to 1½ minutes to reduce slightly. Stir in the capers and cook for 30 seconds. Return the turkey to the pan, turn to coat, and cook for 1 minute to heat through. Remove from the heat and swirl in the butter and remaining ⅛ teaspoon salt and ⅛ teaspoon pepper. Serve hot.

MAKE IT A MEAL

⅔ cup cooked angel hair pasta
150 CALORIES

1 medium steamed artichoke
60 CALORIES

410 CALORIES PER MEAL
★ ★ ★

MAKE IT A MEAL

⅔ cup cooked brown basmati rice
150 CALORIES

2 cups spinach sautéed in 1 teaspoon olive oil
60 CALORIES

410 CALORIES PER MEAL
★ ★

PER SERVING (1 serving = 1 cutlet, 2 tablespoons sauce)

Calories	Total Fat	Saturated Fat	Sodium	Carbohydrate	Dietary Fiber	Protein	Calcium
200	8 g	3 g	460 mg	4 g	0 g	29 g	0%

SMOKED TURKEY AND SHRIMP JAMBALAYA

PREP TIME: 10 MINUTES / **COOK TIME:** 20 MINUTES / **MAKES** 4 SERVINGS

This quicker-cooking version of the Cajun favorite is made with smoked turkey in place of sausage. If you prefer, substitute an equal amount of turkey kielbasa. Adjust the seasonings to your palate's tolerance for spiciness!

1	tablespoon olive oil
1	medium onion, chopped
1	medium green bell pepper, diced
2	ribs celery, chopped
3	cloves garlic, minced
1	can (14.5 ounces) no-salt-added diced tomatoes with Italian seasonings
2	teaspoons Worcestershire sauce
1	teaspoon Cajun seasoning
⅛	teaspoon freshly ground black pepper
2	packages (8.8 ounces each) microwave-ready unseasoned brown rice, or 3½ cups cooked brown rice
1	cup fat-free, reduced-sodium chicken broth
½	pound peeled and deveined shrimp
½	pound thick-sliced (¼") smoked turkey, cubed
	Hot sauce, for serving (optional)

1. HEAT the oil in a large soup pot over medium heat. Add the onion, bell pepper, celery, and garlic. Stir well and cook for 5 minutes, or until the vegetables are softened. Stir in the tomatoes, Worcestershire sauce, Cajun seasoning, and black pepper.

2. STIR in the brown rice and broth. Reduce to a simmer, cover, and cook for 4 minutes. Stir in the shrimp and turkey, re-cover, and cook for 5 to 8 minutes, or until the shrimp are pink and cooked through, and the mixture has thickened.

3. SERVE with hot sauce on the side, if desired.

MAKE IT A MEAL

1 cup juice-packed canned pineapple cubes
80 CALORIES

410
CALORIES PER MEAL

★ ★

MAKE IT A MEAL

Salad made with 1½ cups baby spinach, 1 diced medium tomato, 1 teaspoon olive oil, ½ tablespoon balsamic vinegar
85 CALORIES

415
CALORIES PER MEAL

★ ★ ★

PER SERVING (1 serving = 2 cups)

Calories	Total Fat	Saturated Fat	Sodium	Carbohydrate	Dietary Fiber	Protein	Calcium
330	7 g	1 g	880 mg	37 g	4 g	29 g	6%

ORANGE-GLAZED CORNISH HENS

PREP TIME: 25 MINUTES / **COOK TIME:** 45 MINUTES / **MAKES** 4 SERVINGS

Entertaining? This recipe is easy but impressive. Moist, oven-roasted hens are finished with a fragrant orange glaze.

MAKE IT A MEAL

½ cup wild rice/ brown rice pilaf
140 CALORIES

5 steamed asparagus spears
20 CALORIES

410
CALORIES
PER MEAL
★ ★

MAKE IT A MEAL

1 small (4 ounces) baked potato with 1 teaspoon unsalted whipped butter
135 CALORIES

5 steamed asparagus spears
20 CALORIES

405
CALORIES
PER MEAL
★ ★

2	Cornish hens (1½ pounds each), rinsed and patted dry
½	teaspoon coarse salt
½	teaspoon freshly ground black pepper
½	teaspoon dried thyme
1	teaspoon butter
2	tablespoons minced shallot
¼	cup fresh orange juice
2	tablespoons honey
2	tablespoons fresh lemon juice
1	tablespoon sugar
1	teaspoon Dijon mustard
1	teaspoon grated orange zest
1	navel orange, sectioned

1. PREHEAT the oven to 400°F. Coat a baking sheet with cooking spray.

2. CUT each hen in half lengthwise with a sharp, heavy knife. Place the halves skin-side up on the baking sheet. Sprinkle each half with ⅛ teaspoon of the salt, ⅛ teaspoon of the pepper, and ⅛ teaspoon of the thyme. Bake for 40 to 45 minutes, or until golden and cooked through.

3. MEANWHILE, melt the butter in a medium nonstick skillet. Add the shallot and cook, stirring, for 3 minutes or until softened. Add the orange juice, honey, lemon juice, sugar, and mustard, and whisk until smooth and simmering. Cook for 6 to 8 minutes, or until thick and marmalade-like. Remove from the heat and stir in the orange zest and orange sections.

4. AS soon as the hens are baked, brush each half with some of the glaze. Serve the hens with the remaining glaze and fruit spooned on top.

PER SERVING (1 serving = ½ hen, 2 tablespoons sauce)

Calories	Total Fat	Saturated Fat	Sodium	Carbohydrate	Dietary Fiber	Protein	Calcium
250	7 g	2.5 g	350 mg	20 g	1 g	26 g	4%

DUCK BREAST WITH CHERRY SAUCE

PREP TIME: 10 MINUTES / **COOK TIME:** 15 MINUTES / **MAKES** 4 SERVINGS

Use tart or sweet dried cherries, a combination of the two, or dried cranberries if cherries are hard to find. The sweet and tart sauce counterbalances the rich flavor of the duck breast.

3	teaspoons olive oil
4	boneless, skinless duck breast halves (4 ounces each)
¾	teaspoon salt
¼	teaspoon freshly ground black pepper
⅓	cup finely chopped shallots
⅓	cup port wine
¼	cup cherry preserves
1	tablespoon raspberry vinegar
1	tablespoon sugar
¼	cup dried cherries
2	teaspoons unsalted butter

1. PREHEAT the oven to 200°F.

2. HEAT 2 teaspoons of the oil in a medium nonstick skillet over medium-high heat. Sprinkle the duck with ½ teaspoon of the salt and ⅛ teaspoon of the pepper. Add to the skillet and cook for 4 minutes per side, or until browned and cooked through, but still slightly pink in the center. Transfer to a baking sheet and keep warm in the oven.

3. RETURN the skillet to medium-high heat and add the remaining 1 teaspoon oil. Add the shallots and cook for 1 minute. Stir in the port, preserves, vinegar, and sugar. Cook for 2 minutes to melt the preserves. Stir in the cherries and cook for 2 minutes, or until slightly thickened. Remove from the heat and stir in the butter and remaining ¼ teaspoon salt and ⅛ teaspoon pepper. Stir until the butter has melted. Serve the sauce over the duck breasts.

MAKE IT A MEAL

⅓ cup cooked egg noodles
70 CALORIES

Salad made with 2 cups mixed baby greens and 10 sprays salad dressing spray
30 CALORIES

400 CALORIES PER MEAL
★ ★

MAKE IT A MEAL

⅓ cup cooked mashed potatoes with ½ teaspoon unsalted whipped butter
55 CALORIES

½ cup steamed Brussels sprouts
30 CALORIES

385 CALORIES PER MEAL
★ ★

PER SERVING (1 serving = 1 breast half, about 3 tablespoons sauce)

Calories	Total Fat	Saturated Fat	Sodium	Carbohydrate	Dietary Fiber	Protein	Calcium
300	7 g	2 g	530 mg	28 g	2 g	24 g	2%

DUCK RAGÙ WITH PAPPARDELLE

PREP TIME: 55 MINUTES / **COOK TIME:** 1 HOUR 10 MINUTES / **MAKES** 4 SERVINGS

Roasted duck is swirled with thick, hearty noodles and a rich vegetable sauce. This ingredient list may seem lengthy, but many are common pantry items, and the recipe is quite simple. Get the duck into the oven before prepping the vegetables and it will come together quite easily.

MAKE IT A MEAL

1 small (1 ounce) crusty roll
80 CALORIES

400 CALORIES PER MEAL
★ ★

MAKE IT A MEAL

1 small pear
90 CALORIES

410 CALORIES PER MEAL
★ ★ ★

3 duck leg quarters (10 ounces each)
¾ teaspoon freshly ground black pepper
½ teaspoon dried thyme
1 teaspoon olive oil
2 cloves garlic, minced
2 shallots, finely chopped
4 medium carrots, finely chopped
3 medium ribs celery, finely chopped
1 bulb fennel, finely chopped (about 2 cups)
1 teaspoon dried oregano
½ teaspoon coarse salt
1 bay leaf
½ cup white wine
1 tablespoon tomato paste
1 cup fat-free, reduced-sodium chicken broth

1. PREHEAT the oven to 425°F. Coat a rimmed baking sheet with cooking spray.

2. PLACE the leg quarters skin-side up on the baking sheet and sprinkle evenly with ½ teaspoon of the pepper and the thyme. Bake for 35 to 40 minutes, or until cooked through. When cool enough to handle, discard the skin and cut the meat off the bone. Set the duck meat aside.

3. MEANWHILE, coat a large nonstick skillet with cooking spray and heat over medium-high heat. Add the oil, garlic, shallots, carrots, celery, fennel, oregano, salt, bay leaf, and remaining ¼ teaspoon pepper. Cook for 15 minutes, stirring occasionally, until the vegetables are soft. Add the wine and cook 5 minutes, until almost all of the wine has evaporated. Stir in the tomato paste, broth, and tomatoes. Bring to a simmer, then reduce the heat to medium-low.

4. AT the same time, bring a large pot of water to a boil. Add the pasta and cook according to package directions. Reserve ¾ cup of the cooking water, drain, and return the pasta to the pot.

PER SERVING (1 serving = 1⅓ cups)

Calories	Total Fat	Saturated Fat	Sodium	Carbohydrate	Dietary Fiber	Protein	Calcium
320	7 g	2.5 g	580 mg	41 g	4 g	20 g	15%

2½ cups coarsely chopped canned plum tomatoes

8 ounces pappardelle or tagliatelle pasta

¼ cup thinly sliced fresh basil

2 tablespoons finely chopped fresh parsley

⅓ cup grated Parmesan cheese

5. **ADD** the duck to the sauce and cook for 2 to 3 minutes to blend the flavors and reheat the duck. Pour the vegetables and duck over the pasta. Toss together the basil and parsley until evenly blended. Add about ¼ cup reserved pasta water to thin the sauce, adding more if necessary.

6. **SPOON** 1⅓ cups of pasta and sauce into each of 4 bowls. Garnish each serving with a generous tablespoon of Parmesan.

10

MEATS

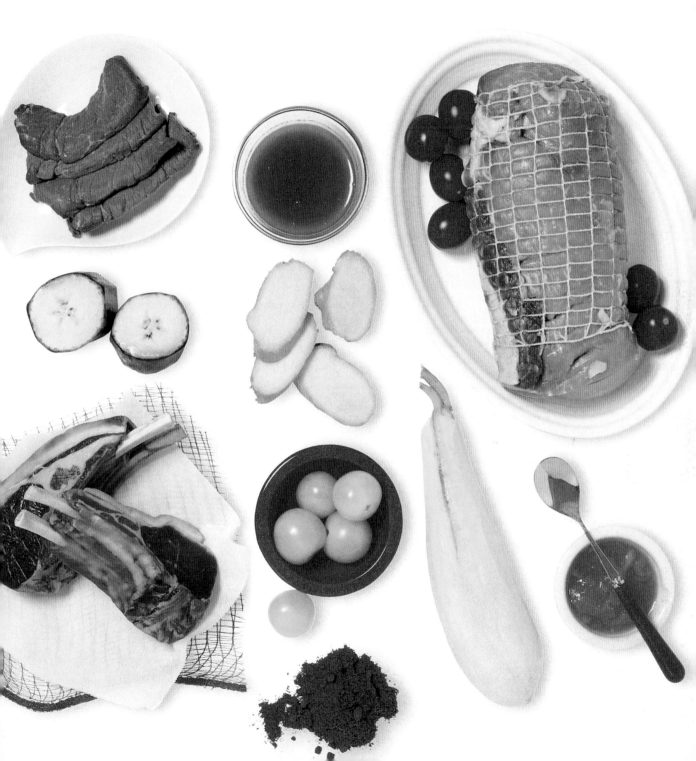

GINGER-APRICOT GLAZED PORK TENDERLOIN

PREP TIME: 5 MINUTES / **COOK TIME:** 30 MINUTES / **MAKES** 4 SERVINGS

Pork tenderloin is extremely lean and therefore prone to dryness if overcooked, so watch the internal temperature carefully. Cherry preserves make a colorful and tasty alternative to apricot.

1	tablespoon toasted sesame oil
3	cloves garlic, minced
2	tablespoons grated fresh ginger
⅛	teaspoon red-pepper flakes
⅔	cup apricot preserves
1	tablespoon reduced-sodium soy sauce
1	pound well-trimmed pork tenderloin
½	teaspoon salt

1. PREHEAT the grill to medium-high.

2. HEAT the sesame oil in a small saucepan over medium-high heat. Add the garlic, ginger, and pepper flakes, and cook for 45 seconds, stirring, until fragrant. Add the preserves and soy sauce, bring to a boil, and cook for 5 minutes, stirring occasionally to thicken slightly. Remove the saucepan from the heat. Measure out 2 tablespoons of the sauce and set aside.

3. SPRINKLE the pork with the salt and set it on a grill rack coated with cooking spray. Grill the pork for 9 minutes, then turn and brush with some of the ginger-apricot mixture. Grill for 9 minutes longer, turn, and brush heavily with ginger-apricot mixture. Grill for 2 minutes, turn, and brush again with the ginger-apricot mixture. Grill for another 2 minutes, brush with any remaining ginger-apricot mixture, and grill until an instant-read thermometer inserted into the thickest part of the tenderloin registers 160°F. Transfer the tenderloin to a cutting board and let rest for 10 minutes before cutting into 12 slices. Top each serving with 1½ teaspoons of the reserved sauce.

PER SERVING (1 serving = 3 slices pork, 1½ teaspoons sauce)

Calories	Total Fat	Saturated Fat	Sodium	Carbohydrate	Dietary Fiber	Protein	Calcium
290	7 g	1.5 g	490 mg	36 g	0 g	23 g	0%

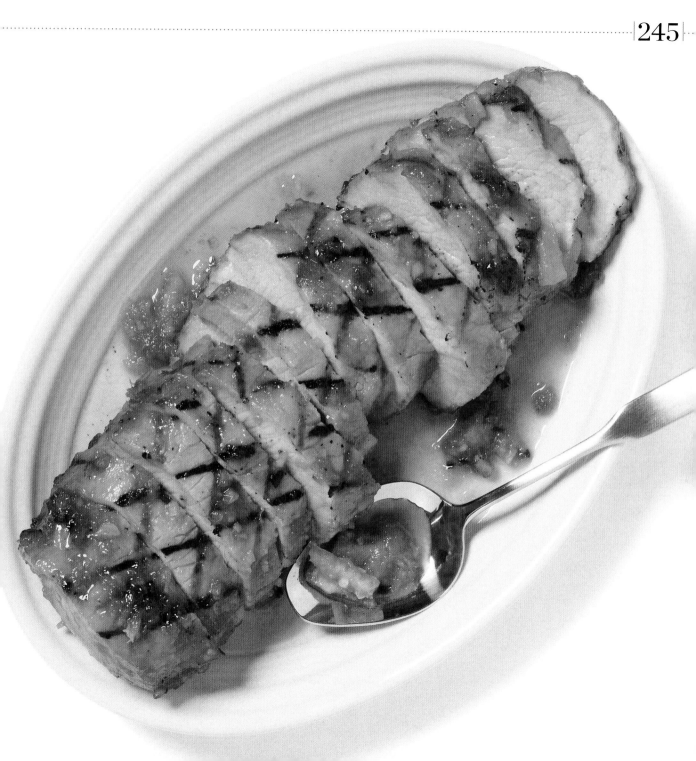

GRILLED TRI-TIP WITH A SMOKY RUB

PREP TIME: 5 MINUTES + 5 MINUTES STANDING / **COOK TIME:** 20 MINUTES / **MAKES** 4 SERVINGS

Tri-tip, also known as bottom sirloin, was virtually unknown outside of California until recently. This moderately lean cut is particularly well suited to grilling. If the steak is uneven in thickness, place the thickest side closest to the heat.

1 tablespoon light brown sugar
1 tablespoon smoked paprika
1 teaspoon mustard powder
1 teaspoon garlic powder
1 teaspoon freshly ground black pepper
½ teaspoon salt
⅛ teaspoon cayenne pepper
1 pound tri-tip steak

1. COMBINE the brown sugar, paprika, mustard powder, garlic powder, black pepper, salt, and cayenne in a small bowl. Rub all over the surface of the steak.

2. SET up a gas or charcoal grill for cooking over indirect heat. For gas, turn the burners on one side to medium-low and leave the other burners off. For charcoal, stack coals on one side only. Place the steak on the cool side of the grill. Cover the grill. Cook the steak for 8 to 10 minutes per side, or until the surface is browned and a thermometer registers 145°F for medium-rare or 160°F for medium.

3. LET sit for 5 minutes before carving into 12 thin slices.

PER SERVING (1 serving = 3 thin slices)

Calories	Total Fat	Saturated Fat	Sodium	Carbohydrate	Dietary Fiber	Protein	Calcium
180	7 g	2 g	350 mg	4 g	1 g	25 g	4%

STEAK WITH CREAMY MADEIRA ONIONS

PREP TIME: 5 MINUTES / **COOK TIME:** 30 MINUTES / **MAKES** 4 SERVINGS

Simple grilled steak gets gussied up with sliced sweet onions in a creamy Madeira wine sauce. The onions take quite a while to cook down, so be sure to get them cooking first.

2	tablespoons + 1 teaspoon olive oil
1	pound sweet onions, thinly sliced
14	ounces beef sirloin tip steak, trimmed of visible fat
½	teaspoon dried thyme
½	teaspoon coarse salt
1	cup fat-free, reduced-sodium beef broth
⅓	cup Madeira wine
1	tablespoon butter
2	tablespoons heavy cream
⅛	teaspoon freshly ground black pepper

1. HEAT 2 tablespoons of the oil in a large nonstick skillet over medium-low heat. Add the onions and cook for 15 to 20 minutes, stirring occasionally, until the onions are soft and quite brown. Be sure to finish cooking down the onions before grilling the steak.

2. MEANWHILE, preheat the grill to medium-high. Cut the steak into 4 equal pieces. Rub the top of the meat with the remaining 1 teaspoon oil. Sprinkle with the thyme and salt. Set aside until the grill is ready.

3. WHEN the grill is hot, place the steak, seasoned-side down, on a grill rack that has been coated with cooking spray. Grill for 7 minutes. (At this point, start the next step in making the onions.) Turn the steak and cook for 7 minutes on the second side, or until cooked to desired doneness (a thermometer inserted sideways in a steak will register 160°F for medium).

4. MEANWHILE, add the broth and wine to the onions in the skillet and increase the heat to medium-high. Cook for 6 minutes, stirring occasionally, until the liquid has reduced by half. Add the butter and cream, and cook for 2 to 3 minutes, until thickened and creamy. Season with the pepper.

5. TRANSFER the steaks to individual plates and spoon the onions alongside. Serve hot.

MAKE IT A MEAL

Salad made with 2 cups mixed baby greens, 1 teaspoon chopped walnuts, ½ teaspoon walnut oil **55 CALORIES**

415 CALORIES PER MEAL
★ ★ ★

MAKE IT A MEAL

1 grilled or broiled peach **60 CALORIES**

420 CALORIES PER MEAL
★ ★

PER SERVING (1 serving = 1 steak, ¼ cup onions)

Calories	Total Fat	Saturated Fat	Sodium	Carbohydrate	Dietary Fiber	Protein	Calcium
360	22 g	8 g	430 mg	12 g	1 g	24 g	4%

LONDON BROIL
WITH CHIMICHURRI SAUCE

PREP TIME: 15 MINUTES + 5 MINUTES STANDING / **COOK TIME:** 12 MINUTES / **MAKES** 4 SERVINGS

London broil is among the leanest cuts of beef. As with all lean cuts, avoid overcooking so that the meat stays moist and tender. Chimichurri is an Argentinean accompaniment for steak that combines shallots or garlic with olive oil and a variety of fresh herbs.

3	tablespoons chopped fresh cilantro
3	tablespoons chopped fresh basil
2	tablespoons red wine vinegar
2	tablespoons finely chopped shallots
5	teaspoons extra-virgin olive oil
½	teaspoon salt
¼	teaspoon freshly ground black pepper
1	pound London broil or flank steak, trimmed of visible fat

1. **PREHEAT** the broiler. Coat a broiler pan with cooking spray.

2. **COMBINE** the cilantro, basil, vinegar, shallots, oil, ¼ teaspoon of the salt, and ⅛ teaspoon of the pepper in a small bowl, and mix well.

3. **SPRINKLE** the steak with the remaining ¼ teaspoon salt and ⅛ teaspoon pepper. Broil the steak 4" from the heat, for 5 to 6 minutes per side for medium-rare or until desired doneness. Transfer to a cutting board and let rest for 5 minutes before slicing across the grain into 16 slices. Serve the chimichurri sauce alongside.

MAKE IT A MEAL

2 small (6")
corn tortillas
120 CALORIES

½ cup diced fresh
tomatoes
20 CALORIES

½ cup raspberries
30 CALORIES

**390
CALORIES
PER MEAL**
★ ★ ★

MAKE IT A MEAL

¼ cup sliced
Hass avocado
60 CALORIES

1 small (1 ounce)
slice Italian bread
80 CALORIES

1 cup cantaloupe
cubes
50 CALORIES

**410
CALORIES
PER MEAL**
★ ★ ★

PER SERVING (1 serving = 4 slices beef, 2 tablespoons sauce)

Calories	Total Fat	Saturated Fat	Sodium	Carbohydrate	Dietary Fiber	Protein	Calcium
220	12 g	3.5 g	340 mg	1 g	0 g	24 g	2%

TEXAS-STYLE BRISKET

PREP TIME: 10 MINUTES / **COOK TIME:** 2 HOURS / **MAKES** 6 SERVINGS

The generous portions in this hearty dish will please meat lovers. But they're relatively high in calories, leaving little room for side dishes like vegetables or dessert. You may prefer to cut down to a 3" slice—saving a bit more than 100 calories—to free up calories for more food, and a more satisfying meal.

BRISKET

- 2 tablespoons packed dark brown sugar
- 1 tablespoon chili powder
- 2 teaspoons ground cumin
- 2 teaspoons garlic powder
- 2 teaspoons smoked paprika
- ½ teaspoon salt
- ½ teaspoon freshly ground black pepper
- 2½ pounds lean center-cut brisket, trimmed

SAUCE

- 1 cup ketchup
- 2 tablespoons cider vinegar
- 2 tablespoons packed dark brown sugar
- 1 tablespoon molasses
- 1 tablespoon chili powder
- 1 teaspoon ground cumin
- 1 teaspoon garlic powder

1. PREHEAT the grill to medium.

2. TO MAKE THE BRISKET: Combine the brown sugar, chili powder, cumin, garlic powder, smoked paprika, salt, and pepper in a small bowl. Rub the mixture over both sides of the brisket to coat. Set the brisket, away from the heat source, on a grill rack that has been coated with cooking spray. Close the lid and cook the brisket, maintaining a 350°F to 375°F temperature, for 2 hours, turning once, until the brisket is cooked through and is moderately tender. Transfer to a cutting board and let stand for 10 minutes before slicing into 4¼" x 1" slices.

3. MEANWHILE, TO MAKE THE SAUCE: Combine the ketchup, vinegar, brown sugar, molasses, chili powder, cumin, and garlic powder in a small saucepan. Bring to a boil over medium-high heat, reduce to a simmer, and cook for 5 minutes, stirring often, until thickened. Serve the sauce at room temperature over the brisket.

MAKE
IT A
MEAL

½ slice Texas Toast*, cut on the diagonal
60 CALORIES

*Traditional Texas Toast is double-thick white bread (about 1¾ ounces per slice)

400
CALORIES
PER MEAL
★

MAKE
IT A
MEAL

½ cup cherries
50 CALORIES

390
CALORIES
PER MEAL
★

PER SERVING (1 serving = 1 slice, 2½ tablespoons sauce)

Calories	Total Fat	Saturated Fat	Sodium	Carbohydrate	Dietary Fiber	Protein	Calcium
340	8 g	2.5 g	790 mg	24 g	1 g	42 g	6%

STUFFED SQUASH WITH MOROCCAN-SPICED BEEF

PREP TIME: 10 MINUTES / **COOK TIME:** 1 HOUR / **MAKES** 4 SERVINGS

Oven-steaming the squash helps make it more tender. In place of acorn squash, you can use butternut, carnival, delicata, or other small-to-medium varieties.

2	teaspoons ground cumin
1	teaspoon ground cinnamon
1	teaspoon paprika
½	teaspoon turmeric
2	acorn squash (1 pound each)
1	pound 90% lean ground beef
1	medium onion, chopped
½	teaspoon salt
¼	teaspoon freshly ground black pepper

1. **PREHEAT** the oven to 400°F.

2. **HEAT** the cumin, cinnamon, paprika, and turmeric in a small skillet over medium heat for 1 minute, or until the spices turn slightly darker in color. Scrape into a medium bowl and set aside.

3. **HALVE** the squash lengthwise. Scoop out and discard the seeds.

4. **ADD** the beef, onion, salt, and pepper to the spices in the bowl, and gently but thoroughly combine.

5. **PACK** one-fourth of the beef mixture (about ¾ cup) into each squash half. Place the squash in a baking dish. Add 1" of water, cover with foil, and bake for 1 hour, or until the squash is tender and a thermometer inserted in the stuffing registers 160°F.

STUFFED SQUASH WITH SOUTHWESTERN PORK *(variation)*

SUBSTITUTE lean ground pork for the ground beef.

SUBSTITUTE 1 tablespoon chili powder for the paprika, cinnamon, and turmeric.

OMIT Step 2.

IN Step 4, combine the pork, onion, salt, pepper, cumin, and chili powder together in a bowl.

MAKE IT A MEAL

½ cup cooked brown rice
110 CALORIES

400 CALORIES PER MEAL
★ ★

MAKE the variation A MEAL

½ cup cooked brown rice
110 CALORIES

½ medium sliced banana
55 CALORIES

415 CALORIES PER MEAL
★ ★ ★

PER SERVING (1 serving = 1 stuffed squash half)
Stuffed Squash with Southwestern Pork (1 serving = 1 stuffed squash half)

Calories	Total Fat	Saturated Fat	Sodium	Carbohydrate	Dietary Fiber	Protein	Calcium
290	12 g	4.5 g	370 mg	22 g	4 g	25 g	10%
250	7 g	2.5 g	380 mg	22 g	4 g	26 g	10%

GREEK-STYLE MEATBALLS

PREP TIME: 25 MINUTES / **COOK TIME:** 22 MINUTES / **MAKES** 4 SERVINGS

These hearty meatballs are topped with a zesty feta and Greek yogurt sauce. Lean ground turkey breast is mixed with the ground lamb to reduce the fat content without sacrificing the flavor.

MEATBALLS
- ½ pound ground lamb
- ½ pound 99% lean ground turkey breast
- 1 large egg, lightly beaten
- 3 scallions, thinly sliced
- 1½ teaspoons grated lemon zest
- 1 tablespoon fresh lemon juice
- 1¼ teaspoons ground cumin
- 1¼ teaspoons dried oregano
- ½ teaspoon coarse salt
- ¼ teaspoon freshly ground black pepper
- ½ cup panko bread crumbs

FETA SAUCE
- 1 pickling cucumber
- 2 tablespoons fresh mint
- 2 tablespoons fresh parsley
- 1 container (6 ounces) fat-free (0%) plain Greek yogurt
- ¼ cup crumbled reduced-fat feta cheese
- ¼ teaspoon ground cumin
- ⅛ teaspoon hot sauce

1. **PREHEAT** the oven to 350°F. Line a baking sheet with foil and coat the foil with cooking spray.

2. **TO MAKE THE MEATBALLS:** Combine the lamb, turkey, egg, scallions, lemon zest, lemon juice, cumin, oregano, salt, pepper, and bread crumbs in a medium bowl, and mix until evenly blended. Divide the mixture in half and form each half into 8 golf ball–sized meatballs.

3. **TRANSFER** the meatballs to the baking sheet and bake for 10 minutes. Turn the meatballs over and bake for 10 to 12 minutes, or until cooked through.

4. **MEANWHILE, TO MAKE THE FETA SAUCE:** Peel and seed the cucumber. Finely chop the cucumber, mint, and parsley. Combine the yogurt, cucumber, feta, mint, parsley, cumin, and hot sauce in a small bowl, and stir until evenly blended.

5. **SERVE** the meatballs with the sauce alongside.

MAKE IT A MEAL

1 small (4") pita
70 CALORIES

2 tomato slices
10 CALORIES

400
CALORIES PER MEAL
★

MAKE IT A MEAL

Salad with 1 cup romaine lettuce, 3 Greek olives, 4 cherry tomatoes, 1 teaspoon olive oil, ½ teaspoon red wine vinegar
90 CALORIES

410
CALORIES PER MEAL
★ ★ ★

PER SERVING (1 serving = 4 meatballs, ¼ cup sauce)

Calories	Total Fat	Saturated Fat	Sodium	Carbohydrate	Dietary Fiber	Protein	Calcium
320	17 g	7 g	480 mg	10 g	2 g	32 g	10%

MOROCCAN LAMB CHOPS WITH ORANGE RELISH

PREP TIME: 15 MINUTES / **COOK TIME:** 8 MINUTES / **MAKES** 4 SERVINGS

Trim the chops well to remove as much extra fat as possible before seasoning and grilling. Look for reasonably priced lamb chops imported from Australia or New Zealand. The Israeli couscous for the side dish is a type of large couscous (sometimes called Moroccan couscous), with spheres the size of split peas. Look for it in the international aisle of your market or substitute regular couscous if it is not available.

MAKE
IT A
MEAL

½ cup cooked
Israeli or Moroccan
couscous
110 CALORIES

390
**CALORIES
PER MEAL**
★

MAKE
IT A
MEAL

½ cup wild rice or
brown rice pilaf
140 CALORIES

420
**CALORIES
PER MEAL**
★

3 navel oranges, peeled and coarsely chopped

3 tablespoons dried currants

3 tablespoons finely chopped red onion

2 tablespoons chopped fresh basil

½ teaspoon salt

¾ teaspoon ground cumin

¼ teaspoon ground allspice

¼ teaspoon ground coriander

¼ teaspoon freshly ground black pepper

⅛ teaspoon ground cinnamon

⅛ teaspoon ground ginger

8 bone-in loin lamb chops (4 ounces each), well trimmed

1. **PREHEAT** the grill to medium-high.

2. **COMBINE** the oranges, currants, onion, basil, and ¼ teaspoon of the salt in a small bowl and mix well.

3. **MIX** the cumin, allspice, coriander, pepper, cinnamon, ginger, and remaining ¼ teaspoon salt in another small bowl. Sprinkle over both sides of the lamb chops to coat.

4. **SET** the lamb on a grill rack coated with cooking spray and grill for 3½ to 4 minutes per side, or until well marked and cooked to medium-rare. Serve with the orange relish.

PER SERVING (1 serving = 2 chops, ¾ cup relish)

Calories	Total Fat	Saturated Fat	Sodium	Carbohydrate	Dietary Fiber	Protein	Calcium
280	10 g	3.5 g	450 mg	19 g	3 g	30 g	8%

SLOW-COOKER MEAT SAUCE WITH POLENTA

PREP TIME: 10 MINUTES / **COOK TIME:** 2 TO 4 HOURS / **MAKES** 4 SERVINGS

The key to lump-free polenta is to pour the polenta in slowly while whisking constantly. For a firm texture, pour the polenta into a small pan, let cool, and cut into rectangles. Warm for 30 seconds in the microwave before topping with sauce.

MEAT SAUCE

- ¾ pound extra-lean ground beef
- 1 medium onion, chopped
- 3 cloves garlic, minced
- 1 teaspoon dried basil
- 1 can (14.5 ounces) no-salt-added diced tomatoes
- ¼ cup tomato paste
- ½ cup water
- ¼ teaspoon salt
- ⅛ teaspoon freshly ground black pepper

POLENTA

- 2 cups fat-free milk
- 1½ cups water
- ¼ teaspoon salt
- ⅛ teaspoon freshly ground black pepper
- ⅔ cup instant polenta
- ½ cup grated Romano cheese

1. TO MAKE THE MEAT SAUCE: Combine the beef, onion, garlic, basil, diced tomatoes, tomato paste, water, salt, and pepper in a slow cooker. Cook for 2 hours on high or 4 hours on low.

2. TO MAKE THE POLENTA: Combine the milk, water, salt, and pepper in a medium saucepan over medium-high heat. Bring just to a boil. Whisking constantly, add the polenta in a slow, steady stream. Cook for 4 to 5 minutes, stirring constantly, until thick and creamy. Remove from the heat and stir in the cheese. Serve the polenta topped with the beef sauce.

MAKE IT A MEAL

Salad made with 2 cups romaine lettuce, 1 tablespoon chopped pecans, 10 sprays salad dressing spray **80 CALORIES**

410 CALORIES PER MEAL ★ ★ ★

MAKE IT A MEAL

Salad made with 2 cups torn escarole, ½ small diced pear, 10 sprays salad dressing spray **70 CALORIES**

400 CALORIES PER MEAL ★ ★ ★

PER SERVING (1 serving = ¾ cup polenta, 1 cup beef sauce)

Calories	Total Fat	Saturated Fat	Sodium	Carbohydrate	Dietary Fiber	Protein	Calcium
330	8 g	4 g	790 mg	34 g	3 g	28 g	35%

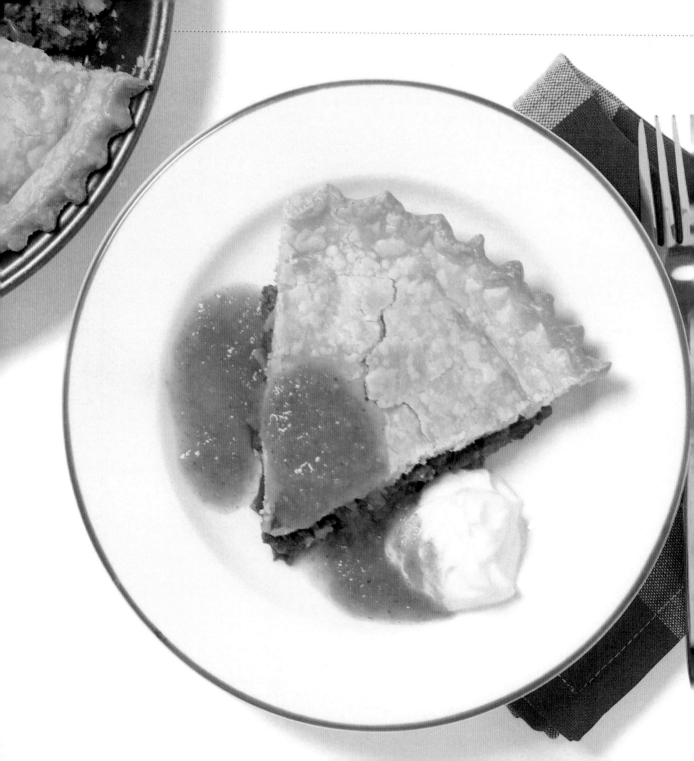

EMPANADA PIE

PREP TIME: 20 MINUTES + 10 MINUTES RESTING / **COOK TIME:** 45 MINUTES / **MAKES** 6 SERVINGS

Empanadas are savory, beef-filled hand pies with a spicy kick, thanks to their South American roots. This pie simplifies the concept for weeknight practicality.

1	tablespoon olive oil
½	onion, chopped
½	green bell pepper, chopped
2	cloves garlic, minced
1	pound 90% lean ground sirloin
1	teaspoon dried oregano
1	teaspoon ground cumin
1	teaspoon green hot pepper sauce
¼	teaspoon coarse salt
⅛	teaspoon ground cinnamon
1	can (10 ounces) diced tomatoes with green chiles (such as Ro-Tel)
1	can (8 ounces) no-salt-added tomato sauce
1	refrigerated pie crust (7.5 ounces)
¾	cup green salsa
¾	cup low-fat plain yogurt

1. **PREHEAT** the oven to 400°F. Coat a 9" pie plate with cooking spray.

2. **HEAT** the oil in a large nonstick skillet over medium heat. Add the onion, bell pepper, and garlic, and cook, stirring, for 3 to 5 minutes, until the onion and pepper have softened. Add the beef and cook, breaking up the meat with a spoon, for 6 to 8 minutes, or until the meat is no longer pink.

3. **ADD** the oregano, cumin, hot sauce, salt, and cinnamon, and stir to combine. Add the diced tomatoes and tomato sauce and stir well. Bring the mixture to a simmer and cook for 5 minutes to thicken slightly and blend the flavors. Pour the meat mixture into the pie plate.

4. **UNROLL** the pie crust and place it over the beef mixture, folding the edges under. Crimp the edges if you desire. With a paring knife, cut 5 slits in the crust to vent. Bake for 25 minutes, or until the beef mixture bubbles around the edges and the crust is nicely browned. Let cool for 10 minutes before cutting into 6 wedges. Serve it with the salsa and yogurt passed at the table.

MAKE IT A MEAL

Broccoli Slaw: 1 cup shredded raw broccoli with 2 tablespoons fat-free ranch dressing **50 CALORIES**

½ cup juice-packed canned pineapple chunks **50 CALORIES**

420 CALORIES PER MEAL ★★

MAKE IT A MEAL

1 cup fresh fruit salad **100 CALORIES**

420 CALORIES PER MEAL ★

PER SERVING (1 serving = one 4½" wedge, 2 tablespoons salsa, 2 tablespoons yogurt)

Calories	Total Fat	Saturated Fat	Sodium	Carbohydrate	Dietary Fiber	Protein	Calcium
320	16 g	6 g	650 mg	27 g	2 g	19 g	8%

HERB-FLECKED THAI BEEF NOODLE STEW

PREP TIME: 30 MINUTES / **COOK TIME:** 15 MINUTES / **MAKES** 4 SERVINGS

With a little bit of chopping you can have restaurant-quality Thai food on your table in less time than it takes to pick up takeout.

MAKE
IT A
MEAL

1 mandarin orange
30 CALORIES

410
CALORIES
PER MEAL
★ ★ ★

MAKE
the variation
A MEAL

1 medium orange
70 CALORIES

420
CALORIES
PER MEAL
★ ★ ★ ★

½ package (8.8 ounces) thin rice noodles, vermicelli-style

6 cups boiling water

2 teaspoons canola oil

2 tablespoons grated fresh ginger

4 cloves garlic, minced

½ pound top round steak, cut into thin 1½"-long strips

1 onion, thinly sliced

1 jalapeño chile pepper, seeded and finely chopped (wear plastic gloves when handling)

1 package (8 ounces) sliced shiitake or white mushrooms

3 carrots, coarsely grated

2 tablespoons reduced-sodium soy sauce

1 tablespoon Thai fish sauce

1 teaspoon light brown sugar

1. **PLACE** the rice noodles in a 13" x 9" baking pan and pour the boiling water over them, making sure they are covered with water.

2. **HEAT** the oil in a large saucepan over medium-high heat. Add the ginger, garlic, and beef. Cook for 2 minutes, stirring, until the beef is medium-rare. Transfer the beef with a slotted spoon to a plate.

3. **ADD** the onion, jalapeño, and mushrooms to the pan. Cook for 6 minutes, stirring, until the mushrooms begin to give off some liquid. Add the carrots, soy sauce, fish sauce, and brown sugar. Simmer for 1 minute to dissolve the sugar.

4. **ADD** the broth and coconut milk. Reduce to a simmer and cook for 3 minutes, then stir in the cilantro, basil, and mint. Return the beef (and any juices accumulated on the plate) to the pan.

PER SERVING (1 serving = ¾ cup noodles, 1½ cups stew, garnishes)
Herb-Flecked Thai Chicken Noodle Stew (1 serving = ¾ cup noodles, 1½ cups stew, garnishes

Calories	Total Fat	Saturated Fat	Sodium	Carbohydrate	Dietary Fiber	Protein	Calcium
380	12 g	5.5 g	1,110 mg	45 g	4 g	21 g	6%
350	8 g	4 g	1,120 mg	45 g	4 g	22 g	6%

2 cups fat-free, reduced sodium beef broth

1 cup light coconut milk

¼ cup finely chopped fresh cilantro

3 tablespoons thinly sliced fresh basil

1 tablespoon finely chopped fresh mint

GARNISHES

1⅓ cups mung bean sprouts

¼ cup chopped dry-roasted unsalted peanuts

1 lime, quartered

Thai chili-garlic sauce (sriracha), optional

5. **DRAIN** the noodles and divide among 4 bowls (about ¾ cup each). Top each bowl with 1½ cups of stew. Garnish each bowl with ⅓ cup bean sprouts, 1 tablespoon peanuts, and a lime quarter. Pass sriracha at the table, if desired.

HERB-FLECKED THAI CHICKEN NOODLE STEW *(variation)*

SUBSTITUTE boneless, skinless chicken breast for the steak. (It will need to cook a few minutes longer than the steak.)

SUBSTITUTE fat-free, reduced-sodium chicken broth for the beef broth.

JERK BEEF WITH GRILLED PLANTAIN SLICES

PREP TIME: 20 MINUTES + 1 HOUR MARINATING / **COOK TIME:** 20 MINUTES / **MAKES** 4 SERVINGS

Scotch bonnet peppers are the traditional pepper used in this dish, but habaneros or other hot peppers can be substituted. Despite the large number of ingredients, the jerk sauce is quick and easy to make.

JERK BEEF

- 2 tablespoons dark rum
- 2 tablespoons white vinegar
- 1 tablespoon olive oil
- 1 tablespoon reduced-sodium soy sauce
- 2 teaspoons light brown sugar
- 1 teaspoon ground allspice
- 1 teaspoon dried thyme
- ¾ teaspoon freshly ground black pepper
- ½ teaspoon ground nutmeg
- ½ teaspoon salt
- ¼ teaspoon ground cinnamon
- Grated zest and juice of 2 limes
- 3 scallions, cut into thirds
- 1 small yellow onion, quartered
- 2 cloves garlic
- 1 fresh Scotch bonnet pepper, seeded

1. TO MAKE THE JERK BEEF: Combine the rum, vinegar, olive oil, soy sauce, brown sugar, allspice, thyme, black pepper, nutmeg, salt, cinnamon, lime zest, lime juice, scallions, onion, garlic, and Scotch bonnet pepper in a blender or food processor. Blend until smooth. Measure out ½ cup of this marinade to use as a sauce. Refrigerate until serving time.

2. PLACE the tri-tip in a bowl or resealable plastic bag. Add the remaining jerk mixture and turn to coat the tri-tip. Refrigerate the beef for at least 1 hour.

3. WHEN ready to cook, set up a gas or charcoal grill for cooking over indirect heat. For gas, turn the burners on one side to medium-low and leave the other burners off. For charcoal, stack the coals on one side only. Discard the marinade and place the tri-tip on the cool side of the grill. Cover the grill and cook for 8 to 10 minutes per side, until the surface is browned and a thermometer inserted in the center registers 145°F for medium-rare or 160°F for medium. Let the meat rest for 5 minutes and then cut into 16 thin slices.

PER SERVING (1 serving = 4 slices beef, 2 tablespoons sauce, 1 piece plantain)

Calories	Total Fat	Saturated Fat	Sodium	Carbohydrate	Dietary Fiber	Protein	Calcium
330	12 g	3 g	510 mg	27 g	3 g	26 g	6%

1   pound tri-tip steak
(bottom sirloin)

1   lime, cut into 4 wedges

GRILLED PLANTAIN

2   teaspoons vegetable oil

2   teaspoons light brown
sugar

⅛   teaspoon cayenne pepper

1   medium plantain,
halved lengthwise
and then crosswise

4. MEANWHILE, TO MAKE THE GRILLED PLANTAIN:
Combine the vegetable oil, brown sugar, and cayenne in a small bowl. Brush the mixture over the flat surface of the plantain pieces. Place, rounded-side down, directly on the grill over indirect heat for 15 minutes, or until the topping is sizzling and the underside of the plantain is browned.

5. TOP each serving of meat with 2 tablespoons of the reserved sauce. Serve with the plantain and garnish with lime wedge.

HUNGARIAN GOULASH

PREP TIME: 20 MINUTES / **COOK TIME:** 1 HOUR 15 MINUTES / **MAKES** 4 SERVINGS

At its core, Hungarian goulash is essentially a beef stew seasoned with paprika and bay leaves. Goulash is traditionally served over egg noodles, but it is equally good over rice.

MAKE
IT A
MEAL

Salad made with
2 cups romaine
lettuce, 1 medium
chopped tomato,
¼ cup grated
carrot, and
10 sprays salad
dressing spray
60 CALORIES

420
CALORIES
PER MEAL
★ ★ ★

MAKE
IT A
MEAL

¼ cup orange
sherbet
50 CALORIES

410
CALORIES
PER MEAL
★

1	teaspoon olive oil
¾	pound lean stew beef (also called round stew beef)
1	medium onion, finely chopped
2	carrots, finely chopped
1	red bell pepper, finely chopped
4	cloves garlic, minced
¼	teaspoon coarse salt
¼	teaspoon freshly ground black pepper
2	tablespoons sweet Hungarian paprika
1	can (14.5 ounces) diced tomatoes
½	cup water
1	large russet (baking) potato (about 14 ounces), peeled and cut into ½" chunks
2	packets (4 grams each) fat-free, salt-free beef bouillon
1	bay leaf
2	cups wide egg noodles (regular or whole wheat)
⅓	cup low-fat plain yogurt
¼	cup thinly sliced fresh chives

1. **HEAT** the oil in a large saucepan over medium-high heat. Add the beef and cook for 5 minutes, stirring, until the beef is seared on all sides. Transfer the beef to a plate with a slotted spoon.

2. **REDUCE** the heat to medium and add the onion, carrots, bell pepper, garlic, salt, and black pepper. Cook for 5 minutes, stirring often, until the onions begin to soften. Add the paprika and cook for 30 seconds, or until fragrant.

3. **STIR** in the tomatoes, water, potato, bouillon, and bay leaf. Bring the mixture to a simmer and return the beef to the pot. Reduce to a gentle simmer, cover, and cook for 1 hour, stirring occasionally.

4. **ABOUT** 15 minutes before the goulash is finished, bring a large pot of water to a boil. Add the noodles and cook according to package directions. Drain.

5. **DIVIDE** the noodles among 4 bowls. Remove the bay leaf from the goulash and top each bowl with 1½ cups goulash. Garnish with a generous tablespoon of the yogurt and sprinkle with 1 tablespoon chives.

PER SERVING (1 serving = 1½ cups goulash, 1 cup noodles)

Calories	Total Fat	Saturated Fat	Sodium	Carbohydrate	Dietary Fiber	Protein	Calcium
360	9 g	3 g	330 mg	47 g	6 g	24 g	10%

CHERRY-GARLIC GLAZED HAM

PREP TIME: 5 MINUTES + 5 MINUTES STANDING / **COOK TIME:** 1 HOUR 20 MINUTES /
MAKES 16 SERVINGS

Read labels carefully when shopping for ham, as many hams are extremely high in fat. The glaze adds a festive touch that makes this ham perfect for a party or holiday meal.

1   96% fat-free honey-roasted dinner ham (3 pounds), such as Hatfield
⅓   cup cherry preserves
2   cloves garlic, minced
2   teaspoons Dijon mustard

1. **PREHEAT** the oven to 400°F.

2. **SET** the ham in a small roasting pan and fill with cold water to come ½" up the sides of the pan. Cover with foil and roast for 1 hour.

3. **MEANWHILE**, combine the preserves, garlic, and mustard in a small bowl.

4. **REMOVE** the ham from the oven and remove the foil. Brush the ham with one-fourth of the cherry mixture, return the ham to the oven and roast for 5 minutes. Repeat 3 more times with the remaining cherry mixture.

5. **TRANSFER** the ham to a cutting board. Let stand for 5 minutes before cutting into 32 slices.

PER SERVING (1 serving = 2 slices)

Calories	Total Fat	Saturated Fat	Sodium	Carbohydrate	Dietary Fiber	Protein	Calcium
130	3 g	1 g	680 mg	12 g	0 g	13 g	0%

MAKE IT A MEAL

1 medium (6½ ounces) baked sweet potato
100 CALORIES

½ cup steamed spinach creamed with 1 wedge Laughing Cow Light cheese spread
55 CALORIES

1 small (1 ounce) crusty roll spread with 1 teaspoon unsalted whipped butter
105 CALORIES

390
CALORIES PER MEAL
★ ★ ★

MAKE IT A MEAL

⅔ cup mashed potatoes with 1 teaspoon unsalted whipped butter
105 CALORIES

1 small (1¼ ounces) buttermilk biscuit
130 CALORIES

½ cup steamed carrots
30 CALORIES

395
CALORIES PER MEAL
★

PASTA WITH SPINACH AND PARSLEY-CHEESE SAUSAGE

PREP TIME: 10 MINUTES / **COOK TIME:** 17 MINUTES / **MAKES** 4 SERVINGS

Greens such as spinach are among the most nutrient-rich of vegetables, as they're packed with beta-carotene and vitamin C. This dish is equally tasty with garden-fresh zucchini in place of the spinach. Because the main recipe and the variation have the same number of calories per serving, you can mix and match the suggested side salads to Make It a Meal.

MAKE IT A MEAL

Salad made with ½ cup diced tomatoes, ½ cup diced cucumber, 1 teaspoon olive oil, and 1½ teaspoons balsamic vinegar
75 CALORIES

385
CALORIES PER MEAL
★ ★

MAKE the variation A MEAL

Salad made with 2 cups mixed baby greens, 4 cherry tomatoes, 1 teaspoon olive oil, and 1½ teaspoons balsamic vinegar
75 CALORIES

385
CALORIES PER MEAL
★ ★ ★

6	ounces spinach fusilli pasta
6	ounces Italian-style parsley-cheese sausage or any Italian-flavored pork sausage (the thin, rope style)
1	cup water
5	teaspoons extra-virgin olive oil
6	cloves garlic, sliced
1	teaspoon dried basil
⅛	teaspoon red-pepper flakes
1	cup cherry tomatoes, halved
4	cups baby spinach
½	cup low-sodium chicken broth
¼	teaspoon salt

1. **BRING** a large saucepan of water to a boil. Add the pasta and cook according to package directions. Drain.

2. **MEANWHILE,** combine the sausage and water in a small nonstick skillet over medium-high heat. Bring to a boil and cook for 10 to 12 minutes, or until the water has evaporated and the sausage is beginning to brown lightly. Remove the pan from the heat and let cool for 5 minutes. Transfer the sausage to a cutting board and cut crosswise into small pieces.

3. **HEAT** the oil in a large nonstick skillet over medium-high heat. Add the sausage, garlic, basil, and pepper flakes, and cook for 45 seconds, stirring often, until fragrant. Add the tomatoes and cook for 1½ minutes, or until they start to wilt. Add the spinach and cook for 1 minute, tossing often, until wilted. Pour in the broth, bring to a boil, and cook for 1 minute. Add the pasta and salt and cook for 1 minute to heat through.

PASTA WITH ZUCCHINI AND PARSLEY-CHEESE SAUSAGE *(variation)*

SUBSTITUTE 4 cups sliced zucchini for the spinach and cook about 5 minutes longer after the zucchini is added.

PER SERVING (1 serving = 2 cups)
Pasta with Zucchini and Parsley-Cheese Sausage (1 serving = 2 cups)

Calories	Total Fat	Saturated Fat	Sodium	Carbohydrate	Dietary Fiber	Protein	Calcium
310	13 g	3 g	510 mg	39 g	5 g	12 g	8%
310	13 g	3 g	440 mg	38 g	4 g	13 g	6%

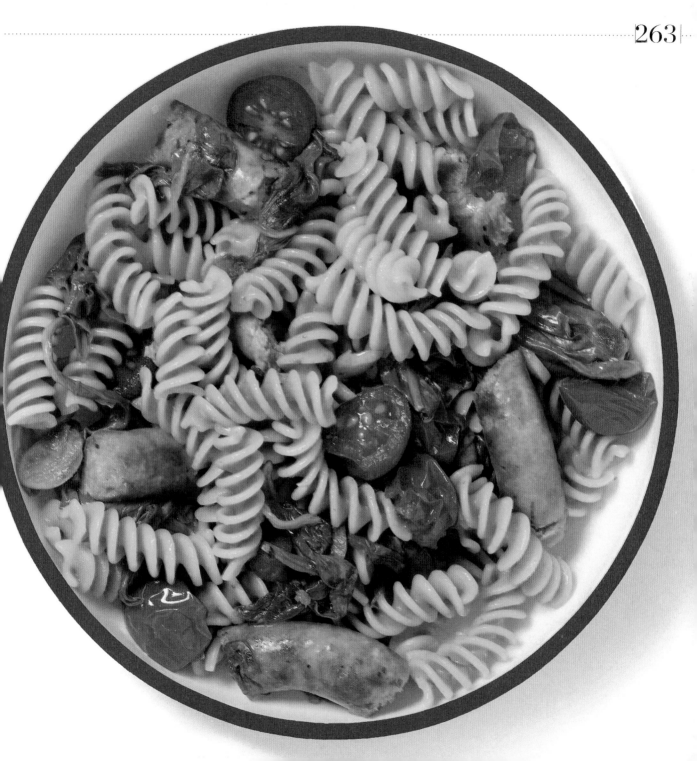

ITALIAN MEATBALLS AND QUICK MUSHROOM RED SAUCE

PREP TIME: 10 MINUTES / **COOK TIME:** 15 MINUTES / **MAKES** 6 SERVINGS

"Meat loaf mix" is a combination of ground chuck, veal, and pork that's frequently on sale at the supermarket. It's perfect for making flavorful meatballs. This recipe calls for baking the meatballs, which requires no extra fat and no hovering over a skillet. Both sauce and meatballs cook at the same time—so convenient.

MEATBALLS

- 1   pound meat loaf mix (or ⅓ pound ground beef, ⅓ pound ground veal, and ⅓ pound ground pork)
- 1   cup soft bread crumbs, preferably from Italian bread
- ½   small onion, finely chopped
- 2   tablespoons finely chopped fresh flat-leaf parsley
- 2   cloves garlic, minced
- ½   cup finely shredded Parmigiano-Reggiano cheese
- 1   large egg
- ¼   teaspoon coarse salt
- ¼   teaspoon freshly ground black pepper

1. TO MAKE THE MEATBALLS: Preheat the oven to 400°F. Combine the meat loaf mix, bread crumbs, onion, parsley, garlic, cheese, egg, salt, and pepper. Gently but thoroughly combine—do not overmix. Form the mixture into 18 meatballs about 1½" in diameter. Place on a baking sheet and bake for 15 minutes or until cooked through.

PER SERVING (1 serving = 3 meatballs, ⅔ cup sauce)

Calories	Total Fat	Saturated Fat	Sodium	Carbohydrate	Dietary Fiber	Protein	Calcium
330	17 g	6 g	670 mg	17 g	3 g	21 g	15%

SAUCE

1	tablespoon olive oil
½	small onion, finely chopped
2	cloves garlic, minced
1	package (8 ounces) sliced portobello mushrooms
1	can (28 ounces) crushed tomatoes with Italian seasoning
1	can (8 ounces) no-salt-added tomato sauce
¼	cup red wine
½	teaspoon Italian seasoning
⅛	teaspoon garlic salt

2. MEANWHILE, TO MAKE THE SAUCE: Heat the oil in a large saucepan over medium heat. Add the onion and garlic, and cook for 3 minutes, stirring, until the onion softens. Add the mushrooms and cook for 4 minutes, stirring occasionally, until the mushrooms have given up their liquid. Stir in the tomatoes, tomato sauce, wine, Italian seasoning, and garlic salt. Reduce the heat to medium-low, cover, and let simmer while the meatballs bake.

3. WHEN the meatballs are done, add them to the sauce and stir to coat.

PORK TAMALES

PREP TIME: 45 MINUTES + 5 MINUTES STANDING / **COOK TIME:** 1 HOUR 52 MINUTES /
MAKES 6 SERVINGS

Homemade tamales are well worth the effort because restaurant tamales are laden with fat, typically lard. There certainly are a lot of steps, but they are all basic and easy. The masa filling can be prepared while the pork roasts. Making the actual tamales is fun and simple enough for children to help.

CORN HUSKS

18   dried corn husks (available at specialty markets or online)

PORK FILLING

1   teaspoon chili powder

1   teaspoon paprika

½   teaspoon ground cumin

½   teaspoon garlic powder

¼   teaspoon freshly ground black pepper

1   pound pork tenderloin

¼   cup fat-free, reduced-sodium chicken or vegetable broth

1. TO PREPARE THE CORN HUSKS: Bring a large pot of water to a boil over high heat. Carefully separate the corn husks. Once the water boils, turn off the heat and add the husks to the pot, pushing them under the water. Allow the husks to sit in the water until ready to make the tamales.

2. TO MAKE THE PORK FILLING: Preheat the oven to 450°F. Combine the chili powder, paprika, cumin, garlic powder, and pepper in a small bowl. Place an 18" length of foil in a 13" x 9" baking pan and set the pork on top of it. Rub the spice mixture all over the pork.

3. CLOSE the foil up around the pork and bake for 45 minutes, until a thermometer inserted into the center of the meat registers 160°F. Open the foil and carefully transfer any cooking juices to a food processor. When cool enough to handle, cut the pork crosswise into ½"-thick slices and add them to the processor along with the broth. Pulse the processor 5 or 6 times to coarsely chop the meat.

4. MEANWHILE, TO MAKE THE MASA FILLING: Heat the broth and butter in a microwaveable bowl for 2 minutes. Whisk the egg and oil together in a small bowl.

5. COMBINE the masa mix, baking powder, salt, and chili powder in the bowl of an electric mixer and whisk to combine. With the mixer on low speed, add the broth

PER SERVING (1 serving = 3 tamales)

Calories	Total Fat	Saturated Fat	Sodium	Carbohydrate	Dietary Fiber	Protein	Calcium
270	8 g	2 g	480 mg	29 g	3 g	22 g	10%

MASA FILLING

2⅓   cups fat-free, reduced-sodium chicken or vegetable broth

1   tablespoon butter

1   large egg, beaten

1   tablespoon canola oil

2   cups instant corn masa mix

¾   teaspoon baking powder

½   teaspoon coarse salt

¼   teaspoon chili powder

mixture to the masa in a slow steady stream. A soft dough will form. Add the egg mixture and mix on medium speed until evenly blended. Set aside until the pork is ready.

6. TO ASSEMBLE AND COOK THE TAMALES: Add about 1" of water to a large pot that can accommodate a steamer insert.

7. LINE up 3 corn husks on the counter with the small tips at the bottom, closest to you. Drop a scant ¼ cup of masa onto the center of each husk. Use the back of a spoon to spread the masa over the center of each husk (the masa should be about ¼" thick).

8. SPOON 1 tablespoon of pork filling into the center of the masa. Fold up the bottom of the husk over the masa and then roll up the husk from right to left over the masa and pork. Repeat with the remaining corn husks, masa, and pork filling. Rest the steamer insert on its side for easier filling. Gently place each tamale in the insert, bottom end first, so that the tamales will stand upright during steaming. If necessary, make a second layer of tamales.

9. BRING the water to a boil. Set the steamer insert in the pan, cover, and reduce the heat to medium-low. Cook for 30 minutes. Check to make sure the pot hasn't boiled dry, add more hot water to the pot if necessary, re-cover, and cook for another 30 minutes.

10. REMOVE the steamer insert. Using tongs, transfer the tamales to a platter and let rest for 5 minutes before serving. To eat, remove the tamale from the husk (discard the husk).

MOUSSAKA

PREP TIME: 40 MINUTES + 10 MINUTES STANDING / **COOK TIME:** 1 HOUR 22 MINUTES /
MAKES 6 SERVINGS

This traditional Greek casserole features layers of savory eggplant, spiced lamb and turkey, and a creamy top layer of white sauce and feta. Moussaka freezes and reheats nicely in the microwave.

1	large eggplant (about 1 pound), peeled and cut crosswise into ½"-thick slices
1	tablespoon unsalted butter
3	tablespoons plain dried bread crumbs
1	teaspoon olive oil
½	cup finely chopped onion
2	cloves garlic, minced
2	teaspoons dried oregano
¾	teaspoon coarse salt
¼	teaspoon freshly ground black pepper
½	pound ground lamb
½	pound 99% lean ground turkey breast
2	teaspoons fresh lemon juice
3	tablespoons no-salt-added tomato paste

1. PREHEAT the oven to 450°F. Line a baking sheet with foil and coat the foil with cooking spray.

2. PLACE the eggplant slices on the baking sheet (they can overlap). Coat the tops with cooking spray. Bake for 18 for 20 minutes, until lightly golden and tender. Remove from the oven. Reduce the oven temperature to 350°F.

3. MEANWHILE, melt the butter in a medium nonstick skillet over medium heat. Add the bread crumbs and cook for 1 minute, stirring, until golden. Transfer the bread crumbs to a plate.

4. COAT the same skillet with cooking spray. Add the oil and warm over medium heat. Add the onion, garlic, oregano, ½ teaspoon of the salt, and the pepper. Cook for 2 minutes, stirring, until the onion begins to soften. Add the lamb and turkey, and cook for 5 minutes, breaking the meat up with a spoon, until cooked through. Add the lemon juice, tomato paste, and diced tomatoes, and cook, stirring, until simmering. Continue to simmer, stirring occasionally, for 5 to 7 minutes, or until the liquid is absorbed. Remove from the heat. Set aside until ready to assemble the casserole.

PER SERVING (1 serving = 2⅔" x 4" piece)

Calories	Total Fat	Saturated Fat	Sodium	Carbohydrate	Dietary Fiber	Protein	Calcium
280	14 g	7 g	550 mg	17 g	4 g	22 g	15%

1   can (14.5 ounces)
    petite-cut diced
    tomatoes, drained
1   cup low-fat (2%)
    evaporated milk
2   teaspoons cornstarch
⅓   cup reduced-fat
    feta cheese

5. WHISK together the evaporated milk, cornstarch, and remaining ¼ teaspoon salt in a small saucepan. Bring to a boil over medium-high heat, stirring constantly. When the sauce boils, it will thicken immediately. Remove from the heat and set the white sauce aside.

6. ASSEMBLE the moussaka: Coat an 8" x 8" baking dish with cooking spray. Make a single layer of eggplant slices in the baking dish (they can overlap), using half the eggplant slices. Top with the meat mixture. Add a second layer of eggplant slices. Pour the white sauce over the eggplant, then sprinkle evenly with the feta and the buttered bread crumbs.

7. BAKE for 25 to 30 minutes, or until bubbling and golden. Let rest for 10 minutes before serving.

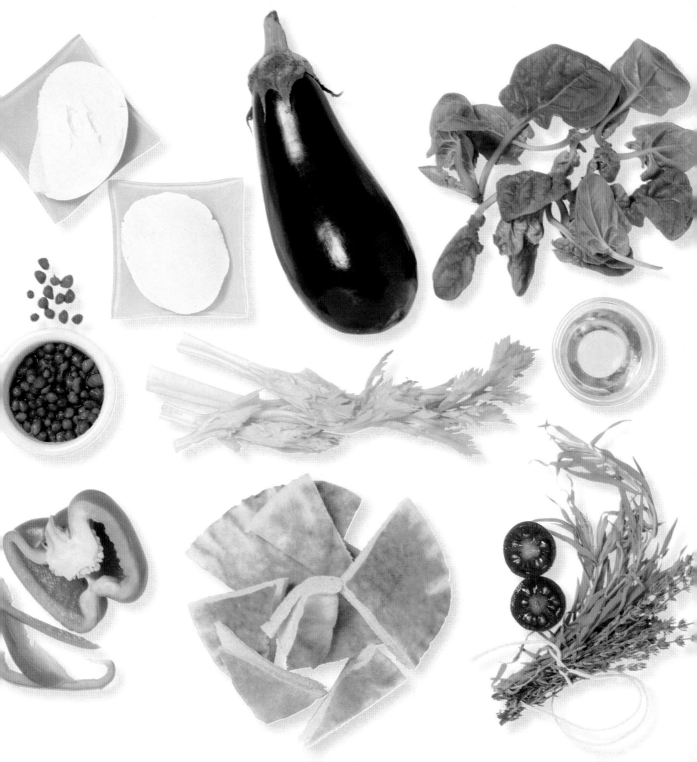

SWEDISH MEATBALLS

PREP TIME: 20 MINUTES / **COOK TIME:** 16 MINUTES / **MAKES** 4 SERVINGS

We cut the fat by using lean ground beef and mixing it with ingredients that add moisture. The portions in this classic appetizer recipe are almost large enough for a full meal. To make room for another appetizer, cut the serving size to 3 meatballs, which increases the total number of servings to 8.

MAKE IT A MEAL

⅔ cup cooked egg noodles
150 CALORIES

410
CALORIES PER MEAL
★

MAKE IT A MEAL

½ cup steamed carrots
30 CALORIES

1 bottle (12 ounces) light beer
100 CALORIES

390
CALORIES PER MEAL
★

2	slices (1 ounce each) day-old whole wheat bread, torn into pieces
1	pound 95% lean ground round beef
1	small onion, finely chopped
1	large egg
¼	teaspoon ground allspice
⅛	teaspoon ground nutmeg
½	teaspoon salt
¼	teaspoon freshly ground black pepper
1	tablespoon + 2 teaspoons Dijon mustard
¾	cup fat-free, reduced-sodium beef broth
2	teaspoons cornstarch
1½	teaspoons Worcestershire sauce
2	teaspoons canola oil
½	cup light sour cream

1. **PLACE** the bread in a food processor and process to fine crumbs. Transfer to a large bowl, Add the beef, onion, egg, allspice, nutmeg, salt, pepper, and 1 tablespoon of the mustard. Mix until well combined and form into 24 meatballs (about 1"). Combine the remaining 2 teaspoons mustard, the broth, cornstarch, and Worcestershire sauce in a bowl and set aside.

2. **HEAT** the oil in a large nonstick skillet over medium heat. Add the meatballs and cook for 12 to 14 minutes, turning occasionally, until browned and almost cooked through. Transfer the meatballs to paper towels to drain.

3. **INCREASE** the heat to medium-high and add the broth mixture to the skillet. Bring to a boil, shaking the pan often, and cook for 2 minutes to thicken. Remove from the heat and stir in the sour cream until well blended. Return the meatballs to the pan and gently turn to coat with the sauce.

PER SERVING (1 serving = 6 meatballs)

Calories	Total Fat	Saturated Fat	Sodium	Carbohydrate	Dietary Fiber	Protein	Calcium
260	11 g	3.5 g	650 mg	11 g	1 g	30 g	8%

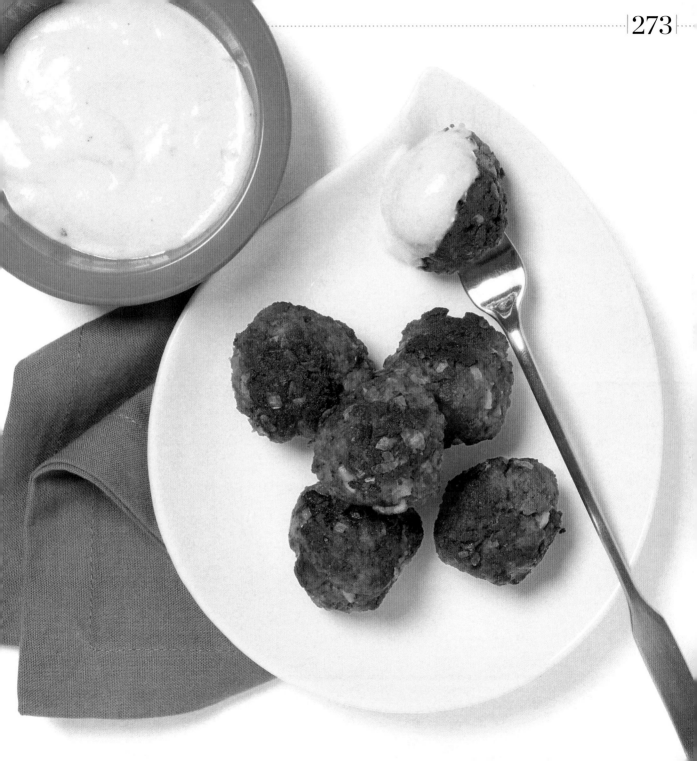

SPINACH DIP IN A SOURDOUGH BOWL

PREP TIME: 10 MINUTES / **MAKES** 6 SERVINGS

Easy to prepare, this light spinach dip is party-friendly in its bread bowl. Since the bread bowl is only decorative and does not get eaten, a second loaf is cut up for dipping. Feel free to substitute rye breads, or skip the dipping bread completely and save the calories for an entrée and dessert.

2	sourdough boule loaves (1 pound each)
1	package (10 ounces) frozen chopped spinach, thawed and squeezed dry
½	cup 1% cottage cheese, preferably small curd
1	medium carrot, grated
1	tablespoon grated Parmesan cheese
1	teaspoon salt-free Italian seasoning
¾	teaspoon dried minced onion
¼	teaspoon garlic salt
2	shakes hot sauce (optional)

1. CAREFULLY cut a 6"- to 8"-diameter circle in the top of one of the sourdough breads. Remove the cut circle and hollow out the bread, leaving enough to provide stability to the bread bowl (you'll remove about 8 ounces of bread total; save for making bread crumbs or discard). Cut the second loaf into small pieces for dipping. Set all bread aside.

2. COMBINE the spinach, cottage cheese, carrot, Parmesan, Italian seasoning, dried onion, garlic salt, and hot sauce (if using) in a medium bowl. Refrigerate the dip until ready to serve. To serve, spoon the dip into the prepared bread bowl and arrange on a platter with bread chunks for dipping.

SPINACH DIP *(without bread chunks) (variation)*
USE the bread bowl to hold the dip, but omit the second sourdough bread for dipping.

PER SERVING (1 serving = ½ cup dip, 1 cup bread chunks) Spinach Dip (1 serving = ½ cup dip)

Calories	Total Fat	Saturated Fat	Sodium	Carbohydrate	Dietary Fiber	Protein	Calcium
270	2.5 g	1 g	690 mg	49 g	4 g	15 g	20%
60	1 g	0.5 g	200 mg	7 g	2 g	6 g	15%

BACON AND CHEDDAR BAKED POTATO SKINS

PREP TIME: 10 MINUTES / **COOK TIME:** 1 HOUR 15 MINUTES (INCLUDES BAKING POTATOES) /
MAKES 4 SERVINGS

This popular restaurant appetizer is easily slimmed down. Use the reserved potato pulp to thicken a vegetable soup or make mashed potatoes at a later date.

- 4 medium russet (baking) potatoes (about 7 ounces each), scrubbed well, baked, and cooled
- 2 teaspoons canola oil
- ½ teaspoon dried minced onion
- ¼ teaspoon garlic salt
- ⅛ teaspoon onion powder
- ⅛ teaspoon smoked paprika
- ⅛ teaspoon freshly ground black pepper
- 3 strips reduced-sodium bacon, cooked and crumbled
- ½ cup shredded reduced-fat sharp Cheddar cheese
- ½ cup light sour cream
- 2 scallions, chopped

1. PREHEAT the oven to 475°F. Coat a baking sheet with cooking spray.

2. HALVE the potatoes lengthwise. Carefully scoop out the potato flesh, leaving enough to form a potato "shell." Place the potato skins, cut-side down, on the baking sheet. Brush each potato skin with a little of the oil, then flip over.

3. IN a small bowl, stir together the dried onion, garlic salt, onion powder, paprika, and pepper. Sprinkle the mixture over the potato skins. Bake the skins for 10 minutes, or until crispy.

4. REMOVE the skins from the oven and top each with one-quarter of the bacon and cheese. Return the skins to the oven and bake for 2 to 3 minutes to melt the cheese. Remove from the oven, and top each with 1 tablespoon of sour cream and a sprinkling of scallions. Serve hot.

BBQ CHICKEN POTATO SKINS *(variation)*

DECREASE the garlic salt to ⅛ teaspoon.

OMIT the bacon, sour cream, and scallions.

MIX 1 cup shredded cooked chicken breast with 2 tablespoons barbecue sauce. In Step 4, fill the potato skins with the chicken mixture. Return to the oven for 5 minutes to heat through. Remove from the oven and sprinkle with the cheese. Serve hot.

MAKE IT A MEAL

1 bottle (12 ounces) light beer
100 CALORIES

380
CALORIES PER MEAL

MAKE the variation A MEAL

12 ounces ginger ale
120 CALORIES

400
CALORIES PER MEAL

PER SERVING (1 serving = 2 potato skins) BBQ Chicken Potato Skins (1 serving = 2 potato skins)

Calories	Total Fat	Saturated Fat	Sodium	Carbohydrate	Dietary Fiber	Protein	Calcium
280	12 g	5 g	280 mg	33 g	4 g	11 g	15%
280	7 g	2.5 g	300 mg	34 g	3 g	18 g	15%

MIDDLE EASTERN HUMMUS

PREP TIME: 15 MINUTES + 2 HOURS CHILLING / **MAKES** 8 SERVINGS

Made from a base of chickpeas, hummus is the perfect dip for crudités and pita. For variety, divide the hummus evenly among 3 bowls. Spice up 1 bowl with ½ teaspoon cayenne pepper and ¼ teaspoon chipotle powder, and drizzle with 1½ teaspoons chili-garlic sauce. Into another bowl, stir in ⅓ cup of chopped roasted red peppers and garnish with 2 additional tablespoons of chopped roasted red peppers. Leave 1 bowl as is for classic hummus.

2	cans (19 ounces each) chickpeas, rinsed and drained
½	cup fresh lemon juice
½	cup tahini (sesame paste)
4	cloves garlic
2	tablespoons extra-virgin olive oil
1½	teaspoons ground cumin
1	teaspoon coarse salt
¼	teaspoon freshly ground black pepper
	Pinch cayenne pepper
⅓	cup water
3	tablespoons chopped fresh parsley

1. **COMBINE** the chickpeas, lemon juice, tahini, garlic, oil, cumin, salt, black pepper, and a pinch of cayenne in a food processor. Puree the mixture until evenly blended, but still somewhat chunky. Add the water and process until smooth.

2. **REFRIGERATE** for at least 2 hours. Garnish with parsley before serving.

PER SERVING (1 serving = a generous ½ cup)

Calories	Total Fat	Saturated Fat	Sodium	Carbohydrate	Dietary Fiber	Protein	Calcium
260	13 g	1.5 g	380 mg	29 g	6 g	8 g	6%

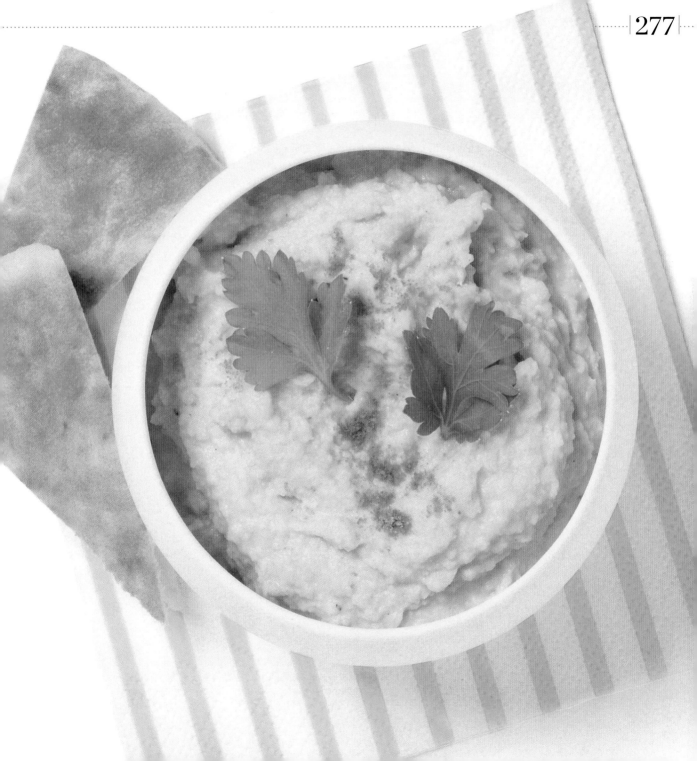

NACHOS

PREP TIME: 10 MINUTES / **COOK TIME:** 10 MINUTES / **MAKES** 6 SERVINGS

Nachos were created by a restaurant owner in Mexico who needed to make a quick meal for a group of guests that arrived after closing time. Legend has it that he used just tortilla chips, cheese, and jalapeño slices. This recipe improves on the original by adding fresh salsa and refried black beans.

2   plum tomatoes, chopped
1   cup chopped fresh pineapple
1   small red onion, chopped
2   tablespoons chopped fresh cilantro
1   tablespoon fresh lime juice
½   teaspoon salt
2   teaspoons olive oil
2   teaspoons chili powder
1   teaspoon ground cumin
½   teaspoon ground coriander
1   can (15 ounces) no-salt-added black beans, rinsed and drained
6   ounces baked tortilla chips
1   cup shredded reduced-fat sharp Cheddar cheese
12   pickled jalapeño pepper slices (wear plastic gloves when handling)

1. PREHEAT the oven to 400°F. Coat a large baking sheet with cooking spray.

2. COMBINE the tomatoes, pineapple, onion, cilantro, lime juice, and ¼ teaspoon of the salt in a bowl.

3. HEAT the oil in a medium nonstick skillet over medium-high heat. Add the chili powder, cumin, and coriander, and cook for 15 seconds, stirring, until fragrant. Add the beans and cook for 3 to 4 minutes, partially mashing with a wooden spoon, until hot. Remove from the heat and stir in the remaining ¼ teaspoon salt. Keep warm.

4. SPREAD the tortilla chips on the baking sheet. Sprinkle the cheese over the chips and bake for 4 to 5 minutes, or until the cheese melts. Remove from the oven and carefully transfer the chips to a serving platter. Top with the bean mixture, tomato-pineapple mixture, and jalapeño slices. Serve hot.

PER SERVING (1 serving = 2 cups)

Calories	Total Fat	Saturated Fat	Sodium	Carbohydrate	Dietary Fiber	Protein	Calcium
250	7 g	3 g	510 mg	37 g	5 g	11 g	35%

CAPONATA OVER GRILLED CROSTINI

PREP TIME: 20 MINUTES / **COOK TIME:** 20 MINUTES / **MAKES** 6 SERVINGS

This versatile spread can be served as an appetizer on crostini, thinned into a salad dressing, or spread on chicken or fish. The sugar and raisins help offset any mild bitterness in the eggplant.

CAPONATA

- 3 tablespoons pine nuts
- 2 tablespoons extra-virgin olive oil
- 1 pound eggplant, cut into ¼" cubes
- 1 medium red bell pepper, finely chopped
- 1 medium onion, finely chopped
- 3 cloves garlic, minced
- 1½ tablespoons white wine vinegar
- 1 tablespoon sugar
- ⅓ cup golden raisins
- 1 tablespoon capers, drained and chopped
- ¼ teaspoon salt
- ⅛ teaspoon freshly ground black pepper

CROSTINI

- 6 ounces baguette, cut on the diagonal into 24 slices

1. TO MAKE THE CAPONATA: Place the pine nuts in a large nonstick skillet and cook over medium-high heat, shaking the pan often, for 3 to 5 minutes, or until lightly toasted. Transfer to a bowl and set aside.

2. ADD the oil to the skillet and heat over medium-high heat. Add the eggplant, bell pepper, onion, and garlic, and cook for 10 to 11 minutes, stirring occasionally, until tender. Stir in the vinegar and sugar, and cook for 1 minute. Stir in the raisins, capers, salt, and black pepper, and cook for 1 minute to warm. Remove from the heat and stir in the pine nuts.

3. TO MAKE THE CROSTINI: Coat a nonstick grill pan with cooking spray and heat over medium-high heat. Add the bread slices, in batches, and grill 1 minute per side or until lightly toasted. Top with the caponata.

PER SERVING (1 serving = ⅓ cup caponata, 4 crostini)

Calories	Total Fat	Saturated Fat	Sodium	Carbohydrate	Dietary Fiber	Protein	Calcium
220	8 g	1 g	330 mg	33 g	4 g	5 g	2%

MAKE IT A MEAL

1 ounce sliced fresh mozzarella and 1 medium sliced tomato drizzled with ½ teaspoon olive oil and sprinkled with slivered fresh basil
120 CALORIES

½ cup seedless grapes
60 CALORIES

400 CALORIES PER MEAL
★ ★

MAKE IT A MEAL

5 ounces Chianti wine
120 CALORIES

1 tablespoon mixed unsalted nuts
50 CALORIES

390 CALORIES PER MEAL
★

OVEN-ROASTED TOMATO BRUSCHETTA

PREP TIME: 15 MINUTES / **COOK TIME:** 1 HOUR 10 MINUTES / **MAKES** 4 SERVINGS

The roasting process caramelizes some of the sugar in the tomatoes, enhancing their natural sweetness. Choose tomatoes that are fully ripe for the best flavor.

¾	pound plum tomatoes, halved lengthwise
1	tablespoon extra-virgin olive oil
¾	teaspoon dried basil
¼	teaspoon dried oregano
¼	teaspoon salt
⅛	teaspoon freshly ground black pepper
4	ounces baguette, cut into 16 slices
2	tablespoons grated Parmesan cheese
1	tablespoon chopped fresh basil

1. PREHEAT the oven to 375°F. Coat a large baking sheet with cooking spray.

2. TOSS the tomatoes with the oil, dried basil, oregano, ⅛ teaspoon of the salt, and the pepper. Arrange cut-side up on the baking sheet. Bake for 1 hour, or until the tomatoes have softened and just hold their shape. Remove from the oven and let cool for 20 minutes.

3. INCREASE the oven temperature to 400°F. Coat another baking sheet with cooking spray. Arrange the bread slices in a single layer and bake for 8 to 10 minutes, or until crisp and lightly golden.

4. MEANWHILE, transfer the cooled tomatoes to a cutting board. Chop and transfer to a bowl. Stir in the Parmesan, fresh basil, and remaining ⅛ teaspoon salt.

5. TO serve, top each toast slice with 1 tablespoon of the tomato mixture.

MAKE IT A MEAL

1 ounce
Parmesan cheese
120 CALORIES

5 ounces
white wine
120 CALORIES

390
**CALORIES
PER MEAL**

MAKE IT A MEAL

1 ounce prosciutto
wrapped around a
honeydew wedge
(⅛ of a 6" melon)
120 CALORIES

5 ounces red wine
120 CALORIES

390
**CALORIES
PER MEAL**

★

PER SERVING (1 serving = 4 bruschetta)

Calories	Total Fat	Saturated Fat	Sodium	Carbohydrate	Dietary Fiber	Protein	Calcium
150	5 g	1 g	400 mg	21 g	2 g	5 g	6%

BOURSIN AND VEGETABLE SPIRALS

PREP TIME: 20 MINUTES / **MAKES** 6 SERVINGS

Perfect party fare, these colorful spirals will satisfy your party guests while you stick to your eating plan. These can be made up to 3 hours in advance and refrigerated until needed.

3	burrito-size whole wheat tortillas (10")
1	package (4.4 ounces) Boursin Light cheese, at room temperature
1	jar (12 ounces) roasted red peppers, drained and patted dry
¾	cup precut carrot matchsticks
½	cucumber, peeled, seeded, and cut into thin strips (about ½ cup)

1. PLACE the tortillas on a work surface. Spread one-third of the cheese over each tortilla (the cheese layer should be thin and just about reach the edges of the tortilla).

2. DIVIDE the peppers among the three tortillas, layering them on one half of each tortilla. Sprinkle ¼ cup of the carrots over the peppers on each tortilla.

3. DIVIDE the cucumber strips among the tortillas, placing them on the top half of each tortilla just above the peppers, but leaving about 2" of cheese along the top edge.

4. TIGHTLY roll up each tortilla starting at the peppers. Place a rolled tortilla seam-side down on a cutting board and cut crosswise into 10 slices, each about 1" wide (the end slices will be slightly larger).

5. ARRANGE the spirals on a serving platter. Serve right away or cover and refrigerate until serving time.

MAKE IT A MEAL

2 tablespoons mixed unsalted nuts
100 CALORIES

10 baby carrots
40 CALORIES

10 cherry tomatoes
30 CALORIES

Spritzer made with 3 ounces white wine and 3 ounces seltzer
70 CALORIES

390 CALORIES PER MEAL
★ ★ ★

MAKE IT A MEAL

5 pimiento-stuffed green olives
40 CALORIES

1 cup raw broccoli florets
20 CALORIES

6 ounces frozen margarita
190 CALORIES

400 CALORIES PER MEAL
★ ★

PER SERVING (1 serving = 5 spirals)

Calories	Total Fat	Saturated Fat	Sodium	Carbohydrate	Dietary Fiber	Protein	Calcium
150	5 g	3 g	560 mg	25 g	2 g	5 g	2%

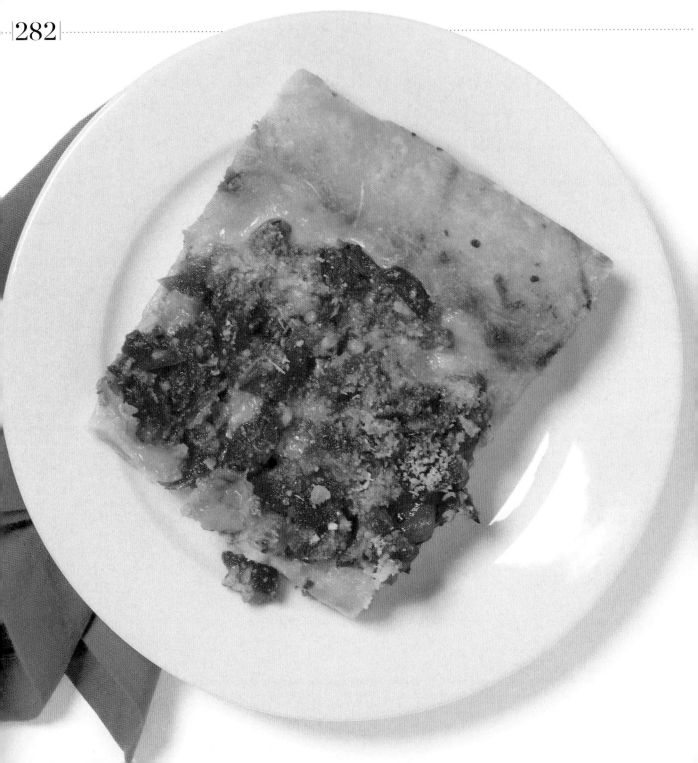

SICILIAN PIZZA "SQUARES"

PREP TIME: 20 MINUTES + 5 MINUTES STANDING / **COOK TIME:** 20 MINUTES / **MAKES** 8 SERVINGS

The difference between regular pizza and Sicilian pizza is that the cheese goes on the dough before the sauce. Traditionally, Sicilian pizza is flavored with anchovies; in this version, we have made that an option.

1	package (20 ounces) refrigerated or frozen whole wheat pizza dough
2	tablespoons all-purpose flour
1½	cups canned crushed tomatoes
2	teaspoons extra-virgin olive oil
½	teaspoon dried oregano
¼	teaspoon coarse salt
2	tablespoons finely chopped fresh basil
1½	tablespoons minced anchovies (optional)
1¼	cups shredded reduced-fat Italian 4-cheese blend
2	tablespoons grated Parmesan cheese

1. **PREHEAT** the oven to 450°F. Coat a rimmed baking sheet (15" x 10") with cooking spray. Set aside.

2. **ALLOW** the dough to come to room temperature. Sprinkle 1 tablespoon of the flour over a work surface and the remaining 1 tablespoon of flour over the top of the dough. Roll the doll into a rectangular shape about ½" thick, using additional flour as needed to prevent sticking. Transfer the dough to the baking sheet and let it rest for 10 minutes.

3. **COMBINE** the tomatoes, oil, oregano, and salt in a small saucepan. Bring to a simmer over medium heat and stir in the basil and anchovies (if using). Remove from the heat.

4. **STRETCH** the dough to fit the baking sheet. (It will be easier to work with now that it has rested.) Coat the top of the dough with cooking spray. Sprinkle the Italian cheese blend evenly over the dough, leaving a ¼" border all around.

5. **DOT** the sauce by tablespoons over the top of the dough. It will not cover the dough and the cheese should be visible. Sprinkle the Parmesan over the entire pizza. Bake for 12 to 15 minutes, or until the crust is crispy and the cheese is bubbling. Let stand for 5 minutes before halving it lengthwise and then cutting it crosswise into fourths (a total of 8 pieces).

PER SERVING (1 serving = 1 piece)

Calories	Total Fat	Saturated Fat	Sodium	Carbohydrate	Dietary Fiber	Protein	Calcium
240	7 g	2.5 g	590 mg	35 g	6 g	11 g	20%

MAKE IT A MEAL

Antipasto plate with 1" cube (generous ½ ounce) provolone cheese, 4 cherry tomatoes, ½ cup pickled vegetables, and 8 almonds (preferably Marcona) **150 CALORIES**

390
**CALORIES
PER MEAL**
★ ★ ★

MAKE IT A MEAL

1 small zucchini brushed with 1 teaspoon olive oil, grilled, then sliced crosswise **60 CALORIES**

5 ounces red wine **120 CALORIES**

420
**CALORIES
PER MEAL**
★

ROASTED PEPPER, BASIL, AND MOZZARELLA QUESADILLAS

PREP TIME: 5 MINUTES / **COOK TIME:** 23 MINUTES / **MAKES** 4 SERVINGS

Quesadillas are among the most versatile of snacks, perfect for feeding hungry friends or family members and well suited to dozens of different fillings. Pick a good melting cheese— here, part-skim mozzarella—for the best results.

MAKE IT A MEAL

¼ cup guacamole for dipping with 1 cup sliced jicama (drizzled with lime juice) and 10 baby carrots
170 CALORIES

400
CALORIES PER MEAL
★ ★ ★

MAKE IT A MEAL

6 ounces frozen margarita
190 CALORIES

420
CALORIES PER MEAL

1½ teaspoons olive oil
1 medium onion, thinly sliced
2 cloves garlic, minced
¼ teaspoon salt
1 roasted pepper, patted dry and thinly sliced
3 flour tortillas (7" or 8")
1 cup shredded part-skim mozzarella cheese
¼ cup thinly sliced fresh basil

1. **HEAT** the oil in a large nonstick skillet over medium-high heat. Add the onion, garlic, and salt, and cook for 5 to 6 minutes, stirring occasionally, until lightly browned. Stir in the roasted pepper and cook for 1 minute. Remove from the heat.

2. **ARRANGE** the tortillas on a work surface. Sprinkle the bottom half (the half nearest you) of each tortilla with 2½ tablespoons of the cheese. Top each with one-third of the onion mixture, basil, and remaining cheese. Fold the top half of the tortilla over the cheese mixture.

3. **WIPE** out the skillet with a paper towel and heat over medium heat. Add 2 quesadillas and cook for 3 to 4 minutes per side, until the cheese melts and the outsides are lightly browned. Transfer to a cutting board and repeat with the remaining quesadilla. Cut each into 4 wedges and serve.

PER SERVING (1 serving = 3 wedges)

Calories	Total Fat	Saturated Fat	Sodium	Carbohydrate	Dietary Fiber	Protein	Calcium
230	10 g	4.5 g	520 mg	23 g	2 g	11 g	25%

ONION GRUYÈRE TART

PREP TIME: 15 MINUTES + 10 MINUTES RESTING / **COOK TIME:** 1 HOUR 5 MINUTES /
MAKES 4 SERVINGS

We turn this elegant (and high-calorie) favorite into a reasonable treat by using only modest amounts of cheese and phyllo dough in place of the more common puff pastry. We like to use Athens Fillo Dough—Twin Pack because it comes in half sheets, which are easy to work with. Although imported Gruyère has the best flavor, you can use any other Swiss-style cheese.

3	teaspoons olive oil
3	medium onions, thinly sliced
1	teaspoon sugar
1/8	teaspoon salt
1/8	teaspoon freshly ground black pepper
1	tablespoon dry sherry
6	sheets (14" x 9") phyllo dough
3	ounces Gruyère cheese, grated

1. **HEAT** 1½ teaspoons of the oil in a large skillet over medium-low heat. Add the onions, cover, and cook for 15 minutes. Mix in the sugar, salt, and pepper. Cook uncovered for 30 minutes, stirring frequently, until the onions are light brown in color. Stir in the sherry and remove from the heat.

2. **PREHEAT** the oven to 350°F. Line a baking sheet with parchment or nonstick liner (or spray with cooking spray).

3. **PLACE** 1 sheet of phyllo dough on the baking sheet. Coat lightly with cooking spray. Repeat with the remaining sheets of phyllo dough. Spread the onion mixture lengthwise down the center of the phyllo dough stack, leaving a 2" border on all sides. Sprinkle with the cheese. Starting with a long side, roll the phyllo dough up to the edge of the filling to form a raised rim. Repeat on all sides. Brush the sides lightly with the remaining 1½ teaspoons oil.

4. **BAKE** for 20 minutes, or until the phyllo is lightly browned and the cheese is bubbling. Let cool for 10 minutes before cutting into 8 pieces.

PER SERVING (1 serving = 2 pieces)

Calories	Total Fat	Saturated Fat	Sodium	Carbohydrate	Dietary Fiber	Protein	Calcium
210	11 g	5 g	230 mg	18 g	2 g	8 g	25%

MAKE IT A MEAL

Salad made with 2 cups arugula, 1 teaspoon olive oil, ½ small diced pear
90 CALORIES

1 small (1 ounce) crusty roll
80 CALORIES

380
CALORIES PER MEAL
★

MAKE IT A MEAL

Salad made with 2 cups arugula, 1 teaspoon olive oil, ½ small diced pear
90 CALORIES

5 ounces white wine
120 CALORIES

420
CALORIES PER MEAL
★

PARTY PLATTER TRIO

TZATZIKI WITH PITA BREAD: **PREP TIME:** 10 MINUTES + 1 HOUR CHILLING / **MAKES** 8 SERVINGS
SMOKED TROUT SPREAD WITH CRACKERS: **PREP TIME:** 10 MINUTES + 2 HOURS CHILLING / **MAKES**
8 SERVINGS WHITE BEAN DIP WITH CRUDITÉS: **PREP TIME:** 10 MINUTES + 2 HOURS CHILLING /
MAKES 8 SERVINGS

*This combination of dips and dippers has something to please all guests. Be sure to start early
enough in the day to allow time for chilling the spreads. If you're running short on time, just
make one or two, though each dip takes only 10 minutes to put together.*

TZATZIKI WITH PITA BREAD

- 1 container (6 ounces) fat-free (0%) plain Greek yogurt
- 1 pickling cucumber, very finely diced (1 cup)
- 1 tablespoon minced red onion
- 1 tablespoon chopped fresh dill
- 1 tablespoon fresh lemon juice
- ¼ teaspoon garlic salt
- 2 large (6½") whole wheat pitas, cut into 8 wedges each

1. TO MAKE THE TZATZIKI: Stir together the yogurt, cucumber, onion, dill, lemon juice, and garlic salt in a small bowl. Cover and refrigerate for at least 1 hour for best flavor. Serve with the pita triangles.

PER SERVING (1 serving = 2 tablespoons tzatziki + 2 wedges pita, 2 tablespoons trout spread + 2 crackers,
3 tablespoons bean dip + 1 cup raw vegetables)

Calories	Total Fat	Saturated Fat	Sodium	Carbohydrate	Dietary Fiber	Protein	Calcium
220	7 g	2.5 g	480 mg	28 g	5 g	12 g	8%

SMOKED TROUT SPREAD WITH CRACKERS

- 3 ounces Neufchâtel cheese, at room temperature
- 4 ounces smoked trout, skin discarded, flaked
- 2 tablespoons light mayonnaise
- 2 tablespoons fat-free plain yogurt
- ½ teaspoon fresh lemon juice
- 1 scallion, very thinly sliced
- 16 whole wheat crackers

WHITE BEAN DIP WITH CRUDITÉS

- 1 can (15.5 ounces) cannellini beans, rinsed and drained
- ¼ cup fat-free cottage cheese
- ⅓ cup fat-free, reduced-sodium chicken broth
- 2 cloves garlic, minced
- ½ teaspoon chili powder
- ¼ teaspoon ground cumin
- ¼ teaspoon coarse salt
- ⅛ teaspoon paprika
- 2 carrots, cut into sticks
- 2 ribs celery, cut into sticks
- 1 Belgian endive, leaves separated
- 1 red bell pepper, cut into strips

2. TO MAKE THE SMOKED TROUT SPREAD: With a fork, mix together the Neufchâtel, trout, mayonnaise, yogurt, and lemon juice in a medium bowl. Transfer the spread to a serving bowl and sprinkle with the scallion. Cover and refrigerate for at least 2 hours for best flavor. Serve with the crackers.

3. TO MAKE THE WHITE BEAN DIP: Combine the beans, cottage cheese, broth, garlic, chili powder, cumin, and salt in a food processor. Process until smooth. Transfer to a serving dish, garnish with the paprika, cover, and refrigerate for at least 2 hours for best flavor. Serve with the carrots, celery, endive, and bell pepper.

SPANAKOPITA WONTONS

PREP TIME: 20 MINUTES / **COOK TIME:** 30 MINUTES / **MAKES** 4 SERVINGS

A twist on Greek spinach pie, we lowered calories and fat by using wonton wrappers instead of butter-brushed phyllo dough. For a different flavor, use plain reduced-fat feta cheese, omit the basil, and add 1 tablespoon of fresh dill.

1	package (10 ounces) frozen chopped spinach, thawed and squeezed dry
½	cup crumbled reduced-fat basil-and-tomato feta cheese
¼	cup pine nuts
3	scallions, finely chopped
1	large egg
½	teaspoon dried basil
20	square or round wonton skins

1. PREHEAT the oven to 350°F. Line a baking sheet with parchment paper or a nonstick liner (or use a nonstick baking sheet).

2. COMBINE the spinach, feta, pine nuts, scallions, egg, and basil in a medium bowl. Place 1 rounded teaspoon of the spinach mixture in the center of a wonton skin. Dampen the edges of the wonton skin with water using a small brush or your fingertip. Fold the wonton skin in half over the filling. Pinch the edges to seal. Repeat with the remaining filling and wonton skins.

3. ARRANGE the wontons on the baking sheet and spray lightly with cooking spray. Bake for 25 to 30 minutes, or until the wontons are light brown and crisp around the edges.

MAKE
IT A
MEAL

½ cup grated cucumber mixed into ½ cup fat-free (0%) plain Greek yogurt
90 CALORIES

5 kalamata olives
50 CALORIES

390
**CALORIES
PER MEAL**
★ ★

MAKE
IT A
MEAL

Salad made with 2 cups romaine lettuce, 1 teaspoon olive oil, ½ teaspoon red wine vinegar, 2 rice-stuffed grape leaves
140 CALORIES

390
**CALORIES
PER MEAL**
★ ★

PER SERVING (1 serving = 5 wontons)

Calories	Total Fat	Saturated Fat	Sodium	Carbohydrate	Dietary Fiber	Protein	Calcium
250	10 g	2 g	530 mg	29 g	4 g	13 g	20%

BUFFALO "WINGS"

PREP TIME: 15 MINUTES / **COOK TIME:** 12 MINUTES / **MAKES** 4 SERVINGS

Chicken wings are extremely high in calories because of the fatty chicken skin. Here, we season chicken breast strips to taste just like the real thing, but with way fewer calories. This recipe calls for two different hot sauces: Louisiana-style, which is made from cayenne peppers, and Tabasco, made from tabasco peppers.

3	tablespoons all-purpose flour
1	teaspoon hot paprika
½	teaspoon ground cumin
1	large egg
1	tablespoon water
1	cup cornflake crumbs
1	pound boneless, skinless chicken breasts, cut into 24 strips
¼	cup Louisiana-style hot sauce (such as Frank's Red Hot)
2	teaspoons red wine vinegar
1	teaspoon Tabasco sauce
½	teaspoon Worcestershire sauce
1	tablespoon unsalted butter

1. PREHEAT the oven to 425°F. Coat a large baking sheet with cooking spray.

2. COMBINE the flour, paprika, and cumin in a bowl. Place the egg in a separate bowl and beat together with the water. Place the cornflake crumbs in a third bowl. Working with a couple of pieces at a time, dredge the chicken in the flour, shaking off the excess. Then dip into the egg mixture to coat and then dredge in the cornflake crumbs. Place the coated strips on the baking sheet.

3. LIGHTLY coat the chicken with cooking spray. Bake for 9 minutes, turn, and bake for 2 minutes, or until crisp and golden.

4. MEANWHILE, combine the Louisiana hot sauce, vinegar, Tabasco sauce, and Worcestershire sauce in a small saucepan over medium heat. Bring to a boil and cook for 1 minute. Remove from the heat and whisk in the butter until melted. Transfer the chicken to a large bowl. Pour the hot sauce mixture over the chicken and toss to coat. Serve hot.

MAKE IT A MEAL

Crudité plate with 10 baby carrots, 1 medium rib celery cut into sticks, and blue cheese dip made with ¼ cup low-fat plain yogurt and 1 tablespoon crumbled blue cheese
120 CALORIES

390 CALORIES PER MEAL
★ ★

MAKE IT A MEAL

1 bottle (12 ounces) of beer
150 CALORIES

420 CALORIES PER MEAL
★

PER SERVING (1 serving = 6 strips)

Calories	Total Fat	Saturated Fat	Sodium	Carbohydrate	Dietary Fiber	Protein	Calcium
270	7 g	3 g	720 mg	24 g	1 g	27 g	2%

GUISA-MOLE AND VEGETARIAN CHOPPED LIVER

GUISA-MOLE: PREP TIME: 15 MINUTES / **MAKES** 6 SERVINGS
VEGETARIAN CHOPPED LIVER: PREP TIME: 15 MINUTES + 10 MINUTES COOLING /
COOK TIME: 10 MINUTES / **MAKES** 6 SERVINGS

For a lighter guacamole-style dip, we used peas (guisantes in Spanish) in place of avocado. Press the pureed peas through a strainer or food mill for a smoother consistency. The nut- and bean-based vegetarian chopped liver is a tasty and hearty alternative to the traditional deli favorite. Peas or asparagus can be substituted for the green beans.

MAKE IT A MEAL

2 tablespoons mixed nuts
100 CALORIES

410
CALORIES
PER MEAL
★ ★

MAKE IT A MEAL

1 bottle (12 ounces) of beer
100 CALORIES

410
CALORIES
PER MEAL
★ ★

GUISA-MOLE

- 1 box (10 ounces) frozen peas, thawed
- 1 medium tomato, chopped
- ⅓ cup finely chopped fresh cilantro
- ¼ cup finely chopped onion
- 2 tablespoons fresh lime juice
- ¾ teaspoon ground cumin
- ¾ teaspoon garlic powder
- ¼ teaspoon salt
- 6 ounces baked tortilla chips

1. TO MAKE THE GUISA-MOLE: Place the peas in a food processor and puree until smooth. Combine the pea puree with the tomato, cilantro, onion, lime juice, cumin, garlic powder, and salt in a medium bowl. Adjust the seasoning to taste. Serve with tortilla chips.

PER SERVING (1 serving = ⅓ cup guisa-mole + 1 ounce baked tortilla chips, ¼ cup vegetarian chopped liver + 2 slices party rye)

Calories	Total Fat	Saturated Fat	Sodium	Carbohydrate	Dietary Fiber	Protein	Calcium
310	11 g	1.5 g	620 mg	45 g	7 g	9 g	10%

VEGETARIAN CHOPPED LIVER

- 1½ teaspoons olive oil
- 1 medium onion, finely chopped
- 1 cup fresh or frozen green beans
- ⅓ cup chopped walnuts
- 1 hard-cooked egg, peeled
- 2 tablespoons light mayonnaise
- ¼ teaspoon salt
- ¼ teaspoon freshly ground black pepper
- 12 slices party rye bread

2. TO MAKE THE VEGETARIAN CHOPPED LIVER: Coat a medium skillet with cooking spray, add the oil and heat over medium-low heat. Add the onion, cover, and cook for 5 minutes, or until softened. Uncover and cook for 3 minutes, or until light brown. Let cool to room temperature, about 10 minutes.

3. MEANWHILE, combine ice and cold water in a medium bowl. Place the green beans in a small microwaveable bowl and microwave for 1 minute (2 minutes for frozen). Transfer to the ice water to stop the cooking.

4. WHEN the onions have cooled, place them in a food processor and add the walnuts, egg, mayonnaise, salt, and pepper. Drain the green beans and add them. Pulse on and off until almost smooth, about 30 pulses. Serve with the rye bread.

CAPRESE STACKS

PREP TIME: 5 MINUTES / **COOK TIME:** 7 MINUTES / **MAKES** 2 SERVINGS

Choose beautiful, ripe tomatoes and fragrant, fresh basil for this satisfying snack. These also make a nice lunch when accompanied with a bowl of soup.

MAKE IT A MEAL

1 cup reduced-sodium tomato soup with 2 tablespoons plain croutons
110 CALORIES

390
CALORIES PER MEAL
★

MAKE IT A MEAL

2 tablespoons unsalted mixed nuts
100 CALORIES

380
CALORIES PER MEAL
★ ★ ★

2	light (100-calorie) English muffins, split
1	medium tomato, cut into 8 thin slices
4	teaspoons sun-dried tomato bruschetta spread
4	slices (1 ounce each) fresh mozzarella cheese
¼	cup fresh basil

1. **PREHEAT** the broiler. Toast the English muffins until lightly browned and quite crispy.

2. **PUT** the toasted muffin halves on a baking sheet. Place 2 slices of tomato on each. Top each with 1 teaspoon of the bruschetta spread and 1 slice of cheese.

3. **BROIL** the muffins for 3 to 5 minutes, or until the cheese is melted and starting to bubble. Garnish each muffin stack with fresh basil. Serve hot.

PER SERVING (1 serving = 2 stacks)

Calories	Total Fat	Saturated Fat	Sodium	Carbohydrate	Dietary Fiber	Protein	Calcium
280	15 g	8 g	420 mg	27 g	9 g	17 g	40%

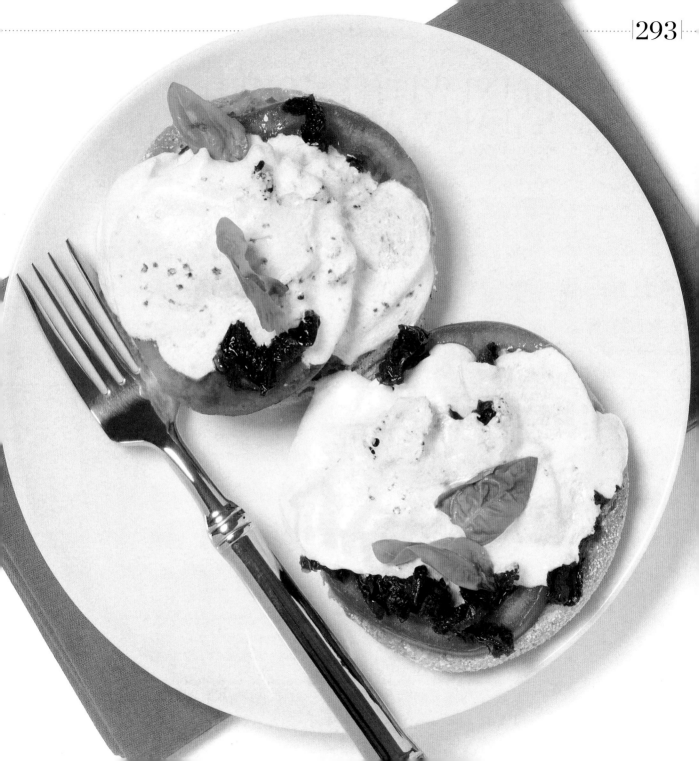

BLINI WITH SMOKED SALMON AND DILL CREAM

PREP TIME: 15 MINUTES / **COOK TIME:** 9 MINUTES / **MAKES** 4 SERVINGS

Serve this festive dish at a party, as an elegant appetizer, or as part of a brunch buffet. Compare sodium levels among different brands of smoked salmon and choose the brand with the lowest amount.

½	cup light sour cream
1	tablespoon chopped fresh dill
2	teaspoons fresh lemon juice
⅔	cup all-purpose flour
3	tablespoons yellow cornmeal
¼	teaspoon baking powder
¼	teaspoon salt
⅛	teaspoon freshly ground black pepper
⅔	cup fat-free milk
1	large egg
4	ounces smoked salmon, cut into 24 pieces

1. COMBINE the sour cream, dill, and lemon juice in a small bowl. Refrigerate until ready to use.

2. MIX the flour, cornmeal, baking powder, salt, and pepper in a medium bowl. Combine the milk and egg in a separate bowl. Stir the milk mixture into the flour mixture until just blended.

3. COAT a large nonstick skillet with cooking spray and heat over medium-high heat. Spoon out about 1 tablespoon of batter per blini. Cook for 2 minutes, or until the tops are covered with bubbles and the edges are almost set. Turn over and cook for 1 minute longer. Transfer to a platter and repeat with the remaining batter.

4. TOP each blini with 1 piece of salmon and a scant teaspoon of the sour cream mixture.

MAKE IT A MEAL

Kir Royale made with 5 ounces Champagne and 1 ounce crème de cassis
210 CALORIES

410 CALORIES PER MEAL ★

MAKE IT A MEAL

Add to the blini: 1 chopped egg yolk, 1 chopped egg white, 1 tablespoon chopped onion, 1 tablespoon capers
85 CALORIES

5 ounces Champagne
110 CALORIES

395 CALORIES PER MEAL ★

PER SERVING (1 serving = 6 blini)

Calories	Total Fat	Saturated Fat	Sodium	Carbohydrate	Dietary Fiber	Protein	Calcium
200	5 g	2 g	450 mg	25 g	1 g	13 g	15%

SWEET AND SPICY MIXED NUTS

PREP TIME: 5 MINUTES / **COOK TIME:** 45 MINUTES / **MAKES** 8 SERVINGS

Nuts taste great with almost any combination of seasonings. The joining of chili powder, chocolate, and cinnamon adds unexpected flavor notes that remind us of Mexican mole sauce. Choose a spicy or a mild chili powder, depending on your preference.

1	large egg white
3	tablespoons sugar
2	teaspoons unsweetened cocoa powder
1	teaspoon chili powder
1	teaspoon ground cinnamon
1	teaspoon water
2	cups lightly salted mixed nuts

1. **PREHEAT** the oven to 300°F. Spray a baking sheet with cooking spray or line with parchment or a nonstick liner.

2. **BEAT** the egg white and sugar in a medium bowl until very frothy. Stir in the cocoa, chili powder, cinnamon, and water. Mix in the nuts until well combined. Spread the nut mixture on the baking sheet. Bake for 45 minutes, or until lightly browned and very crisp. Cool completely before storing in an airtight container.

MAKE IT A MEAL

Fruit and cheese platter with ½ ounce Brie cheese, ½ ounce 50% reduced-fat Cheddar cheese, and ½ cup grapes **150 CALORIES**

390

CALORIES PER MEAL

★

MAKE IT A MEAL

1 bottle (12 ounces) of beer **150 CALORIES**

390

CALORIES PER MEAL

★

PER SERVING (1 serving = ¼ cup)

Calories	Total Fat	Saturated Fat	Sodium	Carbohydrate	Dietary Fiber	Protein	Calcium
240	20 g	3.5 g	120 mg	13 g	2 g	6 g	4%

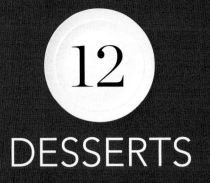

12

DESSERTS

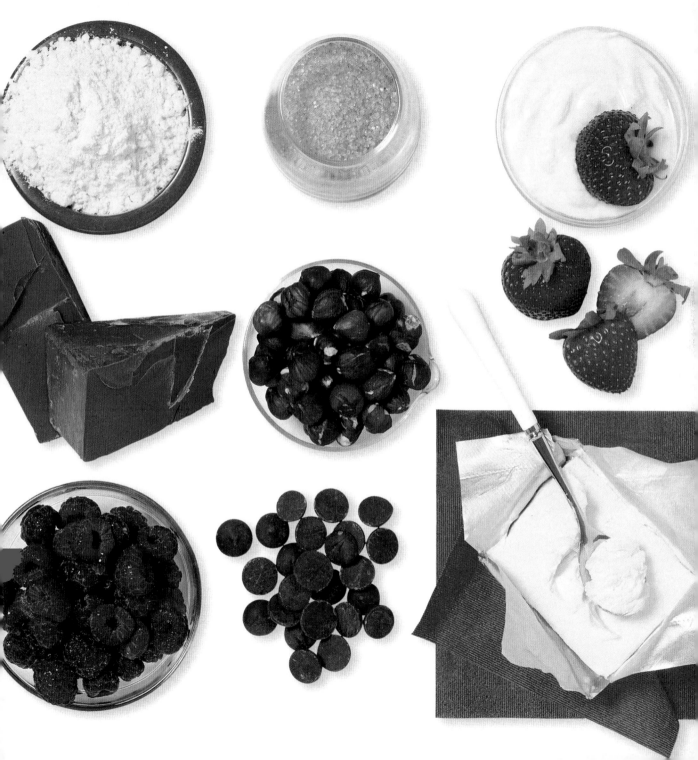

FROZEN WHOOPIE PIES

PREP TIME: 15 MINUTES + 15 MINUTES COOLING / **COOK TIME:** 12 MINUTES / **MAKES** 8 SERVINGS

Whoopie pies are chocolate cakes sandwiched together with a marshmallowy filling. Ours are filled with light vanilla ice cream for a cool and easy treat; peppermint lends a delicious holiday twist. The chocolate cakes can be kept in a tightly covered container for 3 days at room temperature in case you're not serving these all at once. Most whoopies are on the large side; ours are smaller, and therefore easier to work into your eating plan.

MAKE
IT A
MEAL

½ cup vegetarian 3-bean chili topped with 1 tablespoon shredded reduced-fat Cheddar cheese **110 CALORIES**

400
CALORIES
PER MEAL

MAKE
IT A
MEAL

1 cup low-fat milk **100 CALORIES**

390
CALORIES
PER MEAL

6	tablespoons butter, at room temperature
½	cup packed light brown sugar
1	large egg
¾	cup low-fat buttermilk
½	teaspoon instant coffee granules
¼	teaspoon vanilla extract
1	cup all-purpose flour
½	cup whole wheat pastry flour
⅓	cup unsweetened cocoa powder
1	teaspoon baking soda
1½	cups light (100 calories per ½ cup) vanilla ice cream, softened slightly

1. PREHEAT the oven to 350°F. Coat 2 baking sheets with cooking spray.

2. COMBINE the butter and brown sugar together in a medium bowl. Beat with an electric mixer on medium high until blended, about 3 minutes. Add the egg and beat until well incorporated.

3. STIR together the buttermilk, coffee granules, and vanilla in a measuring cup. Stir together the flours, cocoa, and baking soda in a small bowl.

4. ADD half the flour mixture to the butter-egg mixture and beat well. Beat in half the buttermilk. Repeat with the flour and buttermilk mixtures, mixing just until blended.

5. SCOOP the batter onto the baking sheets by rounded tablespoonfuls, making 16 round portions. Bake for 12 minutes. Cool the cakes for 15 minutes on the baking sheet.

6. TO serve, scoop 3 tablespoons softened ice cream onto the flat side of one cake, then top with another cake to make a sandwich. Repeat with remaining cakes and ice cream. Serve immediately or wrap in foil and freeze.

PER SERVING (1 serving = 1 sandwich)

Calories	Total Fat	Saturated Fat	Sodium	Carbohydrate	Dietary Fiber	Protein	Calcium
290	12 g	7 g	280 mg	41 g	2 g	6 g	10%

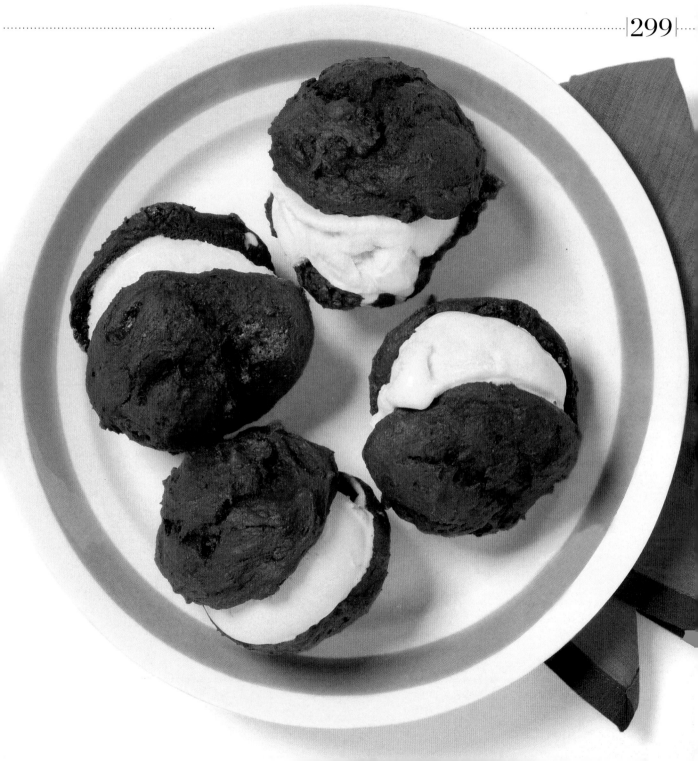

CHOCOLATE HAZELNUT BISCOTTI

PREP TIME: 25 MINUTES + 15 MINUTES COOLING / **COOK TIME:** 45 MINUTES / **MAKES** 10 SERVINGS

Biscotti are Italian twice-baked cookies perfect for dunking into coffee or milk. Feel free to substitute whatever nuts you have on hand—slivered almonds or chopped walnuts are good options. Kept in an airtight container, biscotti can be stored for up to 2 weeks.

½ cup white whole wheat flour
½ cup all-purpose flour
¼ cup unsweetened cocoa powder
¾ teaspoon baking soda
¼ teaspoon coarse salt
⅔ cup packed light brown sugar
2 large eggs
1 tablespoon water
½ teaspoon vanilla extract
¼ cup chopped hazelnuts
⅓ cup semisweet chocolate chips

1. PREHEAT the oven to 350°F. Line a baking sheet with parchment paper.

2. WHISK the flours, cocoa, baking soda, salt, and brown sugar in a medium bowl.

3. LIGHTLY beat the eggs in a small bowl. Measure out 1 tablespoon of beaten egg and set aside in a separate bowl. Whisk the water and vanilla into the remaining eggs. Add the egg mixture to the flour mixture and mix with a wooden spoon until blended, about 2 minutes. The dough should be somewhat stiff and sticky.

4. SHAPE the dough into a single log (4" wide x 12" long x 1" high) on the baking sheet. Gently press the hazelnuts into the top of the dough. Brush the reserved 1 tablespoon egg over the top and sides of the log. Bake for 30 minutes or until the dough is firm to the touch. Remove the cookie log and let cool for 15 minutes. Reduce the oven temperature to 300°F.

MAKE IT A MEAL

Tuna wrap made with 1 whole wheat tortilla (6"), ⅓ cup water-packed light tuna, and 1 tablespoon light mayonnaise
230 CALORIES

½ cup raspberries
30 CALORIES

420 CALORIES PER MEAL
★ ★ ★

MAKE IT A MEAL

1 medium sliced banana
110 CALORIES

½ cup vanilla ice cream
140 CALORIES

410 CALORIES PER MEAL
★ ★

PER SERVING (1 serving = 2 biscotti)

Calories	Total Fat	Saturated Fat	Sodium	Carbohydrate	Dietary Fiber	Protein	Calcium
160	4.5 g	1.5 g	160 mg	28 g	2 g	4 g	2%

5. TRANSFER the cooled cookie log to a cutting board. Using a sharp serrated (bread) knife, cut the log crosswise into 20 biscotti, about ½" wide. Place the cookies on the baking sheet (it's okay if they're touching). Bake for 12 to 15 minutes, or until crisp. Let the cookies cool completely.

6. MELT the chocolate chips in a microwaveable bowl, first for 1 minute on high and then at 12-second intervals, stirring in between, until smooth and fully melted. Dip a fork into the melted chocolate and drizzle it over the biscotti. (You may have to reheat the chocolate if it thickens too much to drizzle.) Let the biscotti sit until the chocolate cools and hardens, then store in an airtight container.

COCONUT BLONDIES

PREP TIME: 10 MINUTES + 30 MINUTES COOLING / **COOK TIME:** 30 MINUTES / **MAKES** 8 SERVINGS

The sweetened flaked coconut gives these bars a chewy texture that can't be achieved with unsweetened coconut. The coconut extract adds extra flavor to these tasty bars.

1	cup all-purpose flour
1¼	teaspoons baking powder
⅛	teaspoon salt
4	tablespoons trans-free margarine, melted
2	large egg whites
1	large egg
1	cup packed light brown sugar
1	teaspoon coconut extract
½	teaspoon vanilla extract
⅔	cup sweetened flaked coconut

1. PREHEAT the oven to 350°F. Coat an 8" x 8" baking pan with cooking spray and dust lightly with flour.

2. COMBINE the flour, baking powder, and salt in a bowl. Mix the margarine, egg whites, whole egg, brown sugar, coconut extract, and vanilla in a separate bowl. Stir the flour mixture into the egg mixture until well combined. Stir in the flaked coconut. Pour into the baking pan.

3. BAKE for 25 to 30 minutes, or until a toothpick inserted in the center comes out with a few moist crumbs. Cool in the pan on a rack for 30 minutes. Cut into 8 bars.

MAKE IT A MEAL

½ peanut butter and jelly sandwich made with 1 slice (1 ounce) whole wheat bread, 2 teaspoons peanut butter, and 2 teaspoons all-fruit jam **150 CALORIES**

400
CALORIES PER MEAL
★

MAKE IT A MEAL

1 tablespoon mini chocolate chips melted and drizzled over a blondie **50 CALORIES**

1 cup low-fat milk **100 CALORIES**

400
CALORIES PER MEAL
★

PER SERVING (1 serving = 1 blondie bar)

Calories	Total Fat	Saturated Fat	Sodium	Carbohydrate	Dietary Fiber	Protein	Calcium
250	8 g	3 g	210 mg	43 g	1 g	4 g	8%

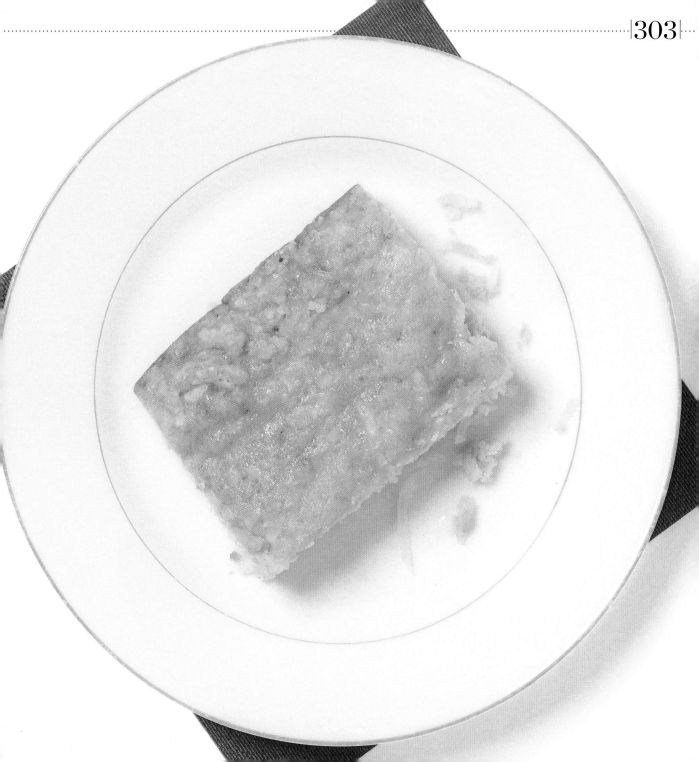

FLOURLESS CHOCOLATE CAKE

PREP TIME: 15 MINUTES + 1 HOUR COOLING / **COOK TIME:** 40 MINUTES / **MAKES** 8 SERVINGS

Serve the cake at room temperature and store leftovers in the refrigerator. Warm leftover cake in the microwave briefly, as it hardens significantly when chilled.

10 ounces bittersweet or dark chocolate, chopped, or 1½ cups dark chocolate chips

4 ounces (1 stick) butter

1 teaspoon vanilla extract

⅛ teaspoon salt

4 large eggs, separated

9 tablespoons sugar

1. **PREHEAT** the oven to 350°F. Coat an 8" to 9" spring-form pan with cooking spray.

2. **MELT** the chocolate and butter in a medium saucepan over low heat. Stir occasionally until the mixture is smooth. Stir in the vanilla and salt. Remove from the heat and set aside to cool slightly.

3. **WHISK** the egg yolks with 5 tablespoons of the sugar in a small bowl until well combined. Set aside.

4. **BEAT** the egg whites with an electric mixer in a medium bowl until frothy. With the mixer on high speed, gradually add the remaining 4 tablespoons sugar, 1 tablespoon at a time, beating until the mixture forms soft peaks, about 10 minutes. Set aside.

5. **STIR** the egg yolk mixture into the cooled chocolate mixture until combined. Gently fold the beaten egg whites into the chocolate mixture—do not overmix. Pour the batter into the pan, smooth the top, and bake for 40 minutes (35 minutes if using a 9" pan) or until the top of the cake appears dry and cracked and the cake is set.

6. **COOL** the cake in the pan for 10 minutes, then run a knife around the inside edge of the pan and release the sides. Cool completely before cutting into 8 wedges. Serve at room temperature.

MAKE
IT A
MEAL

½ cup raspberries
30 CALORIES

400
CALORIES
PER MEAL
★ ★

MAKE
IT A
MEAL

Latte made with ½ cup coffee mixed with ½ cup fat-free milk
40 CALORIES

410
CALORIES
PER MEAL
★

PER SERVING (1 serving = one 3" wedge)

Calories	Total Fat	Saturated Fat	Sodium	Carbohydrate	Dietary Fiber	Protein	Calcium
370	29 g	16 g	75 mg	32 g	3 g	6 g	2%

GINGERBREAD CUPCAKES WITH SPICED FRUIT COMPOTE

PREP TIME: 10 MINUTES / **COOK TIME:** 22 MINUTES / **MAKES** 12 SERVINGS

Any combination of chopped dried fruit works well in this recipe. The spiced fruit compote also makes a tasty topping for oatmeal or yogurt.

MAKE IT A MEAL

3 ounces roasted chicken breast
140 CALORIES

410 CALORIES PER MEAL

★

MAKE IT A MEAL

1 cup steamed low-fat milk flavored with 1 teaspoon honey and ¼ teaspoon vanilla extract
125 CALORIES

395 CALORIES PER MEAL

CUPCAKES

- 1 cup all-purpose flour
- 1 cup white whole wheat flour
- 1 teaspoon baking soda
- 1 teaspoon ground ginger
- ½ teaspoon ground cinnamon
- ½ teaspoon salt
- ¾ cup light molasses
- ⅓ cup sugar
- ¼ cup unsweetened applesauce
- ¼ cup (½ stick) unsalted butter, at room temperature
- 1 large egg
- 1 tablespoon grated fresh ginger
- ⅔ cup hot water

1. TO MAKE THE CUPCAKES: Preheat the oven to 350°F. Coat a 12-cup muffin tin (each cup should hold at least 2 ounces) with cooking spray.

2. WHISK together the flours, baking soda, ground ginger, cinnamon, and salt in a medium bowl.

3. COMBINE the molasses, sugar, applesauce, butter, egg, and fresh ginger in a large bowl. Beat with an electric mixer on medium speed until well combined. Add the flour mixture and mix at medium speed until smooth. Stir in the hot water, mixing until the batter is smooth.

4. FILL the muffin cups about two-thirds full with the batter. Bake for 20 minutes, or until the top springs back when lightly touched and a toothpick inserted in the center of a muffin comes out clean.

PER SERVING (1 serving = 1 cupcake, 2½ tablespoons compote)

Calories	Total Fat	Saturated Fat	Sodium	Carbohydrate	Dietary Fiber	Protein	Calcium
270	4.5 g	2.5 g	220 mg	57 g	3 g	3 g	6%

SPICED FRUIT COMPOTE

- ½   cup dried apple slices
- ½   cup dried apricots, cut into slivers
- ½   cup raisins
- ½   cup dried cranberries
- 2   cups apple juice
- ½   teaspoon ground cinnamon
- ¼   teaspoon freshly ground black pepper
- ⅛   teaspoon ground allspice

5. MEANWHILE, TO MAKE THE SPICED FRUIT COMPOTE: Combine the apples, apricots, raisins, cranberries, apple juice, cinnamon, pepper, and allspice in a medium saucepan. Cover and simmer over medium-low heat for 10 minutes, or until the fruit is soft. Uncover and simmer for 12 minutes, or until the juice thickens slightly.

6. CUT each cupcake into quarters and place on a small plate or in a small bowl. Top each with about 2½ tablespoons of compote.

CARROT CAKE WITH CREAMY FROSTING

PREP TIME: 15 MINUTES + 1 HOUR COOLING / **COOK TIME:** 45 MINUTES / **MAKES** 9 SERVINGS

Moist, spicy, and topped with a generous amount of cream cheese frosting, this carrot cake will cure your craving for an indulgent dessert.

CAKE
- ⅔ cup all-purpose flour
- ⅓ cup whole wheat pastry flour
- 1 teaspoon baking soda
- 1 teaspoon ground cinnamon
- ¼ teaspoon salt
- 1 large egg
- 1 large egg white
- ½ cup granulated sugar
- ¼ cup packed light brown sugar
- ⅓ cup fat-free vanilla yogurt
- 1 tablespoon canola oil
- ½ teaspoon vanilla extract
- 1 can (8 ounces) juice-packed crushed pineapple
- 1 large carrot, grated (about 1 cup)

FROSTING
- 6 ounces Neufchâtel cheese, at room temperature
- ¾ cup confectioners' sugar
- ¼ teaspoon vanilla extract

1. TO MAKE THE CAKE: Preheat the oven to 350°F. Coat an 8" x 8" baking pan with cooking spray.

2. COMBINE the flours, baking soda, cinnamon, and salt in a small bowl.

3. WHISK together the whole egg, egg white, granulated sugar, brown sugar, yogurt, oil, and vanilla in a medium bowl. Stir in the pineapple and grated carrot.

4. STIR the flour mixture into the carrot mixture until just blended. Scrape the batter into the pan and bake for 45 minutes, or until a toothpick inserted in the center comes out clean. Cool the cake in the pan for 30 minutes, then invert the cake onto a plate and let it cool another 30 minutes.

5. MEANWHILE, TO MAKE THE FROSTING: In a small bowl, using a fork or whisk, blend the Neufchâtel, confectioners' sugar, and vanilla until smooth. When the cake is cool, spread the top with the cream cheese frosting. Cut into 9 squares.

PER SERVING (1 serving = 1 square)

Calories	Total Fat	Saturated Fat	Sodium	Carbohydrate	Dietary Fiber	Protein	Calcium
240	7 g	3 g	310 mg	41 g	1 g	4 g	4%

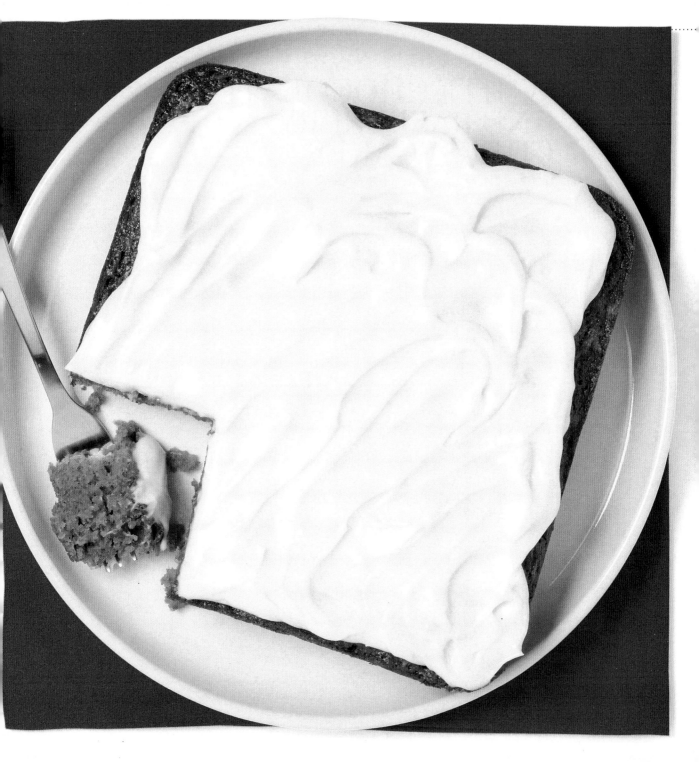

WHITE CHOCOLATE AND RASPBERRY CHEESECAKES

PREP TIME: 15 MINUTES + 1 HOUR 30 MINUTES COOLING + CHILLING / **COOK TIME:** 25 MINUTES / **MAKES** 6 SERVINGS

Individual desserts make portion control so easy! These company-worthy treats feature a chocolate cookie crust, white chocolate cheesecake filling, and a super-easy raspberry topping. Blackberries would be a suitable substitute for the raspberries.

MAKE IT A MEAL

⅔ cup bouillabaisse
160 CALORIES

420 CALORIES PER MEAL
★

MAKE IT A MEAL

1 lobster tail (6 ounces), cooked (4 ounces meat)
110 CALORIES

5 steamed asparagus spears
20 CALORIES

390 CALORIES PER MEAL
★ ★

6	foil cupcake liners
3	chocolate wafer cookies (such as Nabisco Famous Chocolate Wafers)
8	ounces Neufchâtel cheese, at room temperature
¼	cup sugar
¼	teaspoon vanilla extract
1	large egg
⅓	cup white chocolate chips + 1 tablespoon chips, coarsely chopped (for garnish)
¼	cup red raspberry jam or seedless preserves
1	cup fresh raspberries

1. PREHEAT the oven to 350°F. Line a 6-cup muffin pan or a 12-cup muffin pan with the foil liners.

2. PLACE the chocolate wafer cookies in a resealable sandwich-size plastic bag. Close the bag and crush the cookies into fine crumbs with a rolling pin or can. Divide the crumbs among the cupcake liners.

3. COMBINE the Neufchâtel, sugar, vanilla, and egg in a medium bowl. Beat with an electric mixer until smooth, about 4 minutes.

4. MELT ⅓ cup of the white chocolate chips in a small microwaveable bowl at medium power for 1 minute (chips will not appear melted). Stir until smooth. Mix the melted white chocolate into the cheese mixture. Divide the batter evenly among the cupcake liners, being careful not to disturb the cookie crumbs.

PER SERVING (1 serving = 1 cheesecake)

Calories	Total Fat	Saturated Fat	Sodium	Carbohydrate	Dietary Fiber	Protein	Calcium
260	13 g	8 g	190 mg	29 g	1 g	6 g	6%

5. BAKE for 25 minutes. Let cool in the pan for 30 minutes. Refrigerate until chilled, at least 1 hour.

6. JUST before serving, remove the cheesecakes from the liners (peel carefully). Place on dessert plates. Stir the jam in a small bowl or cup until smooth and drizzle about 1 tablespoon over each cheesecake. Sprinkle ¼ cup raspberries over each. Finally, sprinkle each portion with some of the chopped white chocolate chips.

LEMON CHIFFON CAKE AND RASPBERRY SORBET

PREP TIME: 25 MINUTES + 30 MINUTES COOLING / **COOK TIME:** 30 MINUTES / **MAKES** 6 SERVINGS

Chiffon cake is quite similar to angel food cake in texture. This petite version is baked in a loaf pan for portion control ease and features a bright lemon flavor.

1	large egg, separated
1	egg white
¼	teaspoon cream of tartar
½	cup sugar
1	lemon
½	teaspoon vanilla extract
1	tablespoon vegetable oil
½	cup cake flour
½	teaspoon baking powder
¼	teaspoon salt
1	pint raspberry sorbet

1. PREHEAT the oven to 350°F. Coat an 8" x 4" loaf pan with cooking spray.

2. BEAT the two egg whites with an electric mixer on high speed in a medium bowl until foamy. Add the cream of tartar and beat until soft peaks form. With the mixer on high speed, add ¼ cup of the sugar, a little at a time, until stiff peaks form (this may take up to 5 minutes). Set aside.

3. GRATE the zest from the lemon, then juice it (you should have about ¼ cup juice and 1 tablespoon zest). Combine the lemon juice and zest with the egg yolk in a small bowl. Add the vanilla and oil, and blend well with a fork.

4. STIR together the cake flour, baking powder, salt, and remaining ¼ cup sugar in a small bowl. Add the lemon mixture to the flour mixture and blend well with a whisk or fork. Scrape the batter into the bowl with the beaten egg whites. Gently fold the egg whites into the batter, until the whites are incorporated—do not overmix.

5. SCRAPE the mixture into the loaf pan and smooth the top. Bake for 30 minutes, or until the top is golden brown. Let cool in the pan for 15 minutes, then invert onto a cooling rack to cool completely (the cake will sink slightly).

6. TO serve, cut the cake with a serrated knife into 6 slices. Serve each slice topped with a ⅓-cup scoop of raspberry sorbet.

PER SERVING (1 serving = 1 slice cake, ⅓ cup sorbet)

Calories	Total Fat	Saturated Fat	Sodium	Carbohydrate	Dietary Fiber	Protein	Calcium
230	3.5 g	0 g	160 mg	47 g	2 g	3 g	4%

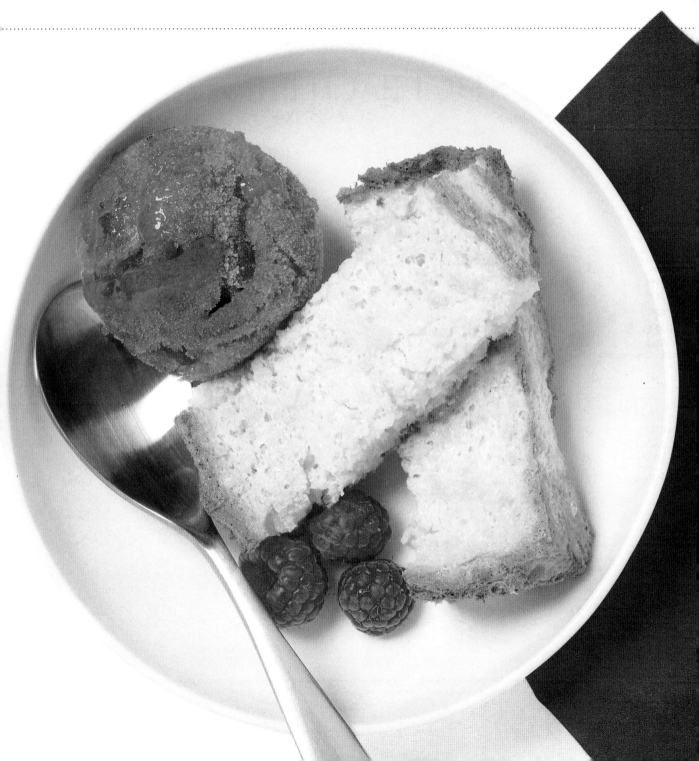

RUSTIC PEACH PIE

PREP TIME: 20 MINUTES + 25 MINUTES STANDING / **COOK TIME:** 48 MINUTES / **MAKES** 6 SERVINGS

Use frozen peaches if fresh are out of season, taking care to thaw fully, drain, and pat dry to remove excess moisture.

2 pounds peaches, sliced
½ cup + 2 teaspoons sugar
1 tablespoon cornstarch
¼ teaspoon ground cinnamon
¼ teaspoon ground ginger
¼ teaspoon almond extract
1 refrigerated pie crust (7½ ounces)
1 egg white, lightly beaten
2 tablespoons peach preserves

1. PREHEAT the oven to 400°F. Coat a large rimmed baking sheet with cooking spray.

2. COMBINE the peaches, ½ cup of the sugar, the cornstarch, cinnamon, ginger, and almond extract in a large bowl and toss well.

3. ROLL out the dough on a lightly floured surface to a 13" circle. Transfer to the baking sheet and pour the peach mixture into the center. Spread the peaches out evenly over the dough, leaving a 1½" border around the edges. Fold the sides of the dough in to partially cover the peach mixture, pleating as you go around. Brush the dough with the beaten egg white and sprinkle with the remaining 2 teaspoons sugar.

4. BAKE in the center of the oven for 45 to 48 minutes, or until the dough is golden and the filling is thick and bubbling. Let stand for 5 minutes. Place the preserves in a microwaveable bowl and warm for 30 to 40 seconds. Brush the peaches with the preserves. Let stand for 20 minutes before cutting into 6 wedges.

MAKE IT A MEAL

½ cup light vanilla ice cream
100 CALORIES

410 CALORIES PER MEAL
★

MAKE IT A MEAL

2 tablespoons whipped cream
50 CALORIES

1 tablespoon toasted sliced almonds
30 CALORIES

390 CALORIES PER MEAL
★ ★

PER SERVING (1 serving = 1 wedge)

Calories	Total Fat	Saturated Fat	Sodium	Carbohydrate	Dietary Fiber	Protein	Calcium
310	10 g	4 g	140 mg	54 g	2 g	3 g	0%

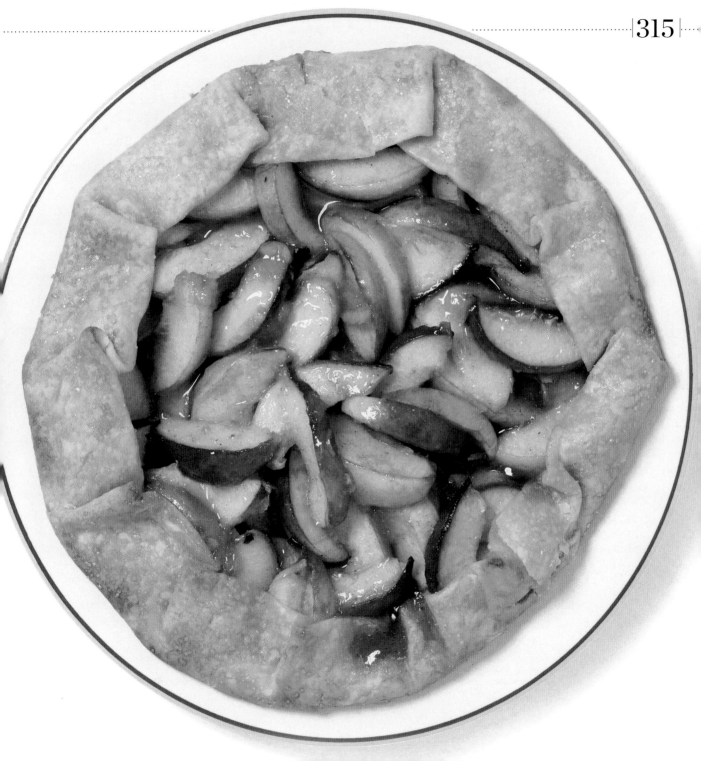

STRAWBERRIES DRIZZLED WITH CHOCOLATE-ALMOND SAUCE

PREP TIME: 5 MINUTES / **COOK TIME:** 5 MINUTES / **MAKES** 4 SERVINGS

Pay a slightly higher price for premium chocolate chips—the flavor is much richer and multi-dimensional. Substitute orange sections or chunks of pineapple when strawberries are out of season.

⅓ cup fat-free milk
1 tablespoon sugar
1 teaspoon unsweetened cocoa powder
⅓ cup semisweet chocolate chips
⅛ teaspoon almond extract
24 large strawberries

1. **COMBINE** the milk, sugar, and cocoa in a small sauce-pan. Cook over medium heat, stirring often, until hot. Add the chocolate chips and cook for 1 minute, stirring, until melted. Remove from the heat and stir in the almond extract.

2. **SERVE** the strawberries drizzled with the chocolate sauce.

PER SERVING (1 serving = 6 strawberries, 2 tablespoons sauce)

Calories	Total Fat	Saturated Fat	Sodium	Carbohydrate	Dietary Fiber	Protein	Calcium
150	6 g	3.5 g	10 mg	25 g	3 g	3 g	4%

GRILLED FRUIT SALAD

PREP TIME: 10 MINUTES / **COOK TIME:** 6 MINUTES / **MAKES** 4 SERVINGS

Choose fruit that is ripe but with enough firmness to stand up to cutting and grilling. During the summer months, nectarines, plums, and apricots can take the place of the pineapple.

1	pineapple, peeled, cored, and cut into 8 slices (½" thick)
2	medium peaches, halved
1	large mango, peeled, pitted, and cut lengthwise into 8 slices (½" thick)
1	tablespoon canola oil
1	quart strawberries, quartered
1	tablespoon fresh lemon juice
1	tablespoon sugar
2	tablespoons sliced fresh basil

1. PREHEAT the grill to medium.

2. BRUSH the pineapple, peaches, and mango with the oil. Grill covered for 3 minutes per side, or until well marked and starting to soften. Transfer to a cutting board. When cool enough to handle, cut into chunks and transfer to a bowl.

3. STIR in the strawberries, lemon juice, and sugar, and let stand for 10 minutes, stirring occasionally. Serve sprinkled with the basil.

MAKE
IT A
MEAL

2 oatmeal raisin cookies (2½")
130 CALORIES

1 cup fat-free milk
80 CALORIES

420
CALORIES
PER MEAL
★ ★

MAKE
IT A
MEAL

S'mores with 2 graham cracker squares, 1 toasted marshmallow, ½ ounce milk chocolate
165 CALORIES

½ cup fat-free milk
40 CALORIES

415
CALORIES
PER MEAL
★ ★

PER SERVING (1 serving = 2 cups)

Calories	Total Fat	Saturated Fat	Sodium	Carbohydrate	Dietary Fiber	Protein	Calcium
210	4.5 g	0 g	0 mg	46 g	7 g	3 g	6%

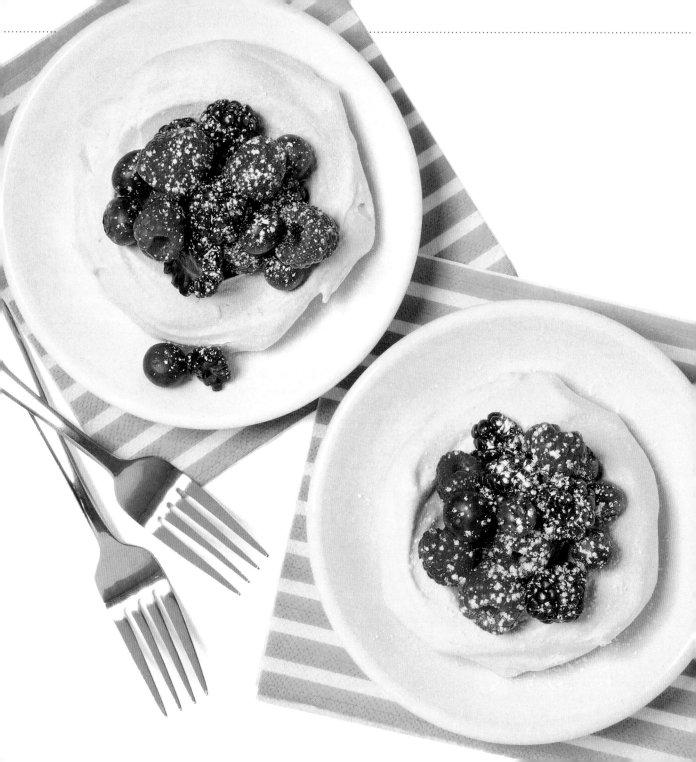

MERINGUE FRUIT TARTS

PREP TIME: 15 MINUTES + 15 MINUTES COOLING / **COOK TIME:** 1 HOUR 30 MINUTES /
MAKES 4 SERVINGS

Filled with berries, these generously-sized, individual meringue tarts are impressive, yet easy to prepare. Feel free to vary the fruit filling (sliced fresh apricots and blackberries would be wonderful) to suit your taste or the season.

2	large egg whites
½	cup sugar
½	teaspoon vanilla extract
½	teaspoon white vinegar
1½	teaspoons cornstarch
2	cups mixed berries (such as blueberries, raspberries, and quartered strawberries)
2	teaspoons confectioners' sugar

1. **PREHEAT** the oven to 250°F. Line a baking sheet with parchment paper. Using a pencil, trace around a 4"-diameter custard cup or can, making 4 circles on the parchment. Flip the parchment over so the pencil marks will not come in contact with the meringues. Set aside.

2. **BEAT** the egg whites with an electric mixer on high speed in a medium bowl until foamy. With the mixer on high speed, add the sugar, 1 tablespoon at a time, and beat until stiff peaks form (this may take up to 5 minutes). Add the vanilla and vinegar, mixing again just to combine. Gently fold in the cornstarch.

3. **DIVIDE** the meringue among the circles on the parchment. Shape the meringue into mounds with a spoon, then use the bottom of the spoon to form a depression in the center of each portion, forming small "bowls."

4. **BAKE** the meringues for 30 minutes, or until lightly browned. Turn the oven off, but leave meringues in the oven to sit and harden for 1 hour. Remove the meringues and let cool completely. (When completely cooled, the meringues can be stored for up to 3 days in a sealed container or resealable plastic bag for later use.)

5. **WHEN** ready to serve, place one meringue on each of 4 dessert plates. Spoon ½ cup of berries into the "bowl" of each tart, then garnish with ½ teaspoon confectioners' sugar.

MAKE IT A MEAL

3 ounces grilled chicken breast
140 CALORIES

Salad made with 2 cups mixed baby greens, 4 pieces melba toast, 10 sprays salad dressing spray
110 CALORIES

400
CALORIES
PER MEAL
★ ★

MAKE IT A MEAL

1 cup low-sodium chicken-vegetable soup
170 CALORIES

1 small piece (1 ounce) store-bought garlic bread
100 CALORIES

420
CALORIES
PER MEAL

PER SERVING (1 serving = 1 tart)

Calories	Total Fat	Saturated Fat	Sodium	Carbohydrate	Dietary Fiber	Protein	Calcium
150	0 g	0 g	30 mg	36 g	2 g	2 g	2%

APPLE STRUDEL WITH CURRANTS, CHERRIES, AND ALMONDS

PREP TIME: 20 MINUTES + 30 MINUTES COOLING / **COOK TIME:** 35 MINUTES / **MAKES** 6 SERVINGS

The half-size phyllo sheets called for in this recipe are much easier to handle than full-size sheets (we used Athens brand). For a drier strudel filling, eliminate the cornstarch and reserved apple juice.

MAKE IT A MEAL

3 ounces grilled boneless pork loin chop
200 CALORIES

1 cup steamed carrots
50 CALORIES

410
CALORIES PER MEAL
★ ★ ★

MAKE IT A MEAL

Cheese and tomato panini made with 2 thin slices (¾ ounce each) Italian bread, 1 ounce fontina cheese, 2 tomato slices
240 CALORIES

400
CALORIES PER MEAL

2	tablespoons currants
2	tablespoons finely chopped dried sour cherries
½	cup apple juice
¼	cup sliced almonds
2	medium Granny Smith apples, peeled and coarsely chopped
1	graham cracker sheet (2 squares), finely crumbled
1	tablespoon light brown sugar
1	teaspoon ground cinnamon
2	teaspoons cornstarch
10	sheets (14" x 9") phyllo dough
2	teaspoons unsalted butter, melted

1. COMBINE the currants, cherries, and apple juice in a small microwaveable bowl. Microwave for 30 seconds. Set aside for 15 minutes to soften.

2. MEANWHILE, toast the almonds in a small skillet over medium heat for 1 minute, or until lightly browned and fragrant. Transfer to a mini food processor to cool, then finely grind. Set aside.

3. PREHEAT the oven to 350°F. Line a baking sheet with parchment paper or a nonstick liner (or use a nonstick baking sheet).

4. COMBINE the apples, graham cracker crumbs, brown sugar, and cinnamon in a medium bowl. Reserve 2 tablespoons of the apple juice and drain the currants and cherries. Add the softened fruit to the apple mixture. Stir the reserved apple juice into the cornstarch and add to the apple mixture. Stir to combine all the ingredients.

PER SERVING (1 serving = ⅓ strudel)

Calories	Total Fat	Saturated Fat	Sodium	Carbohydrate	Dietary Fiber	Protein	Calcium
160	4.5 g	1.5 g	105 mg	28 g	2 g	3 g	2%

5. PLACE the phyllo sheets on a flat surface and cover with a damp towel. Remove one sheet and place on a cutting board with the long side facing you. Spray lightly with cooking spray. Sprinkle with half the ground almonds. Top with a second sheet of phyllo. Coat with cooking spray. Repeat with 3 more sheets (for a total of 5). Do not spray the last sheet.

6. PLACE half the apple mixture lengthwise down the phyllo dough in a 3"-wide strip 1½" in from the side nearest you, and leaving a 1" margin at the short sides. Fold the 1½" margin (the long side) over the apple mixture. Fold the side margins in and over the apple mixture. Gently roll the strudel toward the other long side, tucking in the sides as you roll. Place on the baking sheet, leaving room for the second strudel. Brush with half the melted butter. Cut two evenly spaced slashes in the top of the strudel with a sharp knife or kitchen scissors. Repeat to make the second strudel.

7. BAKE for 35 minutes, or until golden brown. Let cool for at least 30 minutes before cutting each strudel crosswise into thirds.

CHOCOLATE BUTTON MERINGUES

PREP TIME: 15 MINUTES / **COOK TIME:** 1 HOUR + OVERNIGHT / **MAKES** 10 SERVINGS

To vary the flavor of these light cookies, use butterscotch or peanut butter chips in place of the chocolate chips.

60	large extra bittersweet chocolate baking chips (2 ounces, we used Ghirardelli)
2	large egg whites
½	cup sugar
½	teaspoon vanilla extract

1. **PREHEAT** the oven to 275°F. Line a large baking sheet with parchment paper or a nonstick liner.

2. **PLACE** 20 pairs of chocolate chips on the baking sheet, with each pair of chips touching and the pairs positioned 1" apart.

3. **BEAT** the egg whites with an electric mixer on high speed in a medium bowl until foamy. With the mixer running, gradually add the sugar, a little bit a time, until the egg whites are very stiff and glossy, about 10 minutes. Beat in the vanilla.

4. **DOLLOP** the meringue on top of each of the chocolate chip pairs using a rounded tablespoon. Place a chocolate chip on top of each meringue.

5. **BAKE** for 1 hour. Turn the oven off and leave the meringues in the oven overnight or for at least 6 hours.

PER SERVING (1 serving = 2 meringues)

Calories	Total Fat	Saturated Fat	Sodium	Carbohydrate	Dietary Fiber	Protein	Calcium
70	1.5 g	1 g	10 mg	14 g	0 g	1 g	0%

PEANUT BUTTER BUCKEYES

PREP TIME: 20 MINUTES + 25 MINUTES CHILLING / **COOK TIME:** 1 MINUTE / **MAKES** 14 SERVINGS

A familiar, easy, no-bake sweet that fills the bill when you're craving the rich taste of peanut butter and chocolate.

½ cup creamy peanut butter

¼ cup Smart Balance spread

1 cup confectioners' sugar

½ teaspoon vanilla extract

½ cup bittersweet chocolate chips

½ teaspoon shortening

1. **LINE** a baking sheet with waxed paper.

2. **COMBINE** the peanut butter, spread, confectioners' sugar, and vanilla in a medium bowl. Blend well with a fork. Scoop out level tablespoons of the dough and roll into balls. Place the balls on the baking sheet. Move the baking sheet into the refrigerator for 10 minutes.

3. **COMBINE** the chips and shortening in a small microwaveable bowl or cup. Microwave on medium power in 15-second increments, stirring after each, until the mixture is smooth and melted.

4. **SPEAR** a buckeye ball with a toothpick and dip into the melted chocolate until it's about two-thirds covered, leaving some of the peanut butter visible on the top. Place the dipped buckeyes back on the waxed paper. Return the sheet to the refrigerator for 15 minutes to harden the chocolate. Store the buckeyes lightly covered with plastic wrap in the refrigerator.

MAKE IT A MEAL

3 ounces grilled swordfish
130 CALORIES

1 medium (6½ ounces) baked sweet potato
100 CALORIES

380 CALORIES PER MEAL
★ ★ ★

MAKE IT A MEAL

1 cup low-fat milk
100 CALORIES

2 graham cracker squares
60 CALORIES

1 medium banana
110 CALORIES

420 CALORIES PER MEAL
★ ★

PER SERVING (1 serving = 1 buckeye)

Calories	Total Fat	Saturated Fat	Sodium	Carbohydrate	Dietary Fiber	Protein	Calcium
150	10 g	3.5 g	70 mg	14 g	1 g	3 g	0%

HONEY PANNA COTTA WITH PASSION FRUIT SAUCE

PREP TIME: 15 MINUTES + AT LEAST 3 HOURS CHILLING / **COOK TIME:** 5 MINUTES / **MAKES** 6 SERVINGS

Look for passion fruit puree frozen in a flat block in the dessert, fruit, or international section of the freezer case. Other types of fruit can be substituted but do not match the unique flavor of passion fruit.

1½	teaspoons unflavored gelatin
¼	cup water
1	cup half-and-half
¼	cup honey
1	teaspoon vanilla extract
1¼	cups 5% ("classic") plain Greek yogurt
2	tablespoons sugar
½	cup thawed frozen passion fruit puree

1. SPRINKLE the gelatin over the water in a small bowl. Let sit for 10 minutes to soften.

2. COMBINE the half-and-half, honey, vanilla, and gelatin mixture in a small saucepan. Cook for 5 minutes over medium heat, stirring constantly, until the gelatin dissolves and the mixture is simmering but not boiling. Remove from the heat.

3. STIR in the yogurt. Divide among 6 Champagne flutes or wineglasses. Cover and refrigerate for at least 3 hours or until firm.

4. MEANWHILE, stir the sugar into the passion fruit puree until the sugar dissolves. Refrigerate.

5. TO serve, top each panna cotta with 1½ tablespoons of the sweetened passion fruit puree.

PER SERVING (1 serving = scant ½ cup panna cotta + 1½ tablespoons passion fruit sauce)

Calories	Total Fat	Saturated Fat	Sodium	Carbohydrate	Dietary Fiber	Protein	Calcium
200	8 g	5 g	50 mg	26 g	0 g	7 g	10%

SWEET POTATO TART

PREP TIME: 25 MINUTES + 2 HOURS COOLING / **COOK TIME:** 43 MINUTES / **MAKES** 8 SERVINGS

Perfect for fall and winter festive occasions, this pretty tart features a tasty gingersnap crust filled with a creamy nutmeg-and-cinnamon-spiked sweet potato filling. If you prefer, substitute $1\frac{1}{3}$ cups canned pumpkin or squash puree for the sweet potato.

1	large sweet potato (about 1 pound), peeled and cut into ½" chunks
5	ounces small gingersnap cookies (about 25)
3	tablespoons butter, melted
⅓	cup fat-free sweetened condensed milk
¼	cup low-fat (2%) evaporated milk
3	tablespoons sugar
½	teaspoon ground cinnamon
½	teaspoon vanilla extract
½	teaspoon fresh lemon juice
⅛	teaspoon ground nutmeg
2	large eggs
1	cup pressurized light whipped cream

1. PREHEAT the oven to 350°F. Coat an 8" springform pan with cooking spray.

2. PLACE the sweet potato in a small saucepan and add water to cover. Bring to a boil over high heat and cook for 8 to 10 minutes, until the sweet potato is very tender. Drain and set aside.

3. MEANWHILE, add the gingersnaps to a food processor and pulse to break up the cookies. Process the cookies further until fine crumbs form. Add 2 tablespoons of the melted butter and process to evenly blend. Transfer the crumb mixture to the springform pan and press into an even layer over the bottom. Bake for 6 to 8 minutes, or until crisped.

4. WIPE out the processor and add the drained sweet potatoes, condensed milk, evaporated milk, sugar, cinnamon, vanilla, lemon juice, nutmeg, and the remaining 1 tablespoon butter. Process until smooth. Add the eggs and process to blend.

5. POUR the filling over the crust and spread into an even layer. Place the springform pan on a baking sheet and bake for 25 minutes, or until the filling is set. Let the tart cool for 2 hours before removing the sides and slicing into 8 wedges. Serve each wedge with 2 tablespoons whipped cream.

MAKE IT A MEAL

2 ounces roasted turkey breast
80 CALORIES

2 tablespoons cranberry sauce
50 CALORIES

390
CALORIES PER MEAL
★

MAKE IT A MEAL

½ cup frozen yogurt
100 CALORIES

½ cup hot apple cider
60 CALORIES

420
CALORIES PER MEAL
★

PER SERVING (1 serving = 1 wedge + 2 tablespoons whipped cream)

Calories	Total Fat	Saturated Fat	Sodium	Carbohydrate	Dietary Fiber	Protein	Calcium
260	9 g	4.5 g	220 mg	40 g	2 g	5 g	10%

DRIED CHERRY BROWNIES

PREP TIME: 10 MINUTES + 30 MINUTES COOLING / **COOK TIME:** 37 MINUTES / **MAKES** 8 SERVINGS

This recipe keeps calories under control by calling for less fat—here, trans-free margarine—and sugar than traditional recipes. The tartness of the cherries nicely offsets the sweetness of the chocolate.

MAKE
IT A
MEAL

½ cup
frozen yogurt
100 CALORIES

410
**CALORIES
PER MEAL**
★

MAKE
IT A
MEAL

Latte made with
¾ cup low-fat milk
80 CALORIES

390
**CALORIES
PER MEAL**
★

4 ounces semisweet chocolate, chopped

4 tablespoons trans-free margarine

2 large eggs

¾ cup sugar

1 teaspoon vanilla extract

¾ cup all-purpose flour

¼ cup unsweetened cocoa powder

¾ teaspoon baking powder

⅛ teaspoon salt

⅔ cup dried tart cherries

1 tablespoon confectioners' sugar

1. PREHEAT the oven to 325°F. Coat an 8" x 8" baking pan with cooking spray and dust lightly with flour.

2. COMBINE the chocolate and margarine in a small bowl set over a saucepan of barely simmering water. Cook, stirring occasionally, until the mixture is melted and smooth. Remove from the heat and let cool for 2 minutes.

3. MEANWHILE, combine the eggs, sugar, and vanilla in a medium bowl. Combine the flour, cocoa, baking powder, and salt in a separate medium bowl. Whisk the slightly cooled chocolate mixture into the egg mixture until smooth. Add the flour mixture, stirring until combined. Gently fold in the cherries. Pour the batter into the pan.

4. BAKE for 30 to 35 minutes, or until a toothpick inserted in the center comes out nearly clean. Let cool in the pan for 10 minutes. Remove from the pan and cool completely on a rack. Cut into 8 bars and sprinkle with the confectioners' sugar before serving.

PER SERVING (1 serving = 1 brownie bar)

Calories	Total Fat	Saturated Fat	Sodium	Carbohydrate	Dietary Fiber	Protein	Calcium
310	12 g	5 g	160 mg	47 g	5 g	5 g	4%

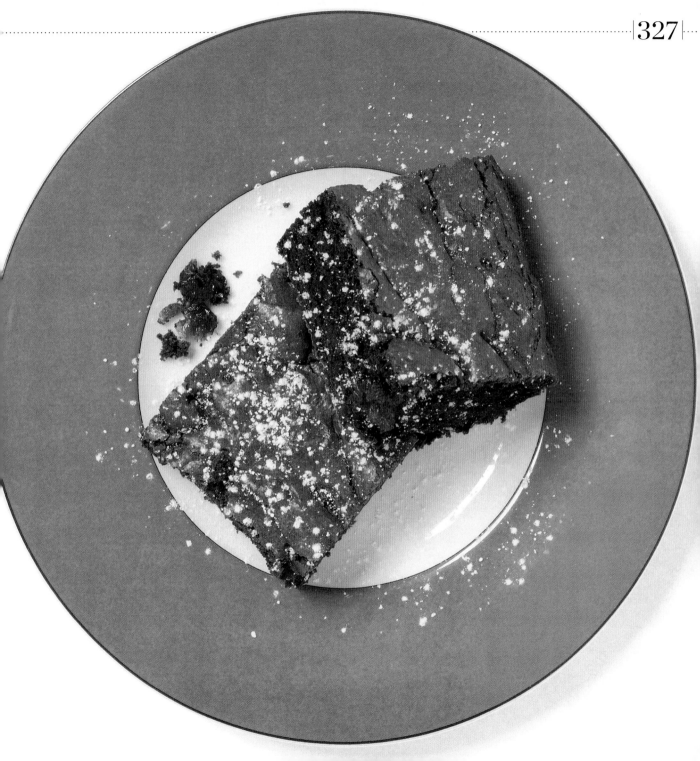

GRAND MARNIER–SPIKED SOUFFLÉS

PREP TIME: 20 MINUTES / **COOK TIME:** 30 MINUTES / **MAKES** 6 SERVINGS

Delicate and decadent, these orange-kissed soufflés are a lovely way to finish a meal. They are surprisingly easy to make and rarely collapse—no need to tiptoe around the kitchen while they are baking. Just take care to avoid getting even a drop of yolk into the whites or they will not whip properly. For lemon soufflés, substitute finely grated lemon zest for the orange zest and limoncello liqueur for the Grand Marnier.

2 tablespoons butter

2 tablespoons all-purpose flour

1 cup low-fat (2%) evaporated milk

1½ teaspoons finely grated orange zest

4 teaspoons Grand Marnier or other orange liqueur

4 large eggs, separated, at room temperature

½ teaspoon cream of tartar

¼ cup granulated sugar

2 tablespoons confectioners' sugar

1. PREHEAT the oven to 400°F. Coat six 1-cup ramekins or custard cups with cooking spray and place them on a baking sheet.

2. HEAT the butter in a small saucepan over medium heat. Stir in the flour and cook until the mixture is bubbling and evenly blended. Slowly whisk in the evaporated milk and bring to a simmer (it will thicken quickly). Transfer the mixture to a small bowl. Stir in the orange zest and Grand Marnier. Set aside to cool slightly.

3. COMBINE the egg whites and cream of tartar in a medium bowl. Beat with an electric mixer on medium speed until frothy. Increase the speed to high and beat until soft peaks form.

4. COMBINE the egg yolks and granulated sugar in another medium bowl. Beat with an electric mixer on high speed for 2 minutes, or until pale and doubled in volume. Stir the orange mixture into the yolk mixture until smooth.

PER SERVING (1 serving = 1 soufflé)

Calories	Total Fat	Saturated Fat	Sodium	Carbohydrate	Dietary Fiber	Protein	Calcium
180	8 g	4 g	120 mg	19 g	0 g	7 g	15%

5. STIR one-third of the beaten egg whites into the orange mixture to lighten it. Add the remaining egg whites and gently fold in until just combined—do not overmix.

6. DIVIDE the soufflé mixture among the 6 ramekins. Place the baking sheet in the oven and immediately reduce the oven temperature to 350°F. Bake for 20 to 25 minutes, or until the soufflés are very puffed and golden.

7. PLACE the confectioners' sugar in a fine-mesh sieve and tap the sieve to sprinkle the sugar evenly over the tops of the soufflés.

COSMO GRANITA

PREP TIME: 5 MINUTES + UP TO 4 HOURS FREEZING / **MAKES** 4 SERVINGS

This deliciously refreshing dessert is a twist on the popular cosmopolitan cocktail. Vodka does not freeze solid in a home freezer, so it prevents the granita from becoming too grainy. If you prefer to use sweetened cranberry juice cocktail (not diet), reduce the sugar to ¼ cup.

1	cup 100% unsweetened cranberry juice (we used Trader Joe's)
½	cup orange juice
⅓	cup vodka or water
⅓	cup sugar

1. COMBINE the cranberry juice, orange juice, vodka or water, and sugar in a medium bowl and stir until the sugar dissolves. Pour into ice cube trays and freeze until almost solid.

2. PLACE the cubes in a food processor or blender and process until slushy. Return to the freezer until ready to serve.

PER SERVING (1 serving = ⅔ cup)

Calories	Total Fat	Saturated Fat	Sodium	Carbohydrate	Dietary Fiber	Protein	Calcium
150	0 g	0 g	0 mg	28 g	0 g	0 g	0%

SORBET WITH LACE COOKIES

PREP TIME: 10 MINUTES / **COOK TIME:** 10 MINUTES / **MAKES** 6 SERVINGS

Bake the lace cookies until the entire center is bubbling so that the cookie will crisp up as it cools. Any combination of sorbet and fruit works well.

¼ cup packed light brown sugar

2 tablespoons light corn syrup

2 tablespoons unsalted butter, melted

¼ cup + 1 tablespoon all-purpose flour

2 tablespoons finely chopped almonds

⅛ teaspoon salt

¼ teaspoon almond extract

¾ cup chocolate sorbet

¾ cup raspberry sorbet

1½ cups raspberries

1. PREHEAT the oven to 375°F. Line 2 large baking sheets with parchment paper or foil. Coat with cooking spray.

2. COMBINE the brown sugar, corn syrup, and butter in a medium bowl. Stir in the flour, almonds, and salt. Mix until thoroughly combined. Stir in the almond extract.

3. PLACE the dough in scant tablespoons on the baking sheets, spacing them about 6" apart. You should get 12 cookies total. You may have to bake the cookies in two batches. Bake for 10 minutes, until the cookies are completely flat and the dough is bubbling. Allow the cookies to cool on the baking sheet for 2 minutes. Carefully transfer the cookies to a rack using a thin metal spatula.

4. PLACE a cookie on each of 6 small plates. Top each cookie with a 1-ounce scoop of each sorbet and with ¼ cup raspberries. Place the second cookie standing up between the two sorbet scoops.

MAKE IT A MEAL

3 ounces grilled mahi mahi
90 CALORIES

1 medium (6½ ounces) baked sweet potato
100 CALORIES

390
CALORIES PER MEAL
★ ★ ★

MAKE IT A MEAL

3 ounces grilled London broil
170 CALORIES

1 cup steamed green beans
40 CALORIES

410
CALORIES PER MEAL
★ ★ ★

PER SERVING (1 serving = 2 cookies, ¼ cup sorbet, ¼ cup raspberries)

Calories	Total Fat	Saturated Fat	Sodium	Carbohydrate	Dietary Fiber	Protein	Calcium
200	5 g	2.5 g	75 mg	38 g	3 g	2 g	2%

400 CALORIE FIX FOODS

Once you understand the principles of putting together 400-calorie meals, try making your own. Here's a list of some foods you can use, marked according to the 4 Star Nutrition System described on pages 9 through 11. Meat, poultry, and some types of fish earn a blue protein star if they provide at least 20 grams of protein in a 3-ounce cooked portion. The orange fiber star appears next to foods with at least 7 grams of fiber per serving. To earn a red good fats star, a food item must supply monounsaturated or omega-3 fatty acids. A 1-cup serving of a fruit or vegetable earns a green star.

Food	Star	Standard Serving Size	Calories
MEAT (portions are cooked amounts unless otherwise noted)			
Bacon		1 slice (½ oz)	50
Flank steak	Protein ★	3 oz	170
Ham, deli, lean		3 oz	90
Hamburger patty, extra-lean (95%)	Protein ★	3 oz	130
Hamburger patty, 90% lean	Protein ★	3 oz	180
Pork chop	Protein ★	3 oz	200
Pork tenderloin	Protein ★	3 oz	120
Prosciutto		1 slice	30
Roast beef	Protein ★	3 oz	180
Sausage, smoked, low-fat		3 oz	90
Steak, London broil, lean	Protein ★	3 oz	170
POULTRY (portions are cooked amounts unless otherwise noted)			
Chicken breast, boneless, skinless	Protein ★	3 oz	140
Chicken drumstick or thigh, skinless	Protein ★	1	110
Turkey bacon		1 slice	20
Turkey breast, deli		3 oz	90
Turkey breast, roasted	Protein ★	3 oz	110
Turkey, ground, extra-lean	Protein ★	3 oz	110
Turkey, ground, 92% or 93% lean	Protein ★	3 oz	140

Food	Star	Standard Serving Size	Calories
FISH AND SEAFOOD (portions are cooked amounts unless otherwise noted)			
Clams, steamed		10 medium	110
Cod		3 oz	90
Crab cake		3 oz	130
Lobster meat		3 oz	80
Salmon, burger or fillet	Good fats ★	3 oz	180
Salmon, smoked	Good fats ★	3 oz	130
Scallop wrapped in bacon		1	50
Shrimp cocktail		3 shrimp, ½ cup sauce	50
Shrimp, grilled		3 oz	60
Sole	Protein ★	3 oz	100
Sushi—California roll	Good fats ★	4 pieces	170
Sushi—spicy tuna roll		4 pieces	140
Tilapia	Protein ★	3 oz	110
Trout	Good fats ★	3 oz	110
Tuna	Protein ★	3 oz	120
Tuna, canned, light, water-packed	Protein ★	3 oz	90
Tuna salad, reduced-fat	Protein ★	½ cup	130
BEANS & MEATLESS PROTEINS (portions are cooked amounts unless otherwise noted)			
Black beans		½ cup	110
Cannellini beans		½ cup	110
Chickpeas		½ cup	140
Egg, large		1	80
Egg whites		2	30
Falafel balls		2	110
Hummus		½ cup	210
Kidney beans		½ cup	100

Food	Star	Standard Serving Size	Calories
Lentils		½ cup	120
Soybeans (edamame)	Good fats ★	½ cup	100
Three-bean salad		½ cup	90
Tofu, extra-firm	Good fats ★	3 oz	80
Tofu, silken	Good fats ★	3 oz	50
Soy burger	Good fats ★	1 patty	100
Vegetarian chili, canned		½ cup	90
DAIRY & DAIRY ALTERNATIVES			
American cheese		1 slice (⅔ oz)	70
Asiago cheese, grated		2 Tbsp	60
Blue cheese, crumbled		2 Tbsp	60
Cheddar cheese, reduced-fat, shredded		2 Tbsp	40
Cottage cheese, 1%		½ cup	80
Cream cheese, light		2 Tbsp	60
Feta cheese, reduced-fat, crumbled		2 Tbsp	40
Goat cheese, soft		2 Tbsp	80
Greek yogurt, fat-free (0%), plain		6 oz	90
Half-and-half		2 Tbsp	40
Mexican cheese, reduced-fat, shredded		2 Tbsp	40
Milk, fat-free		1 cup	80
Milk, low-fat		1 cup	100
Monterey Jack cheese, shredded		2 Tbsp	50
Monterey Jack cheese, reduced-fat, shredded		2 Tbsp	40
Mozzarella, fresh		1 oz	80
Mozzarella, part-skim, grated		2 Tbsp	40
Nondairy creamer, flavored		2 Tbsp	50
Parmesan cheese, grated		2 Tbsp	40

Food	Star	Standard Serving Size	Calories
Provolone cheese		1 oz	100
Rice milk		1 cup	120
Ricotta cheese, part-skim		¼ cup	70
Sour cream, light		2 Tbsp	40
Soymilk		8 fl oz	110
Swiss cheese, reduced fat		1 slice (1 oz)	90
Whipped cream, fresh		2 Tbsp	50
Whipped cream, pressurized		2 Tbsp	20
Yogurt, light fruit-flavored		6 oz	80
Yogurt, low-fat plain		6 oz	120
BREADS			
Bagel, plain, 4"		1	290
Biscuit, small, 2½"		1	130
Bran muffin, mini		1 oz	70
Bread, 100% whole wheat		1 slice (1 oz)	70
Bread, crusty Italian		1 medium slice (2 oz)	150
Bread, French		1 medium slice (2 oz)	160
Bread, garlic		1 medium slice (2 oz)	210
Bread, rye		1 slice (1 oz)	80
Bread, white		1 slice (1 oz)	70
Bread, whole grain		1 slice (1 oz)	70
Corn muffin, mini		1 oz	90
Croutons, plain		2 Tbsp	15
Croutons, seasoned		2 Tbsp	25
English muffin		1	130

Food	Star	Standard Serving Size	Calories
Hamburger bun		1	120
Hot dog bun		1	120
Pita, 6½", white or whole wheat		1	170
Pita Pocket Bread, WeightWatchers 100% Whole Wheat	Fiber ★	1	100
Roll, dinner, white or whole wheat		1 small (1 oz)	80
Sandwich Thins, Arnold Multi-Grain		1 piece	100
Toast, whole wheat, with 1 tsp butter		1 slice (1 oz)	100
Toast, whole wheat, with 1 tsp jam		1 slice (1 oz)	90
Tortilla, corn, 6"		1	60
Tortilla, flour, 6"		1	140
Tortilla, flour, 10"		1	220
Tortilla, whole wheat, 6"		1	120
CEREALS			
Cheerios		1 cup	100
Cornflakes		1 cup	100
Granola, low-fat		½ cup	190
Muesli, five-grain		½ cup	140
Oatmeal, cooked		½ cup	80
Raisin bran	Fiber ★	1 cup	190
Wheat germ		1 Tbsp	30
PASTA AND GRAINS (portions are cooked amounts unless otherwise noted)			
Barley		½ cup	100
Bulgur wheat		½ cup	80
Couscous		½ cup	90
Couscous, Moroccan or Israeli		½ cup	110
Pasta, white		½ cup	110

Food	Star	Standard Serving Size	Calories
Pasta, whole wheat		½ cup	90
Quinoa		½ cup	110
Rice, brown		½ cup	110
Rice, fried		½ cup	200
Rice pilaf		½ cup	140
Rice, white		½ cup	100
Soba noodles		½ cup	60
Tortellini salad (deli or salad bar)		½ cup	190
FRUITS			
Apple	Fruits/veggies ★	1 medium	100
Applesauce, unsweetened	Fruits/veggies ★	1 cup	100
Apricots, dried	Fruits/veggies ★	4 whole or 8 halves	70
Avocado, Hass, cubed	Good fats ★	¼ cup	60
Avocado, Hass	Good fats ★	1	320
Banana	Fruits/veggies ★	1 medium	110
Banana, sliced	Fruits/veggies ★	1 cup	130
Berries, mixed, frozen	Fruits/veggies ★	1 cup	60
Blackberries, frozen	Fruits/veggies ★	1 cup	100
Blueberries	Fruits/veggies ★	1 cup	80
Cantaloupe, cubed	Fruits/veggies ★	1 cup	50
Cherries, dried		2 Tbsp	60
Cherries, fresh	Fruits/veggies ★	1 cup	100
Cranberries, dried		2 Tbsp	50
Fig, dried		1	20
Fruit, dried, chopped		2 Tbsp	60
Fruit salad	Fruits/veggies ★	1 cup	100
Grapefruit		½ medium	50

Food	Star	Standard Serving Size	Calories
Grapes, seedless, red or green	Fruits/veggies ★	1 cup	110
Honeydew melon, cubed	Fruits/veggies ★	1 cup	60
Kiwifruit		1 medium	50
Mango, sliced	Fruits/veggies ★	1 cup	110
Orange	Fruits/veggies ★	1 medium	70
Papaya, cubed	Fruits/veggies ★	1 cup	50
Peach		1 medium	60
Peaches, juice-packed, canned	Fruits/veggies ★	1 cup	110
Pear	Fruits/veggies ★	1 medium	100
Pear, juice-packed, canned	Fruits/veggies ★	1 cup	120
Pineapple, juice-packed, canned	Fruits/veggies ★	1 cup	110
Pineapple chunks, fresh	Fruits/veggies ★	1 cup	80
Raisins		2 Tbsp	50
Raspberries	Fruits/veggies ★	1 cup	60
Strawberries	Fruits/veggies ★	1 cup	50
Watermelon, cubed	Fruits/veggies ★	1 cup	50
VEGETABLES			
Alfalfa sprouts, raw	Fruits/veggies ★	1 cup	10
Artichoke, cooked		1 medium	60
Arugula, raw	Fruits/veggies ★	1 cup	5
Asparagus, cooked	Fruits/veggies ★	5 spears	20
Beets, cooked	Fruits/veggies ★	2 medium	40
Bok choy, cooked	Fruits/veggies ★	1 cup	20
Broccoli, cooked	Fruits/veggies ★	1 cup	50
Broccoli, raw	Fruits/veggies ★	1 cup	20
Carrots, baby, raw		10	40
Carrots, sliced, cooked	Fruits/veggies ★	1 cup	50
Cauliflower, cooked	Fruits/veggies ★	1 cup	30
Celery, raw	Fruits/veggies ★	1 cup	20

Food	Star	Standard Serving Size	Calories
Coleslaw, deli style		½ cup	170
Collard greens, cooked	Fruits/veggies ★	1 cup	50
Corn kernels, canned	Fruits/veggies ★	1 cup	130
Corn kernels, frozen	Fruits/veggies ★	1 cup	160
Corn on the cob		1 medium	80
Cucumber, sliced	Fruits/veggies ★	1 cup	15
Escarole, raw	Fruits/veggies ★	1 cup	10
Green beans, cooked	Fruits/veggies ★	1 cup	40
Green peas, cooked	Fruits/veggies ★	1 cup	130
Guacamole	Good fats ★	1 Tbsp	20
Jicama, sliced	Fruits/veggies ★	1 cup	50
Lettuce, mixed greens	Fruits/veggies ★	1 cup	10
Mixed veggies, frozen	Fruits/veggies ★	1 cup	40
Mushrooms, raw, sliced	Fruits/veggies ★	1 cup	15
Olives, whole	Good fats ★	5	50
Onion, red		1 slice	10
Onion, white		1 slice	15
Pepper, bell, green	Fruits/veggies ★	1 medium	20
Pepper, bell, red	Fruits/veggies ★	1 medium	40
Peppers, red, roasted	Fruits/veggies ★	1 cup	80
Potato, baked		1 small (4 oz)	110
Potato salad, deli		½ cup	150
Potatoes, roasted		½ cup	90
Potatoes, mashed		½ cup	60
Scallion, chopped		2 Tbsp	5
Spinach, raw or baby	Fruits/veggies ★	1 cup	10
Squash, acorn, cooked	Fruits/veggies ★	1 cup	110
Squash, butternut, cooked	Fruits/veggies ★	1 cup	80
Sweet potato, cooked	Fruits/veggies ★	1 medium (6½ oz)	100

Food	Star	Standard Serving Size	Calories
Tomato		2 slices	10
Tomato		1 medium	20
Tomatoes, cherry	Fruits/veggies ★	10	30
Water chestnuts	Fruits/veggies ★	1 cup	90
Zucchini	Fruits/veggies ★	1 cup	20
OILS			
Olive oil		1 tsp	40
Sesame oil		1 tsp	40
Vegetable oil		1 tsp	40
CONDIMENTS, SAUCES, AND SPREADS			
Broth, chicken, fat-free, reduced-sodium		1 cup	5
Butter		1 tsp	30
Chutney		1 Tbsp	30
Duck sauce		1 Tbsp	20
Gravy, turkey		1 Tbsp	10
Honey		1 Tbsp	60
Jam, all fruit		1 tsp	10
Ketchup		1 Tbsp	15
Margarine, trans-free		1 tsp	30
Mayonnaise, light		1 Tbsp	50
Miracle Whip Light		1 Tbsp	40
Mustard, deli		1 tsp	5
Mustard, Dijon		1 tsp	5
Mustard, honey		1 tsp	10
Pasta sauce, tomato-based		½ cup	80
Peanut sauce	Good fats ★	1 Tbsp	50
Pesto	Good fats ★	1 Tbsp	80

Food	Star	Standard Serving Size	Calories
Pickles, bread and butter		1 Tbsp	10
Pickle slices		2	0
Salad dressing, Caesar, light		1 Tbsp	20
Salad dressing, Italian, light		1 Tbsp	25
Salad dressing, ranch, fat-free		1 Tbsp	20
Salad dressing spray		10 sprays	10
Salsa		1 Tbsp	5
Soy sauce, reduced-sodium		1 tsp	5
Sugar, brown		1 tsp	15
Sugar, white		1 tsp	15
Syrup, chocolate		1 Tbsp	60
Syrup, maple		1 Tbsp	50
Tahini	Good fats ★	1 Tbsp	50
Teriyaki sauce, low-sodium		1 Tbsp	15
Vinegar, balsamic		1 Tbsp	10
Vinegar, red wine		1 Tbsp	0
NUTS			
Almond butter	Good fats ★	1 Tbsp	100
Almonds, sliced	Good fats ★	1 Tbsp	30
Almonds, whole roasted	Good fats ★	10	80
Cashews, unsalted	Good fats ★	1 Tbsp	50
Coconut, shredded		1 Tbsp	30
Peanut butter	Good fats ★	1 Tbsp	90
Peanuts	Good fats ★	1 Tbsp	50
Pecans, chopped	Good fats ★	1 Tbsp	50
Pine nuts	Good fats ★	1 Tbsp	60
Pistachios, chopped	Good fats ★	1 Tbsp	40

Food	Star	Standard Serving Size	Calories
Sunflower seed kernels, unsalted	Good fats ★	1 Tbsp	50
Trail mix	Good fats ★	¼ cup	170
Walnut halves	Good fats ★	1 Tbsp	40
Walnuts, chopped	Good fats ★	1 Tbsp	50
CAKES, COOKIES, AND CANDY			
Angel food cake		1 slice (1/12 of a 9" cake)	70
Apple pie		1 slice (⅛ of a 9" pie)	300
Biscotti		2 (⅔ oz each)	180
Candy-coated peanuts	Good fats ★	20 pieces	210
Caramel rice cakes		4	200
Cheesecake		1 slice (2½ oz)	260
Chocolate chip cookies		2 (⅜ oz each)	110
Chocolate chips, mini	Good fats ★	1 Tbsp	50
Chocolate, dark	Good fats ★	½ oz	70
Chocolate, milk		½ oz	80
Chocolate mousse cake		3 oz (about ⅔ slice)	330
Cupcake, yellow, with chocolate frosting		Small (2½ oz) cupcake with 2 Tbsp frosting	380
Fortune cookie		1	30
Gingersnaps		3	90
Graham cracker squares		2	60
M&Ms		30 pieces	100
Oatmeal cookies		2 (⅓ oz each)	90
Peanut butter cookies		2 (⅜ oz each)	120

Food	Star	Standard Serving Size	Calories
Peanut butter cups, mini	Good fats ★	5 pieces	180
Pound cake		1 slice (2 oz)	220
CHIPS AND CRACKERS			
Brown rice crackers		10	70
Doritos		1 oz	150
Fritos		1 oz	160
Lay's Potato Chips		1 oz	150
Lay's Potato Chips, baked		1 oz	110
Oyster crackers		10	40
Popcorn, microwave, 94% fat-free		2 cups	30
Rice cakes		2	70
RyKrisp crackers		2	60
Tortilla chips		1 oz	140
Tortilla chips, baked		1 oz	120
Triscuits		6	120
Wheat Thins		16	150
DESSERTS			
Frozen whipped topping, light		2 Tbsp	20
Frozen yogurt		½ cup	100
Fudge Bar, Skinny Cow		1 bar	100
Ice cream, light		½ cup	100
Ice cream, premium		½ cup	250–290
Ice cream, regular		½ cup	130–140
Pudding, fat-free		1 mini cup (3½ oz)	90–100
Pudding, fat-free, sugar-free		½ cup	25

Food	Star	Standard Serving Size	Calories
Sorbet, lemon		½ cup	110
Sorbet, other flavors		½ cup	80
BEVERAGES			
Apple juice	Fruits/veggies ★	1 cup	110
Beer		8 fl oz	100
Beer, light		8 fl oz	70
Bloody Mary		8 fl oz	160
Cappuccino (made with 1 cup fat-free milk)		16 fl oz	80
Champagne		8 fl oz	180
Cranberry juice cocktail		1 cup	140
Cocoa, hot, sugar-free		1 packet	50
Coffee with half-and-half		1 cup with 1 Tbsp half-and-half	20
Cosmopolitan		8 fl oz	400
Gatorade		8 fl oz	60
Grapefruit juice	Fruits/veggies ★	1 cup	90
Iced tea, sweet		8 fl oz	60
Lemonade		1 cup	100
Martini		8 fl oz	450
Orange juice	Fruits/veggies ★	1 cup	110
Pomegranate-cranberry juice drink		1 cup	100
Sake		8 fl oz	320
Sangria		8 fl oz	160
Tomato juice	Fruits/veggies ★	1 cup	40
V8, low-sodium	Fruits/veggies ★	1 cup	50
Wine, red		8 fl oz	190
Wine, white		8 fl oz	190

ACKNOWLEDGMENTS

FIRST, OUR GRATITUDE TO THE RODALES. For generations, the family who founded and runs *Prevention* magazine has remained committed to its mission of inspiring people to live their whole lives. Our most heartfelt thanks to CEO Maria Rodale for her leadership, friendship, and support throughout this project.

Very special thanks to Karen Rinaldi and Gregg Michaelson for their enthusiasm, wisdom, and guidance always. And to Janine Slaughter, Sindy Berner, Matt Neumaier, and Lori Magilton, who took our vision and communicated it to the masses. To Mary Murcko, whose passion for the *Prevention* reader and the stories we give her knows no bounds. To Robin Shallow, who makes everything at Rodale better, then tells the world and takes no credit. To Bethridge "I-booked-you-again" Toovell and Lauren Paul, for their huge talents and herculean efforts on behalf of all of *Prevention*'s many products.

We must acknowledge the inspiration of *Prevention*'s brilliant creative director, Jill Armus, who loved *Flat Belly Diet!* and suggested a whole book of 400-calorie meals. Her vision for this project is reflected in every page of this gorgeous, energetic, and infinitely useful book.

Endless gratitude to Marlea Clark and Andrea Au Levitt, who have kept the *400 Calorie Fix* so close to their hearts and been careful, caring stewards of this project every step of the way. This book would not have been possible without Andrea or her team, including Marielle Messing, Hope Clarke, Chris Krogermeier, Sara Cox, JoAnn Brader, Carol Angstadt, and Jenelle Wagner.

A zillion thanks to this project's unsung heroes: Rebecca Simpson Steele, who directed the photo shoots with style and grace; Katie Kackenmeister, who organized the recipe development like the pro she is; Alyson Cameron, Sunny Stafford, and Kerrie Keegan, who channeled Jill's vision; David Bonom and Kitty Broihier, who helped to develop the most delicious 400-calorie recipes ever. Thanks also to Alyssa Shaffer, Teresa Dumain, Diana Kelly, Marisa Bardach,

Amanda Junker, Lisa Schnettler, and Deborah Wilburn, who've all touched and shaped this brand in many vital ways.

We're thrilled that we were able to feature the brilliant photography of Ted Morrison in the book. Thanks as well to his team, including food stylist extraordinaire Mariana Velasquez and prop stylist Philip Shubin.

We'd like to extend our gratitude to our *400 Calorie Fix* test panel, which was conducted in the summer of 2009. Thank you, Sandi (Fagan) Hill, Patti Robbins, Janet Sartorius, Donna Agajanian, Virginia Simpson, Judi Herrmann, Denise Bernstein, Gladys DiSisto, Melody Rubie, Bill Berkowsky, Jordan and Ronni Metzger, Francesca Minerva, Kristin Lewandowski, Helen Cannavale, and Lisa Frankel for providing us with the essential insights that helped us develop this book into a diet plan any type of eater can love.

As always, thanks to Courtenay Smith, Polly Chevalier, Jonathan Bigham, Fotoulla Euripidou, and Bill Stump for their counsel and work on all things *Prevention* and, of course, for all the laughs. To the smartest photo and art team in the business, including *Prevention*'s Helen Cannavale, Leah Vinluan, Maureen O'Brien, Jessica Sokol, Donna Agajanian, and Mallory Craig. And a hug for the lovely Susan Graves for keeping the entire *Prevention* team sane and centered (and running on time).

—Liz & Mindy

CONVERSION CHART

THESE EQUIVALENTS HAVE BEEN SLIGHTLY ROUNDED TO MAKE MEASURING EASIER.

Volume Measurements

US	Imperial	Metric
$\frac{1}{4}$ tsp	–	1 ml
$\frac{1}{2}$ tsp	–	2 ml
1 tsp	–	5 ml
1 Tbsp	–	15 ml
2 Tbsp (1 oz)	1 fl oz	30 ml
$\frac{1}{4}$ cup (2 oz)	2 fl oz	60 ml
$\frac{1}{3}$ cup (3 oz)	3 fl oz	80 ml
$\frac{1}{2}$ cup (4 oz)	4 fl oz	120 ml
$\frac{2}{3}$ cup (5 oz)	5 fl oz	160 ml
$\frac{3}{4}$ cup (6 oz)	6 fl oz	180 ml
1 cup (8 oz)	8 fl oz	240 ml

Weight Measurements

US	Metric
1 oz	30 g
2 oz	60 g
4 oz ($\frac{1}{4}$ lb)	115 g
5 oz ($\frac{1}{3}$ lb)	145 g
6 oz	170 g
7 oz	200 g
8 oz ($\frac{1}{2}$ lb)	230 g
10 oz	285 g
12 oz ($\frac{3}{4}$ lb)	340 g
14 oz	400 g
16 oz (1 lb)	455 g
2.2 lb	1 kg

Length Measurements

US	Metric
$\frac{1}{4}$"	0.6 cm
$\frac{1}{2}$"	1.25 cm
1"	2.5 cm
2"	5 cm
4"	11 cm
6"	15 cm
8"	20 cm
10"	25 cm
12" (1')	30 cm

Pan Sizes

US	Metric
8" cake pan	20 × 4 cm sandwich or cake tin
9" cake pan	23 × 3.5 cm sandwich or cake tin
11" × 7" baking pan	28 × 18 cm baking tin 180°
13" × 9" baking pan	32.5 × 23 cm baking tin
15" × 10" baking pan	38 × 25.5 cm baking tin (Swiss roll tin)
1$\frac{1}{2}$ qt baking dish	1.5 liter baking dish
2 qt baking dish	2 liter baking dish
2 qt rectangular baking dish	30 × 19 cm baking dish
9" pie plate	22 × 4 or 23 × 4 cm pie plate
7" or 8" springform pan	18 or 20 cm springform or loose-bottom cake tin
9" × 5" loaf pan	23 × 13 cm or 2 lb narrow loaf tin or pâté tin

Temperatures

Fahrenheit	Centigrade	Gas
140°	60°	–
160°	70°	–
80°	–	
225°	105°	$\frac{1}{4}$
250°	120°	$\frac{1}{2}$
275°	135°	1
300°	150°	2
325°	160°	3
350°	180°	4
375°	190°	5
400°	200°	6
425°	220°	7
450°	230°	8
475°	245°	9
500°	260°	–

INDEX

UNDERSCORED PAGE REFERENCES INDICATE BOXED TEXT.
BOLDFACED PAGE REFERENCES INDICATE PHOTOGRAPHS.